Strategies for Sustainable Urban Development—Addressing the Challenges of the 21st Century

Strategies for Sustainable Urban Development—Addressing the Challenges of the 21st Century

Editors

Liyin Shen
Jorge Ochoa
Haijun Bao

MDPI • Basel • Beijing • Wuhan • Barcelona • Belgrade • Manchester • Tokyo • Cluj • Tianjin

Editors
Liyin Shen
Hangzhou City University
China

Jorge Ochoa
University of South Australia
Australia

Haijun Bao
Hangzhou City University
China

Editorial Office
MDPI
St. Alban-Anlage 66
4052 Basel, Switzerland

This is a reprint of articles from the Special Issue published online in the open access journal *Buildings* (ISSN 2075-5309) (available at: https://www.mdpi.com/journal/buildings/topical_collections/Sustainable_Urban).

For citation purposes, cite each article independently as indicated on the article page online and as indicated below:

LastName, A.A.; LastName, B.B.; LastName, C.C. Article Title. *Journal Name* **Year**, *Volume Number*, Page Range.

ISBN 978-3-0365-7356-4 (Hbk)
ISBN 978-3-0365-7357-1 (PDF)

Cover image courtesy of Jose Jorge Ochoa Paniagua

Contents

About the Editors

Liyin Shen

Professor Liyin Shen is a Qiantang Distinguished Professor and the Chief Scientist at the Research Institute for Planning and Sustainability at Hangzhou City University. He is also the Director of the International Research Centre for Sustainable Built Environment at Chongqing University. Professor Shen has been focusing on the research discipline of sustainable built environment with a specific interest in low carbon city, urban carrying capacity and experience mining for sustainable urban development. He is on the lists of Highly Cited Researcher International published by Clarivate, The Most Cited Chinese Research Scholar published by Elsevier, and The World's Top 2% Scientists (Career and Single-year) published by Stanford University. Professor Shen was the Founding President of the Chinese Research Institute of Construction Management (CRIOCM) and the Founding Editor-in-Chief of the International Journal of Construction Management (IJCM). He holds a number of external appointments as Honorary Professor and Visiting Professor internationally.

Jorge Ochoa

Dr Jorge Ochoa is a Senior Lecturer at the University of South Australia. He is a leading scholar in the field of sustainable transformation of built environments. His research is focused on developing systems and decision support tools that leverage cutting-edge technologies such as big data analytics, artificial intelligence, and visualizations to address challenges in the built environment. Dr Ochoa collaborates closely with industry partners and end-users to develop innovative solutions with real-world impact beyond the academic sphere. As a result, his work has been widely recognized and adopted by prestigious organizations, including the United Nations Human Settlements Program (UN-Habitat), the European Commission DG Environment, the United Nations World Water Assessment Program, and the New York City Panel on Climate Change. Dr Ochoa's contributions to the field have also earned him numerous external appointments as a Visiting Professor, and he has been invited to deliver keynote addresses at prominent industry and academic forums, such as Rio+20 and the World Urban Forum.

Haijun Bao

Prof Haijun Bao is a Professor and the Head of School of Spatial Planning and Design at Hangzhou City University. He is also the Director of the Research Institute of Planning and Sustainability at the University. He obtained his PhD degree and Postdoctoral training at the College of Environmental and Resources Sciences at Zhejiang University. Professor Bao's research interests include spatial planning and urban and rural governance. He has been focusing on the issues of new urbanization and rural revitalization, land space governance and common prosperity. He is the Director of the Special Committee on Quality of Urban Green and Low Carbon Development in the China Association of Building Energy Efficiency (CABEE). In the capacity of Principal Investigator, Professor Bao has headed four national-level projects from National Natural Science Foundation of China and the National Social Science Foundation of China, and ten provincial- and ministerial-level projects. He has published more than 40 academic papers in top international journals, including Land Use Policy, Cities, Journal of Rural Studies, and Habitat International. He has received the 20th Outstanding Achievement Award of Philosophy and Social Sciences of Zhejiang Province and the 19th Outstanding Achievement Award of Philosophy and Social Sciences of Zhejiang Province.

buildings MDPI

Editorial

Strategies for Sustainable Urban Development—Addressing the Challenges of the 21st Century

Liyin Shen [1], J. Jorge Ochoa [2,*] and Haijun Bao [1]

1 Research Institute of Urban Planning and Sustainability, School of Spatial Planning and Design, Hangzhou City University, Hangzhou 310000, China; shenliyin@zucc.edu.cn (L.S.); baohaijun@zucc.edu.cn (H.B.)
2 UniSA STEM, University of South Australia, Adelaide, SA 5000, Australia
* Correspondence: jorge.ochoa@unisa.edu.au

Urbanisation has been one of the most transformative processes of our time, and in recent decades has led to significant changes in the way we live, work, and interact with the world around us. With more people moving to cities, there is a growing need for sustainable urban development strategies that balance economic growth, environmental protection, and social well-being. At the same time, the field of urban studies and planning is rapidly evolving, and so are the challenges that cities face in the 21st century. From climate change and resource depletion to pandemics and social inequality, the complex and interconnected nature of urban systems requires innovative approaches for planning and design.

This Special Issue brings together a diverse range of scholars and practitioners who share a commitment to advancing sustainable urban development. The collection of papers presents cutting-edge research on a wide range of topics, including resilience, value creation, blockchain architecture, decarbonisation, COVID-19, street network efficiency, vulnerable communities, transit-oriented development, green roofs, and post-occupancy evaluation. Each study offers a unique perspective on the challenges and opportunities of sustainable urban development, highlighting innovative strategies and best practices that can inform future urban planning and policy.

The interdisciplinary and international scope of this publication reflects the complex and diverse nature of sustainable urban development, as well as the urgent need for collaboration and exchange across disciplines and borders. By presenting ten original research studies, this publication aims to foster a more informed and productive conversation about the future of our cities and the challenges we face in building sustainable, equitable, and resilient urban communities. As such, this Special Issue is intended to serve as a valuable resource for researchers, practitioners, policymakers, and students who seek to advance the cause of sustainable urban development in the 21st century.

Citation: Shen, L.; Ochoa, J.J.; Bao, H. Strategies for Sustainable Urban Development—Addressing the Challenges of the 21st Century. *Buildings* **2023**, *13*, 847. https://doi.org/10.3390/buildings13040847

Received: 14 March 2023
Accepted: 20 March 2023
Published: 23 March 2023

Wang et al. [1] evaluated the resilience level of cities in the Chengdu–Chongqing urban agglomeration of China, using multiple interdisciplinary methods such as the entropy weight method, Theil index, and geographically and temporally weighted regression. The research shows that urban resilience has evolved from a low to high level, with significant spatial differences in resilience levels. The study also identified several factors that positively impact urban resilience, including administrative level, marketisation level, industrial structure, population density, urbanisation level, and the level of emergency facilities, which have spatial and temporal heterogeneity. The study proposes strategies from the perspective of sustainable urban development to improve the resilience level of urban agglomerations in western China. These findings provide new theoretical support and decision-making reference for sustainable urban development in China.

The academic study by Li et al. [2] focused on the value creation of public–private partnerships (PPPs) in the development of urban rail transit (URT) projects in China. PPPs are adopted in URT projects to benefit both public and private sectors due to the heavy investment and abundant construction and management experience required. However, achieving basic project objectives is no longer sufficient for value creation, and partner synergy is necessary to achieve added value. This study adopts a grounded theory approach to identify the influencing factors of value creation of URT PPP projects in China. Resource complementarity among stakeholders, cooperation environments, and partnership synergy were identified as the main influencing factors. The study establishes a theoretical model to describe how these factors promote value creation during the implementation of URT PPP projects, providing a model for further empirical examination.

Lv et al. [3] examined the potential use of blockchain technology as a solution to security and privacy issues in the context of the Internet of Things (IoT), with a focus on smart homes. The authors propose a classification-based blockchain architecture with a hierarchical proof-of-work mechanism to reduce storage consumption and decrease latency. This involves dividing IoT devices into child nodes by data classification and adjusting the difficulty of the proof-of-work to set moderate-cost security grades. The proposed architecture is shown to offer significant improvements in terms of storage and efficiency compared to traditional methods and current technology, while maintaining security. This research provides valuable insights into the development of secure and efficient blockchain-based solutions for IoT applications.

Salazar et al. [4] explored the challenges of reducing greenhouse gas (GHG) emissions in the building sector, which is one of the main emitters contributing to climate change. Governments have developed nationally determined contributions (NDCs) and roadmaps to establish measures to achieve net-zero emissions. However, stakeholder integration is a significant barrier to implementing these measures, especially in the building sector. This research employs social network analysis (SNA) concepts to explore the roles of actors required to achieve net-zero emissions in the Colombian building sector. The study uses the results of semi-structured interviews led by the Colombian Green Building Council (CGBC) within the framework of the Zero Carbon Building Accelerator (ZCBA) project. The findings reveal highly interconnected networks characterised by redundant connections among actors. Three types of actors are identified within each enabler network: prominent actors, second-level actors, and perimeter actors. The study emphasises the importance of stakeholder integration in the transition to net-zero emissions in the building sector.

Kim S. and Kim H. [5] investigated the night-time economy (NTE) of Seoul, Korea, and explored the relationship between NTE vitality (NTEV), COVID-19, and credit card sales. The research aims to empirically identify the characteristics of Korea's NTE and derive an indicator of NTEV by considering the NTE in urban regions. The study evaluates NTEV using indicators of nightly floating population, night-lighting value, and the number of entertainment facilities. The results suggest that the NTEV can boost the consumption economy of the entire city. Additionally, the impact of COVID-19 on the economy differed depending on the density of facilities to which the social distancing policy was applied, and an increase in the number of confirmed COVID-19 patients decreased credit card sales, thereby deteriorating the urban economy. The study highlights the importance of NTEs in promoting economic recovery in the wake of the COVID-19 pandemic.

Anabtawi and Scoppa [6] employed quantitative methods to assess the effectiveness of street connectivity policies implemented by Abu Dhabi's Urban Planning Council (UPC) in newly developed projects. The study measured efficiency by analysing the directness of pedestrian routes between residential and non-residential destinations in twelve neighbourhoods of the Capital District project. The results indicated that over 58% of the neighbourhoods failed to connect residential plots efficiently, and more than 40% of residential plots could not connect efficiently to non-residential plots. The study provides recommendations for policymakers and project developers to enhance street infrastructure using the sikkak alleyway system found in other neighbourhoods in the city, aligning with Estidama's walkability standards. The study's rigorous quantitative analyses can be utilised in real-world projects, improving the connection between policy and practice.

The study by Giorgi et al. [7] examined the vulnerability of communities, cities, and territories due to current changes and the potential for urban architectural interventions to mitigate these vulnerabilities. However, these interventions require sustained and transversal visions that consider the temporal context of the coming decades. To address this issue, the study describes the research project "Design for Vulnerables", which aims to define methodologies for reducing urban vulnerabilities in the future. The project involved a design workshop in a vulnerable community in northern Mexico, which was analysed using a research-by-design methodology. The study identifies current issues that affect urban vulnerabilities and generates a set of principles for Design for Vulnerables, graphically represented by a re-interpretation of the Krebs cycle. This multidisciplinary approach demonstrates the potential for urban design to reduce vulnerabilities and support social initiatives.

Huang et al. [8] studied the challenges in promoting Transit-Oriented Developments (TODs) through urban design and proposed a new framework that integrates generative design methods and data-driven decision-making approaches. The authors argue that the traditional design decision making, which is based on designers' experience, lacks quantitative feedback on design schemes and therefore fails to promote progress in urban design. The proposed framework incorporates urban design intelligence for TODs and employs parametric tools and models to evaluate generative urban design proposals, providing timely feedback to support design decisions. A case study was conducted to demonstrate the feasibility of the proposed approach, which successfully selects optimal TOD design solutions. This study highlights the significance of integrating quantitative and qualitative assessment in experience-based decision making and emphasises the role of designers' decision making in generative urban design.

Alqahtany [9] investigated the major effects and challenges faced in implementing the green roof technique in Riyadh, Saudi Arabia. The implementation of green roofs is crucial for achieving urban sustainability, as they are energy-efficient, eco-friendly, and cost-effective in the long run. Despite their benefits, there is a reluctance to adopt green roofs in Saudi Arabia, and the reasons for this have not been reported. To address this gap in knowledge, a survey questionnaire was designed to explore the level of awareness among the public and the challenges they face in installing green roofs. An extensive literature review and reconnaissance survey were conducted to identify the key factors and challenges to include in the questionnaire. The findings indicate a high level of support for green roofs among the people of Riyadh, with aesthetic enhancement and air quality control being the most commonly cited benefit; however, the climate of the region was identified as the biggest challenge in implementing green roofs. The study concludes with recommendations for local authorities to take action and assist building owners and policy makers in overcoming the challenges associated with green roofs.

Wu and Li [10] examined the significance of sports parks for physical activity in China in the context of the COVID-19 epidemic. The study reviewed national fitness policies and identifies different types of sports parks to investigate the usage and preferences of urban dwellers in sports parks using a questionnaire, behavioural observation, and interviews as research methods. The study examined the Beijing Olympic Forest Park, Sun Park, and Huilongguan Park as examples and found that participants exhibited high overall satisfaction with the sports parks. Furthermore, the study identified Sports Facilities and Maintenance and Management as the two most significant factors that influence residents' willingness to use sports parks. The findings of this study can guide future planning and construction of sports parks in China.

In conclusion, this Special Issue presents a comprehensive and insightful examination of new research in sustainable urban development, highlighting the associated challenges and opportunities. The studies emphasise the crucial role of community engagement and the pressing need to address the specific challenges, particularly confronting vulnerable communities. It is our firm belief that this publication will constitute a noteworthy contribution to the ongoing dialogue on sustainable urban development and foster the development of more efficacious and comprehensive strategies for urban planning and design. Such efforts are essential to address the multifaceted challenges that confront our cities today and in the future.

We are grateful to the authors for their valuable contributions and dedication to advancing knowledge in this field. We also extend our appreciation to the peer reviewers for their critical evaluation and feedback, which has helped ensure the quality and rigour of the papers included in this publication. We aspire that this compilation of works will inspire further research and dialogue on sustainable urban development and facilitate the development of more sustainable urban communities worldwide.

Conflicts of Interest: The authors declare no conflict of interest.

References

1. Wang, B.; Han, S.; Ao, Y.; Liao, F. Evaluation and Factor Analysis for Urban Resilience: A Case Study of Chengdu–Chongqing Urban Agglomeration. *Buildings* **2022**, *12*, 962. [CrossRef]
2. Li, X.; Yuan, J.; Liu, X.; Ke, Y.; Jia, S. Identifying Critical Influencing Factors of the Value Creation of Urban Rail Transit PPP Projects in China. *Buildings* **2022**, *12*, 1080. [CrossRef]
3. Lv, W.; Wang, N.; Xie, X.; Hong, Z. A Classification-Based Blockchain Architecture for Smart Home with Hierarchical PoW Mechanism. *Buildings* **2022**, *12*, 1321. [CrossRef]
4. Salazar, J.; Guevara, J.; Espinosa, M.; Rivera, F.; Franco, J.F. Decarbonization of the Colombian Building Sector: Social Network Analysis of Enabling Stakeholders. *Buildings* **2022**, *12*, 1531. [CrossRef]
5. Kim, S.-A.; Kim, H. Structural Relationship between COVID-19, Night-Time Economic Vitality, and Credit-Card Sales: The Application of a Formative Measurement Model in PLS-SEM. *Buildings* **2022**, *12*, 1606. [CrossRef]
6. Anabtawi, R.; Scoppa, M. Measuring Street Network Efficiency and Block Sizes in Superblocks—Addressing the Gap between Policy and Practice. *Buildings* **2022**, *12*, 1686. [CrossRef]
7. Giorgi, E.; Cattaneo, T.; Serrato Guerrero, K.P. The Principles of Design for Vulnerable Communities: A Research by Design Approach Overrunning the Disciplinary Boundaries. *Buildings* **2022**, *12*, 1789. [CrossRef]
8. Huang, X.; Yuan, W.; White, M.; Langenheim, N. A Parametric Framework to Assess Generative Urban Design Proposals for Transit-Oriented Development. *Buildings* **2022**, *12*, 1971. [CrossRef]
9. Alqahtany, A. Green Roofs as an Approach to Enhance Urban Sustainability: A Study of Public Perception in Riyadh, Saudi Arabia. *Buildings* **2022**, *12*, 2202. [CrossRef]
10. Wu, X.; Li, X. Post-Occupancy Evaluation of Sports Parks during the COVID-19 Pandemic: Taking Sports Parks in Beijing as Examples. *Buildings* **2022**, *12*, 2250. [CrossRef]

buildings

MDPI

Article

Evaluation and Factor Analysis for Urban Resilience: A Case Study of Chengdu–Chongqing Urban Agglomeration

Bo Wang [1], Shan Han [1,*], Yibin Ao [2,*] and Fangwei Liao [3]

1 School of Civil Engineering and Architecture, Southwest University of Science and Technology, Mianyang 621010, China; boy@swust.edu.cn
2 College of Environmental and Civil Engineering, Chengdu University of Technology, Chengdu 610059, China
3 School of Management, University of Science and Technology of China, Hefei 230026, China; lfw377801@163.com
* Correspondence: hanshan2020@mails.swust.edu.cn (S.H.); aoyibin10@mail.cdut.edu.cn (Y.A.)

Abstract: Resilient cities provide a new operating mechanism for sustainable urban development and can effectively reduce urban disaster losses. Urban resilience has become an important research topic, but few scholars focus on the urban resilience of urban agglomerations in western China. Therefore, this paper takes the Chengdu–Chongqing urban agglomeration of China as the study area and aims to evaluate the resilience level of cities in typical regions of western China. This study uses multiple interdisciplinary methods, such as the entropy weight method, Theil index, and geographically and temporally weighted regression, to evaluate the resilience levels of 16 cities in the region and discuss the influencing factors of regional urban resilience. The results show that the urban resilience of cities in the Chengdu–Chongqing urban agglomeration has evolved from a low to high level. Additionally, there are significant spatial differences in urban resilience in the Chengdu–Chongqing urban agglomeration, and the resilience levels of cities in the east and west of the region are relatively high, while the resilience levels of cities in the south and north are relatively low. Further research found that factors such as administrative level, marketization level, industrial structure, population density, urbanization level, and emergency facility level all have a significant positive impact on the improvement of urban resilience, but this impact has spatial and temporal heterogeneity. Based on the above research results, the strategies have been proposed from the perspective of sustainable urban development to provide a new theoretical support and decision-making reference for improving the resilience level of urban agglomerations in western China.

Keywords: sustainable urban development; urban resilience; influencing factors; Chengdu–Chongqing urban agglomeration

Citation: Wang, B.; Han, S.; Ao, Y.; Liao, F. Evaluation and Factor Analysis for Urban Resilience: A Case Study of Chengdu–Chongqing Urban Agglomeration. *Buildings* **2022**, *12*, 962. https://doi.org/10.3390/buildings12070962

Academic Editors: Liyin Shen, Jorge Ochoa and Haijun Bao

Received: 1 June 2022
Accepted: 4 July 2022
Published: 6 July 2022

1. Introduction

The city is an important part of human society and an important carrier of human activities, and its sustainable development is an important guarantee for the progress of human society. As a complex system integrating economy, society, ecology, and infrastructure, urban sustainable development means that a city can better solve the problems encountered in the process of development, and its core lies in coordinating the relationship between urban development and urban resources, environment, and security [1]. However, the continuous expansion of urban scale and the high concentration of the population make the contradiction between urban development and urban resources, environment, and security increasingly prominent [2]. High-intensity economic activities and frequent emergencies have caused excessive consumption of urban resources and substantial damage to the environment, which has brought serious challenges to the sustainable development of cities [3]. The potential impact and catastrophic consequences of emergencies such as earthquakes, floods, and COVID-19 in recent years have become increasingly significant, severely restricting the sustainable urban development [4].

Fortunately, due to the direct relationship between urban resilience and sustainable urban development, the proposal of resilient cities provides a new operating mechanism for sustainable urban development [5]. Resilient cities aim for the sustainable development of cities, can improve the speed of disaster response, and reinforce the disaster operation mechanism of cities through the preparation work before emergencies [6]. Therefore, resilient cities can quickly adapt to and absorb the hazards of disasters, effectively reduce the potential impact of disasters, reduce the disaster losses of cities, and enhance the sustainable development capacity of cities [7].

In recent years, facing the threat of escalating emergencies, building resilient cities has become a key issue of international concern [8]. China established the Ministry of Emergency Management and included resilient cities in its long-term development plan [9]. The United Nations [10], the Rockefeller Foundation [11], and other relevant international institutions are also constantly promoting the development of resilient cities. Simultaneously, urban resilience research has also become the theme of current urban governance research [12], but few scholars have paid attention to urban resilience in relatively backward areas in western China.

Therefore, we take the Chengdu–Chongqing urban agglomeration in western China as the research area and aim to explore the resilience improvement strategies and enhance the sustainable development capabilities of cities. In this study, we summarize the current research progress on urban resilience in Section 2, and present the general research area, framework, and methodology of this paper in Section 3. We analyze the level of urban resilience and the influencing factors of urban resilience in the Chengdu–Chongqing urban agglomeration in Section 4. In Section 5, We discuss theoretical contributions and development proposals. In Section 6, we summarize the main conclusions of this study and point out aspects that can be further explored by subsequent research.

2. Research Review

At the end of the last century, resilience theory was first used to study the problem of complex urban systems responding to natural disasters [13] and emergencies [14]. At the beginning of this century, the International Council for Local Environmental Initiatives (ICLEI) first proposed the concept of urban resilience and incorporated it into urban sustainable and healthy development policies, promoting the application of resilience theory in urban ecosystem research [15]. By reviewing the existing international research on urban resilience, it is found that domestic and foreign scholars have carried out rich research on urban resilience from multiple backgrounds, multiple perspectives, and multiple regions. These studies mainly concentrate on three aspects: theoretical research on the concept and features of urban resilience; empirical research on the evaluation and evolution mechanism of urban resilience; and exploratory research on the improvement paths of urban resilience level.

In terms of theoretical research, existing research first discusses the connotation of urban resilience. Due to different research perspectives, the definition of urban resilience can be divided into two categories: anti-stress protection theory and capacity improvement theory. The theory of anti-stress protection defines urban resilience as the ability of a city to achieve public environmental security, social order stability, and normal operation of the economic system when faced with internal and external sudden disasters [16,17]. The theory of capacity improvement defines urban resilience as a sustainable development ability of a city to protect the normal operation of internal systems during disasters and reorganize internal systems to improve overall resilience after disasters [18,19]. Second, in terms of theoretical research, scholars also discussed the characteristics of resilience cities. Scholars have discussed the characteristics of resilient cities in terms of their premise [20], effect [21], mechanism [7], and purpose [22].

In terms of empirical research, scholars mainly evaluate the resilience level of cities in specific regions from three perspectives: the disaster response perspective, urban composition perspective, and urban resilience characteristics perspective [23]. From the perspective of disaster response, scholars have mainly evaluated the disaster response capacity of different urban systems with the background of specific disasters, such as climate change [24], earthquakes [25], flood disasters [26], and economic crises [27]. From the perspective of urban composition, relevant scholars mainly evaluate the level of urban resilience from four dimensions: society, economy, ecology, and organization [28]. On this basis, related scholars continue to expand the evaluation dimension, such as system and culture [29]. From the perspective of urban resilience characteristics, scholars mainly evaluate the urban resilience level of a specific region based on the combination characteristics, such as the combination characteristics of "scale density form" [30], the combination characteristics of "response, recovery and adaptability" [31] and the combination characteristics of "prediction, adaptation and recovery" [32].

In terms of exploratory research, scholars mainly focus on the research theme of analyzing the influencing factors of urban resilience and explore ways and methods to improve urban resilience [33]. Das et al. (2020) [34] found through a questionnaire survey that the education level, economic development level, and infrastructure level of local people are important factors affecting the urban resilience of the east coast of the Indian Ocean, and put forward urban resilience improvement strategies, such as improving insurance policies and smart asset investment. Liu et al. (2021) [35] used a spatial econometric model to study and discover that factors such as urbanization rate and administration all had an important impact on urban resilience in Henan, China, and proposed urban resilience improvement ways, such as continuously promoting the level of new urbanization and optimizing the industrial structure. Khan et al. (2021) [36] used structural equation modeling to study and discover that geographic location, government decision-making, and urban financial conditions have a significant impact on urban resilience and gave related methods to improve urban resilience. Moradi (2021) [37] used the expert scoring method to find that economic indicators and physical environment conditions are all important factors for improving the urban resilience of Iran's second-largest city, and also put forward suggestions for improving urban resilience.

However, due to the late start of the research on urban resilience, the existing research still has some limitations. In the selection of a study area, the existing research is mainly limited to the relatively developed coastal areas of the global economy, and lacks the resilience research of relatively backward inland cities. In terms of research methods, exploratory research is mostly limited to econometric methods such as linear regression, structural equations, and spatial econometric models, and new research methods need to be introduced. In terms of research content, most studies are limited to the measurement and evolution mechanism of urban resilience, lacking more in-depth research on regional spatial optimization and coordinated improvement of regional urban resilience.

Compared with existing research, this paper is the first to comprehensively evaluate the urban resilience level of the Chengdu–Chongqing urban agglomeration in western China, which provides a decision-making reference for enhancing the urban resilience of the area and driving the improvement of urban governance level in western China. Second, this paper combines the methods of econometrics and geography, improves the traditional entropy weight method by adding time variables, and introduces the geographically and temporally weighted regression model into the field of urban governance research, which innovates the research method. Finally, on the basis of evaluating the level of regional urban resilience, this study analyzes and puts forward the improvement strategy of urban resilience coordinated development, which broadens the theoretical boundary and scope of application.

3. Materials and Methods

3.1. Study Area

This study chooses the Chengdu–Chongqing urban agglomeration in western China as the study area, which consists of 16 cities as shown in Figure 1. It has the unique advantage of connecting southwest and northwest China and connecting East Asia, Southeast Asia, and South Asia [38]. Firstly, it is the region with the strongest industrial foundation, the broadest market space, and the highest degree of openness in western China. In 2021, the total economic volume of the Chengdu–Chongqing urban agglomeration will account for 6.5% of the national total and 30.8% of the western region [39]. Secondly, it is another major coordinated development area following the three major coordinated development areas along the eastern coast of China. It is an important economic center with national influence and has a unique strategic position in driving the overall development of western China. Thirdly, the Chengdu–Chongqing urban agglomeration is adjacent to many countries in Southeast Asia, and is also inhabited by ethnic minorities. The geographical environment is special and complex, and public events occur frequently. According to the data of the Ministry of National Emergency Management, in recent years, the incidence of earthquake disasters, traffic accidents, man-made damage, and public emergencies in the study area has remained high, showing the characteristics of complex composition, widespread, and severe social impact, which seriously threaten the safety and the sustainable development of regional cities [40].

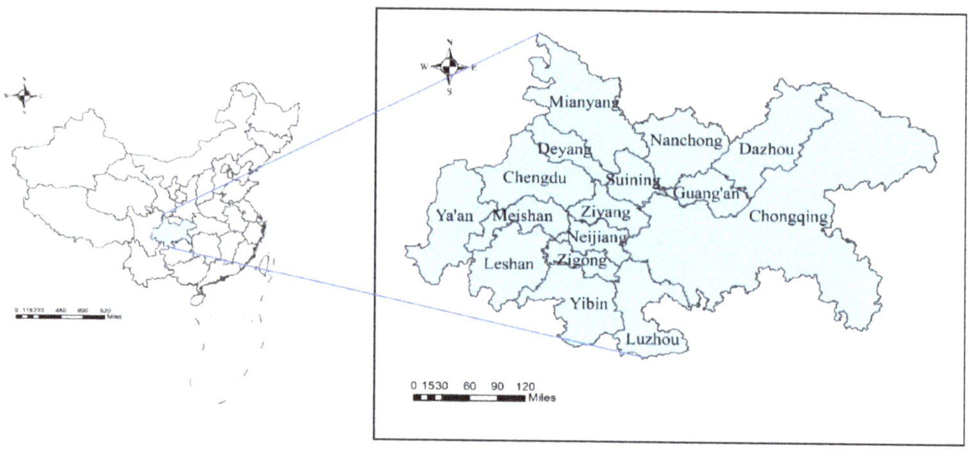

Figure 1. Study area.

3.2. Data Sources

3.2.1. Statistical Data

This study takes the statistical data of 16 cities in the study area from 2005 to 2019 as the study sample. The data mainly come from the relevant statistical yearbooks and statistical bulletins of the country, province, and city. For individual missing and wrong values, this paper uses the mean value method of adjacent years to interpolate and correct, so as to guarantee the completeness and authenticity of the data.

3.2.2. Geographic Data

The geographic data in this paper are mainly from the National Basic Geographic Information Center of China and the National Geographic Information Resource Catalog Service System of China. After screening and processing, the geographic data conforming to the study area are obtained. Meanwhile, in this paper, after processing, the resolution of the processed geographic data is 1000, which can better present the research content.

3.3. *Methodology*

3.3.1. Entropy Weight Method

The entropy weight method (EWM) is a weight calculation and evaluation method. Compared with the subjective weighted scoring methods, the entropy weight method can make a more objective and real evaluation of the object, and it is simple and easy to operate [41]. Based on the traditional entropy weight method, this paper adds the time variable of different years for improvement, which makes the evaluation of urban resilience more accurate and comprehensive. This paper uses MATLAB (Version 2018a, MathWorks, Natick, Massachusetts, United States), a programming calculation software, for calculation and the specific process is as follows:

(1) Assuming there are n cities, m years, and s indicators, the original indicator matrix is $X = \{X_{aij}\}\ m \times n \times s\ (0 < i < n,\ 0 < a < m,\ 0 < j < s)$. Then, the j-th index of the city i in the a-th year can be expressed as X_{aij}, and in this paper n, m, and s are 16, 15, and 25, respectively.

(2) Indicator data standardization:

1. Positive indicator:

$$X'_{aij} = \frac{X_{aij} - \min\{X_j\}}{\max\{X_j\} - \min\{X_j\}} \tag{1}$$

2. Negative indicator:

$$X'_{aij} = \frac{\max\{X_j\} - X_{aij}}{\max\{X_j\} - \min\{X_j\}} \tag{2}$$

(3) Indicator data normalization:

$$Y_{aij} = \frac{X'_{aij}}{\sum\limits_{a=1}^{m}\sum\limits_{i=1}^{n} X'_{aij}} \tag{3}$$

(4) Calculating the entropy value of the indicator:

$$e_j = -\frac{1}{\ln(mn)}\sum_{a=1}^{m}\sum_{i=1}^{n} Y_{aij}\ln(Y_{aij}) \tag{4}$$

(5) Calculating the redundancy of the index entropy value:

$$g_i = 1 - e_j \tag{5}$$

(6) Calculating indicator weights:

$$W_j = \frac{g_j}{\sum\limits_{j=1}^{s} g_j} \tag{6}$$

(7) Calculating urban resilience scores:

$$R = \sum_{j=1}^{s} X'_{aij} W_j \tag{7}$$

3.3.2. Theil Index

The Theil index is an indicator that uses the concept of entropy in information theory to evaluate the development gap between individuals or regions [42]. This study takes the

Theil index to describe the spatial imbalance characteristics of urban resilience development in the study area.

$$T = \sum_{i=1}^{n} P_i \frac{x_i}{u} \ln\left(\frac{x_i}{u}\right) \quad (8)$$

Among them, n refers to the number of cities, P_i represents the proportion of the population of the i-th city to the total urban population, x_i represents the resilience level of the i-th city, and u represents the weighted average of all observed urban resilience levels.

3.3.3. Geographically and Temporally Weighted Regression

It is a local linear regression model, which can combine temporal information and spatial information and consider both time and space non-stationarity. It can estimate the effect of influencing factors in different regions and different times, so that the relationship between variables can change with the change of time and spatial position, and the result is more in line with the objective reality [43]. This paper uses ArcGIS10.7 (Version 10.7, Environmental Systems Research Institute, Redlands, CA, USA), a geographic data analysis software, for calculation and analysis, and its model structure is as follows:

$$Y_i = \beta_0(u_i, v_i, t_i) + \sum_k \beta_k(u_i, v_i, t_i) X_{ik} + \varepsilon_i \quad (9)$$

Among them, Y_i is the explained variable and (u_i, v_i, t_i) is the spatiotemporal dimension coordinate, where u_i is the longitude coordinate, v_i is the latitude coordinate and t_i is the time coordinate of the i-th sample point. $\beta_0(u_i, v_i, t_i)$ is the constant term (intercept), while $\beta_k(u_i, v_i, t_i)$ is the regression coefficient of the k-th explanatory variable.

Among them, the regression coefficient adopts the local weighted least squares estimation, and the method is as follows:

(1) Calculating the space–time distance:

$$d_{ij}^{ST} = \sqrt{\lambda\left[(u_i - u_j)^2 - (v_i - v_j)^2\right] + \mu(t_i - t_j)^2} \quad (10)$$

where d_{ij}^{ST} is the space–time distance and λ and μ are the weights of the Gaussian function method.

(2) Calculating the space–time weight function:

$$W_{ij} = \exp\left[-\frac{\left(d_{ij}^{ST}\right)^2}{h^2}\right] \quad (11)$$

where W_{ij} is the space–time weight function and d_{ij}^{ST} is the space–time distance. h is the spatiotemporal bandwidth, selected according to the minimum cross-validation (CV) value, and is the sum of the squared errors between the actual value y_i and the predicted value $\hat{y}_i(h)$, and the formula is as follows:

$$CV(h) = \sum_i (y_i - \hat{y}_i(h))^2 \quad (12)$$

(3) Constructing the space–time weight matrix:

$$W(u_i, v_i, t_i) = diag(W_{i1}, W_{i2}, \cdots, W_{ij}, \cdots W_{in}) \quad (13)$$

where the space–time weight matrix $W(u_i, v_i, t_i)$ is an $n \times n$ diagonal matrix, where $W_{ij}(1 \le j \le n)$ is the space–time weight function.

(4) Calculating the regression coefficient:

$$\hat{\beta}(u_i, v_i, t_i) = \left[X^T W(u_i, v_i, t_i) X\right]^{-1} X^T W(u_i, v_i, t_i) Y \quad (14)$$

3.4. Index System and Weight

3.4.1. Index System

Through the above review of existing research, this paper considers urban resilience as the degree to which a city can endure, adapt, and absorb hazards when faced with various disasters, and as the recovery capability after the disaster. From the perspective of urban resilience composition and urban resilience characteristics, this paper designs an evaluation index system with three levels: target level, criterion level, and index level [44]. This paper takes overall resilience as the target layer and chooses economic resilience, social resilience, ecological resilience, and infrastructure resilience as the criterion layers from the perspective of urban resilience composition and characteristics. Additionally, combined with domestic and foreign urban resilience evaluation index systems [45], this paper selects 25 specific indicators to build the evaluation index system (as in Table 1).

Table 1. Evaluation Index System.

Target Layer	Criterion Layer	Indicator Layer	Indicator Nature
Overall resilience	Economic resilience	Per capita GDP (CNY) [46]	+
		Proportion of tertiary industry in GDP (%) [28]	+
		Per capita investment in fixed assets (CNY) [47]	+
		Dependence on foreign trade (%) [31]	+
		Proportion of fiscal revenue in GDP (%) [47]	+
		Per capita disposable income of urban residents (CNY) [37]	+
	Social resilience	Urbanization level (%) [48]	+
		Proportion of non-agricultural employed population (%) [29]	+
		Urban registered unemployment rate (%) [49]	-
		Number of college students per 10,000 (person) []	+
		Proportion of employees in public management and social organizations (%) [50]	+
		Number of hospital beds per 10,000 people (piece) [51]	+
	Ecological resilience	Greening coverage rate of built-up area (%) [52]	+
		Per capita green space area in municipal area (m^2) [53]	+
		Industrial wastewater discharge per unit GDP (t) [54]	-
		Industrial sulfur dioxide emission per unit GDP (t) [54]	-
		Industrial smoke (dust) emission per unit GDP (t) [54]	-
		Centralized treatment rate of domestic sewage (%) [55]	+
		Comprehensive utilization rate of industrial solid waste (%) [52]	+
	Infrastructure resilience	Per capita water consumption (m^3) [56]	-
		Per capita electricity consumption (kW·h) [56]	-
		Fixed Internet users per 10,000 people (households) [50]	+
		Gas penetration rate (%) [52]	+
		Per capita Road area (m^2) [53]	+
		Density of drainage pipeline in built-up area (km/km^2) [51]	+

3.4.2. Indicator Weight

Based on the assessment file framework built over, this study employs the improved entropy weight method to compute the weight value of the urban resilience evaluation index of the study area after collecting the data. Through MATLAB calculation, the weight coefficients of the criterion layer and indicators are obtained, as appeared within the taking after Table 2:

Table 2. Weights of Evaluation Indicators.

Target Layer	Criterion Layer	Weight	Indicator Layer	Weight
Overall resilience	Economic resilience	0.3549	Per capita GDP (CNY)	0.0818
			Proportion of tertiary industry in GDP (%)	0.0431
			Per capita investment in fixed assets (CNY)	0.0854
			Dependence on foreign trade (%)	0.0103
			Proportion of fiscal revenue in GDP (%)	0.0632
			Per capita disposable income of urban residents (CNY)	0.0711
	Social resilience	0.2979	Urbanization level (%)	0.0305
			Proportion of non-agricultural employed population (%)	0.0297
			Urban registered unemployment rate (%)	0.0286
			Number of college students per 10,000 (person)	0.1389
			Proportion of employees in public management and social organizations (%)	0.0112
			Number of hospital beds per 10,000 people (piece)	0.059
	Ecological resilience	0.1005	Greening coverage rate of built-up area (%)	0.0161
			Per capita green space area in municipal area (m^2)	0.0287
			Industrial wastewater discharge per unit GDP (t)	0.0109
			Industrial sulfur dioxide emission per unit GDP (t)	0.0049
			Industrial smoke (dust) emission per unit GDP (t)	0.0045
			Centralized treatment rate of domestic sewage (%)	0.0245
			Comprehensive utilization rate of industrial solid waste (%)	0.0109
	Infrastructure resilience	0.2467	Per capita water consumption (m^3)	0.0127
			Per capita electricity consumption (kW·h)	0.0099
			Fixed Internet users per 10,000 people (households)	0.1059
			Gas penetration rate (%)	0.0218
			Per capita Road area (m^2)	0.0355
			Density of drainage pipeline in built-up area (km / km2)	0.0609

3.5. Study Variables and Test

3.5.1. Study Variables

(1) Explained Variable.

This paper takes the urban resilience level as the explained variable. Based on the previous construction of an urban resilience level evaluation index system, this study will utilize the improved entropy weight method to evaluate the urban resilience level of 16 cities in the study area from 2005 to 2019, which will be used as the explanatory variable.

(2) Explanatory Variables.

After comprehensively considering the connotation and characteristics of urban resilience, combined with existing investigations, this paper selects the explanatory variables from the aspects of society, environment, economy, population, and facilities that affect the urban resilience. The explanatory variables selected in this paper are as follows: (1) administrative level. Government departments are the direct leading departments of urban planning and development. The administrative level of government departments is directly related to the urban resilience. This paper uses the extent of public monetary use to GDP to measure the urban administrative level. (2) Open level. The opening level of the city will affect the development of the industry, technology, economy, and employment of the city; therefore, the level of urban openness has a great impact on the urban resilience of the city. This paper uses the proportion of the total import and export trade to GDP to measure the opening level of the city. (3) Marketization level. The market level reflects the consumption power and economic vitality of the city, can invigorate the development of the city's economy to a certain degree, and also has an imperative effect on the resilience. This paper adopts the marketization level of the per capita retail quota of social consumer goods. (4) Science and education level. The level of science and education is the driving drive for the sustainable improvement of cities and has an imperative effect on the level of urban resilience. This paper selects the extent of science and instruction uses in fiscal expenditures to measure the level of science and education in cities. (5) Industrial structure. Industrial structure is the embodiment of the city's economic and social stability and is an important guarantee for the city to resist shocks. This paper selects the extent of the tertiary industry in GDP to measure the city's industrial structure. (6) Credit level. The credit level reflects the financial development potential of the city and has a great effect on the city's ability to resist economic shocks. This paper uses the ratio of the total deposits and loans of financial institutions to GDP to measure the city's credit level. (7) Population density. Population density directly affects the distribution and use of urban labor resources and plays an important role in urban economic and social development. This paper uses the proportion of population to urban area to measures population density. (8) Urbanization level. Urbanization can better integrate market resources, create a better urban development environment, and play an important role in the level of urban resilience. This study selects the urbanization rate to measure the urbanization level of a city. (9) Emergency facility level. The level of urban emergency facilities is an important criterion to measure the urban emergency response capability and determines the level of urban resilience. In this paper, the level of urban emergency facilities is measured by the urban per capita infrastructure investment quota.

3.5.2. Variable Test

In the geographically and temporally weighted regression model, when the variance inflation factor (VIF) of the explanatory variable is higher than 10, the model will become unstable. Before performing regression, it is necessary to verify the correlation and multicollinearity between variables. In this paper, the urban resilience scores of 16 cities in the study area from 2005 to 2019 are used as explanatory variables, and the data of the nine explanatory variables collected are standardized at the same time, so that the effect of influencing factors can be directly compared. Based on the statistical data analysis software SPSS (Version 25.0, IBMCorp, Armonk, New York, United States), the correlation and multicollinearity between variables were tested by the Pearson correlation coefficient and variance inflation factor, and key explanatory variables were screened. As can be seen from Table 3, among the nine explanatory variables selected in this study, except for the science and education level, which has no significant correlation with urban resilience, the rest of the explanatory variables are significantly related to urban resilience, and there is no multicollinearity.

Table 3. Explanatory Variable Correlation and Multicollinearity Tests (Note: 1. The dependent variable is urban resilience; 2. ** implies critical at the level of 0.01; 3. According to the score of correlation coefficient, (0.7, 1) is strong correlation, (0.3, 0.7) is medium correlation, (0, 0.3) is weak correlation; 4. Referring to the judgment of ArcGIS on multicollinearity, when VIF > 10, the data index has multicollinearity).

Variable	Correlation		Multicollinearity		
	Pearson Coefficient	Relevance Judgment	Tolerance	VIF	Multicollinearity Diagnostics
Administrative level (X_1)	0.171 **	Significantly weak correlation	0.527	1.896	No collinearity
Open level (X_2)	0.475 **	Significant moderate correlation	0.326	3.066	No collinearity
Marketization level (X_3)	0.934 **	Significant strong correlation	0.133	7.520	No collinearity
Science and education level (X_4)	−0.013	No significant correlation	0.754	1.327	No collinearity
Industrial structure (X_5)	0.750 **	Significant strong correlation	0.303	3.305	No collinearity
Credit level (X_6)	0.735 **	Significant strong correlation	0.205	4.875	No collinearity
Population density (X_7)	0.271 **	Significantly weak correlation	0.436	2.294	No collinearity
Urbanization level (X_8)	0.867 **	Significant strong correlation	0.137	7.303	No collinearity
Emergency facility level (X_9)	0.898 **	Significant strong correlation	0.170	5.896	No collinearity

4. Results

4.1. Evaluation Results of the Urban Resilience

This paper uses the interval taxonomy way to divide the urban resilience score into four grades between (0, 1): less than 0.25 is the low resilience level, between 0.25–0.50 (including 0.25) is the general resilience level, between 0.50–0.75 (including 0.50) is the medium resilience level, and greater than 0.75 (including 0.75) is the high resilience level. Based on this division of urban resilience levels, this study analyzes the urban resilience level and its influencing factors in the Chengdu–Chongqing urban agglomeration.

4.1.1. Urban Resilience Level

From the statistics of the urban resilience score in Table 4, it can be seen that, from 2005 to 2019, the resilience level of the 16 cities in the area showed a continuous upward trend. The urban resilience of Chengdu and Chongqing has increased from a general level of resilience to a high level of resilience, and the urban resilience of the remaining 14 cities has also increased from a low level of resilience to a medium level of resilience. Among them, Guang'an has the largest increase, and its urban resilience level rose from 0.131 in 2005 to 0.577 in 2019, and the annual growth rate reached 22.7%. As Guang'an is a low-resilience city, it is relatively easy to improve its resilience, and it is adjacent to Chongqing, which is driven by the radiation of Chongqing, and the growth rate is obvious. However, the resilience levels of cities such as Chengdu and Chongqing have improved relatively slowly, with a yearly increasing rate of only 6.7% and 8.9%, respectively. This is mainly due to Chengdu and Chongqing being provincial capitals with relatively large scales, and the improvement of urban resilience is affected by various factors, making it relatively difficult. In terms of rankings, the two provincial capitals, Chengdu and Chongqing, are firmly in the top two resilience levels, leading the construction and development of resilient cities in the area. Cities such as Mianyang, Deyang, Zigong, and Ya'an have also been ranked at the forefront, and they are the core forces for the construction and development of resilient cities in the region. The rankings of cities such as Luzhou, Yibin, and Guang'an are also rising, and their role in the construction and development of resilient cities in the region is becoming more and more important.

Table 4. Urban Resilience Scores in the Chengdu–Chongqing Urban Agglomeration.

City	2005		2010		2015		2019	
	Scores	Rank	Scores	Rank	Scores	Rank	Scores	Rank
Chongqing	0.334	2	0.514	2	0.674	2	0.781	2
Chengdu	0.414	1	0.564	1	0.744	1	0.829	1
Zigong	0.322	3	0.392	3	0.462	6	0.62	6
Luzhou	0.189	8	0.283	8	0.452	7	0.578	7
Deyang	0.215	5	0.346	6	0.473	5	0.668	4
Mianyang	0.229	4	0.381	4	0.534	3	0.676	3
Suining	0.151	10	0.264	13	0.406	13	0.529	12
Neijiang	0.15	13	0.24	16	0.369	15	0.508	15
Leshan	0.173	9	0.306	7	0.42	10	0.575	10
Nanchong	0.201	7	0.283	9	0.416	12	0.522	14
Meishan	0.151	11	0.276	10	0.451	8	0.578	8
Yibin	0.151	12	0.275	11	0.393	14	0.536	11
Guang'an	0.131	16	0.262	14	0.418	11	0.577	9
Dazhou	0.133	15	0.257	15	0.309	16	0.443	16
Ya'an	0.211	6	0.357	5	0.513	4	0.655	5
Ziyang	0.14	14	0.268	12	0.434	9	0.523	13

4.1.2. Temporal Evolution Characteristics of Urban Resilience

This paper uses the average resilience of 16 cities to measure the overall resilience level of the region. As shown in Figure 2, from 2005 to 2019, the overall regional resilience level of the Chengdu–Chongqing urban agglomeration grew from 0.206 to 0.6, and the resilience of the economy, society, ecology, and infrastructure also increased significantly. During the period, the ecological resilience level was obviously higher than that of other subsystems such as economy and society in the area, mainly because the urban agglomeration was located in western China, the economic and social level was relatively backward and increase slow, and the ecological environment was not overused, making the ecological resilience level in the region relatively high. In recent years, due to the rapid development of cities in western China, the Chengdu–Chongqing urban agglomeration has been utilizing a large amount of ecological and environmental resources, which has slowed down the improvement of regional ecological resilience, but the resilience of the regional economy, society, and infrastructure has improved rapidly. At the same time, the state has put forward a coordinated development plan for the Chengdu–Chongqing urban agglomeration, which means the overall resilience of the region still has a lot of room for improvement. In the future, the overall resilience of the area will continue to improve.

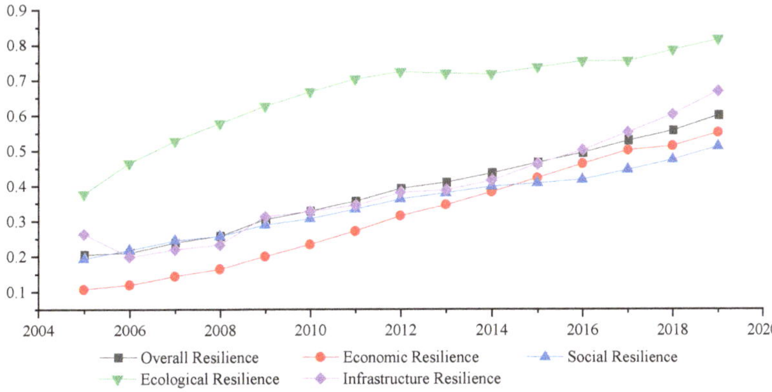

Figure 2. Average value of regional overall resilience and subsystem resilience of the Chengdu–Chongqing urban agglomeration from 2005 to 2019.

4.1.3. Spatial Evolution Characteristics of Urban Resilience

Influenced by geographical location, resource endowment, development level, and other factors, the urban resilience of the 16 cities in the region has significant spatial differences. Based on ArcGIS 10.7 software, this study conducted a spatial representation of the urban resilience of the 16 cities in 2005, 2010, 2015, and 2019. As can be seen from Figure 3: (1) the resilience level of Chengdu, Deyang, Mianyang, and Ya'an in the northwest of the region is relatively high, while the cities with low resilience level are concentrated in the southwest and northeast of the region, mainly Yibin, Zigong, Dazhou, and Guang'an, showing significant spatial differences. (2) In the region, the urban resilience level of Chengdu and Chongqing is much higher than that of other cities, and the core position of the two cities is obvious. Chongqing is located in the east of the region, bordering on the Central Plains urban agglomeration, and Chengdu is located in the west of the region, respectively leading and radiating the construction and development of resilient cities in the region. (3) The resilience level of the surrounding cities of Chengdu is also relatively high, with a good radiation-driven development effect. However, the resilience level of the surrounding cities of Chongqing is relatively low, showing a strong siphon effect, which is related to the fact that Chongqing lacks coordinated development with other cities.

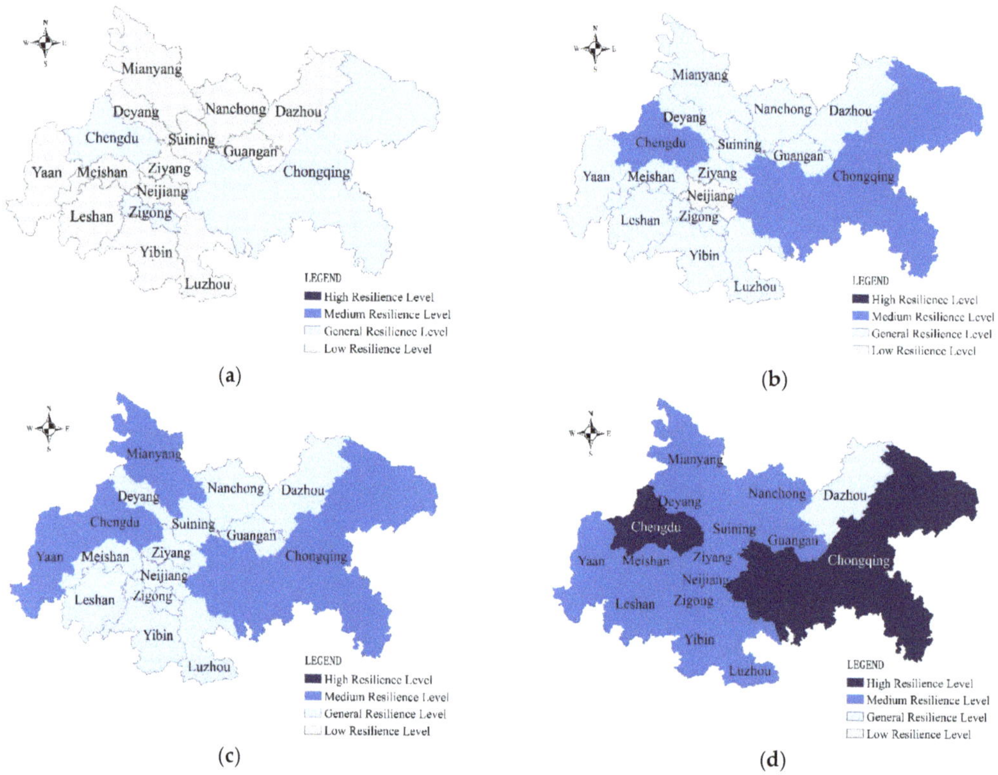

Figure 3. Spatial evolution of urban resilience in the Chengdu–Chongqing urban agglomeration. (**a**) 2005. (**b**) 2010. (**c**) 2015. (**d**) 2019.

In this paper, the Theil index of urban resilience is calculated as shown in Figure 4. It can be found that while the urban resilience of the cities is continuously improving, the gap in resilience levels between cities is decreasing, and the spatial differences and development imbalances are constantly weakening. Among them, the spatial difference between urban ecological resilience and infrastructure resilience is small, and the fluctuation changes are small, but the spatial differences of urban social and economic resilience are large, and the fluctuation changes are obvious, which makes the overall resilience level of regional cities have significant spatial differences and large changes. During the period, the Theil index of regional urban economic and social resilience dropped from 0.538 and 0.47 to 0.219 and 0.182, respectively, and the Theil index of overall urban resilience dropped from 0.205 to 0.117. Spatial differences in urban resilience are shrinking, mainly because of the implementation of the relevant strategies and plans, which accelerate regional economic and social development. Led by Chengdu and Chongqing, the social and financial level of each city has been continuously improved, narrowing the social and economic gap between the cities, and making the unbalanced development of the overall urban resilience weaken. Although the gap still exists, the gap still has a decreasing trend.

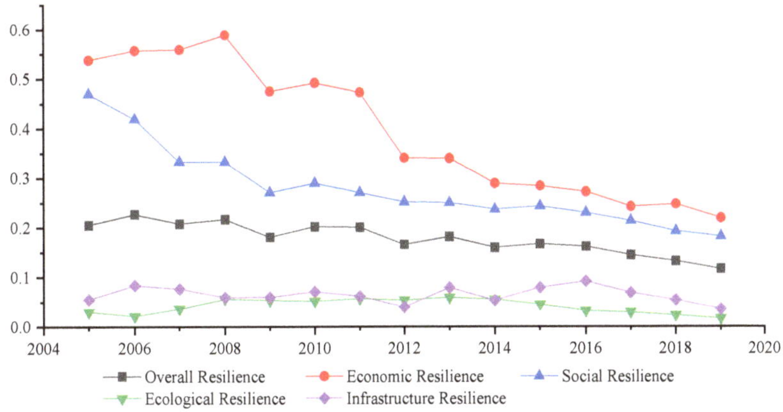

Figure 4. Theil index of urban resilience in the Chengdu–Chongqing urban agglomeration from 2005 to 2019.

4.2. Results of Influencing Factors on Urban Resilience

4.2.1. Analysis of the Action Results of Influencing Factors

From the regression results in Table 5, we can see that for the overall resilience, apart from the level of openness and the level of credit that inhibit the improvement of urban resilience, other explanatory variables have obvious impacts on the improvement of urban resilience. (1) Among them, the marketization level has the most noteworthy effect on urban resilience, mainly because the area is located inland and the economic development is relatively backward, so that improving the level of economic development is a viable way to make strides in the level of urban resilience. (2) The impact of the urbanization level on urban resilience is second. In the study area, where the level of urbanization is relatively backward, the improvement of the urbanization level enables cities to more rationally allocate resources such as population, capital, technology, and information, and improve urban resilience. (3) Industrial structure also has a positive influence on the resilience of the city. The research object as a traditional agricultural area, optimizing the industrial structure can promote urban economic and social development, thereby enhancing urban resilience. (4) Simultaneously, the administrative level and the level of emergency facilities also have positive effects on urban resilience. Since the research object is located in an area prone to natural disasters, the improvement of the administrative level and the level of emergency facilities can promote the level of urban management, improve the speed of urban emergency response, and directly affect the improvement of urban resilience. (5) The study area is rich in population resources, but because of the backward economic and social level there is an excess of labor resources, so population density has little effect on the improvement of urban resilience. (6) The opening level and credit level have negative impacts on urban resilience, which shows that the economic system of the study area inland is relatively fragile and vulnerable to external factors, and it needs to adjust and innovate the opening-up mechanism and development mode to enhance urban resilience.

Table 5. Statistics of the effect of explanatory variables.

	Average Value	Minimum Value	Lower Quartile	Median	Upper Quartile	Maximum Value
X_1	0.1224868	−0.3816324	−0.0135089	0.0544626	0.2102124	0.3274534
X_2	−0.0596576	−0.5084665	−0.2144015	−0.0717284	0.0514928	0.4990566
X_3	0.4984856	−0.6077710	0.1169416	0.3406415	0.7409104	0.9372762
X_5	0.1629620	−0.2222558	0.0421896	0.1616027	0.2609606	0.7530721
X_6	−0.0913039	−0.3589074	−0.2115222	−0.0324012	0.0446096	0.3195433
X_7	0.0390264	−0.4329643	−0.1227017	−0.0217110	0.0767105	0.3949507
X_8	0.4631614	−0.0654836	0.2203307	0.4260468	0.6425338	0.8057922
X_9	0.1612041	−0.0727728	0.0466173	0.1468703	0.2966193	0.5434512
Bandwidth	0.114996	N/A	N/A	N/A	N/A	N/A
AICc	−271.289	N/A	N/A	N/A	N/A	N/A
R^2	0.9507	N/A	N/A	N/A	N/A	N/A

4.2.2. Temporal and Spatial Heterogeneity of the Results

From the statistical results in Table 5, it can be seen that there is obvious temporal and spatial heterogeneity within the effect of the influencing factors of urban resilience in the Chengdu–Chongqing urban agglomeration. This paper uses ArcGIS 10.7 software to spatially characterize the effect of the marketization level, industrial structure, urbanization level, and emergency facility level on urban resilience. As we can see in Figure 5: (1) the level of emergency facilities has a high degree of effect on the urban resilience of Chengdu and Chongqing in the eastern and western of the region, while it has a low degree of effect on the resilience of cities, such as Luzhou and Dazhou in the north and south; (2) the effect of industrial structure on the resilience of regional cities gradually weakens from southwest to northeast, and the impact on cities close to the Central Plains urban agglomeration is relatively low; (3) the urbanization level has a higher degree of impact on cities with higher resilience levels in the eastern and western of the area, and a lower degree of impact on cities with lower resilience levels in the northern of the area; and (4) the marketization level has a lower degree of impact on cities with higher resilience levels in the eastern and western regions, but has a higher degree of impact on cities with lower resilience levels in northern and southern cities.

In this paper, the effect of each influencing factor on cities with different resilience levels was calculated to analyze the temporal heterogeneity of the influencing factors of urban resilience. In Table 6, it can be found that with the improvement of urban resilience, the impact of urbanization level and emergency facilities' level on urban resilience continues to increase, while the impact of the marketization level will gradually decrease with the improvement of urban resilience, which is consistent with the conclusion of spatial heterogeneity of influencing factors. The impact of administrative level, industrial structure, and population density on urban resilience fluctuates little with the improvement of the urban resilience level. However, with the improvement of the urban resilience level, the opening-up level and credit level have an increasingly obvious inhibitory effect on urban resilience. For sustainable urban development in the area, it is imperative to adjust the opening-up mechanism and development mode to improve the overall resilience of regional cities.

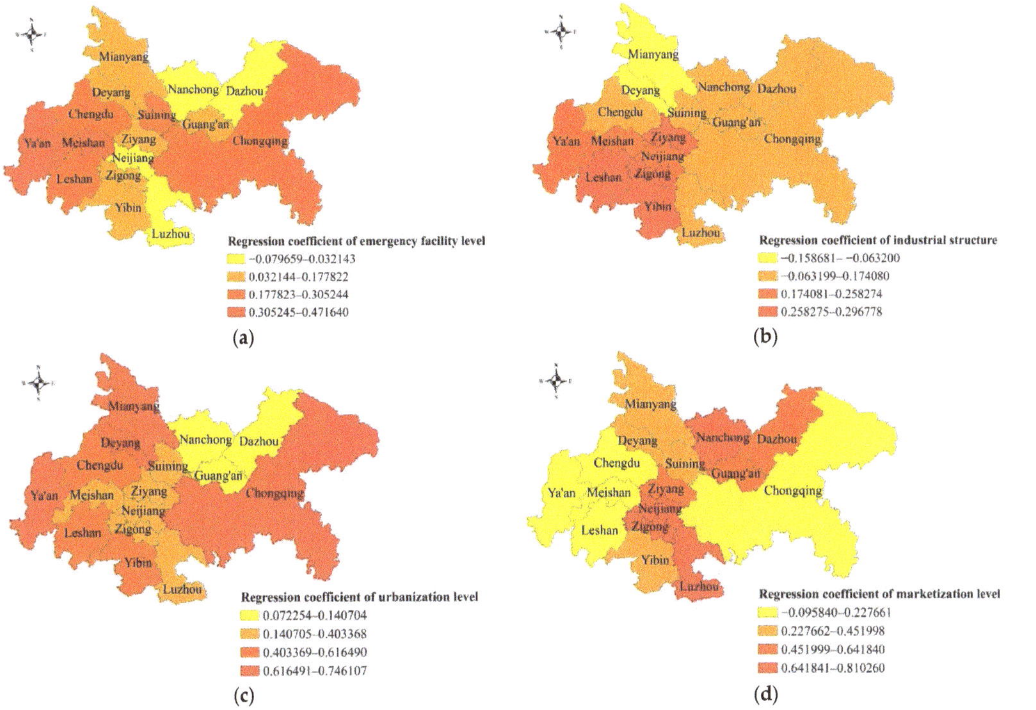

Figure 5. Spatial distribution of the mean value of regression coefficients of influencing factors from 2005 to 2019. (**a**) Emergency facility level. (**b**) Industrial structure. (**c**) Urbanization level. (**d**) Marketization level.

Table 6. Mean Values of Regression Coefficients of Influencing Factors for Different Resilience Levels.

	Low Resilience Level	General Resilience Level	Medium Resilience Level	High Resilience Level
X_1	0.16033	0.14411	0.14294	0.11298
X_2	0.05192	−0.05359	−0.18342	−0.27803
X_3	0.63693	0.47339	0.10429	0.12712
X_5	0.20246	0.13812	0.17777	0.25834
X_6	−0.09513	−0.07018	−0.13833	−0.15987
X_7	0.00500	0.08721	−0.05280	0.04182
X_8	0.20684	0.43747	0.79880	0.72370
X_9	0.17099	0.18069	0.19208	0.26274

5. Discussion

5.1. Theoretical Contribution

With the continuous increase of urban disaster events and the increasing threat risk, building resilient cities and improving the level of urban resilience are becoming a new direction for the current sustainable development of cities. This study comprehensively evaluates the urban resilience level of the Chengdu–Chongqing urban agglomeration and explores the influencing factors of urban resilience. This can verify and enrich the related research on urban resilience of inland cities to a certain extent and broaden the theoretical boundary and application scope of urban resilience.

Firstly, through the measurement of the resilience level of the cities in the study area, this study finds that the level of economic resilience and social resilience is the key to determining the overall resilience level of the city. This confirms the research of Zheng et al. (2018) [57] and Ma et al. (2020) [58], arguing that economic and social levels are the main determinants of urban resilience. Cities with higher economic and social levels have relatively large resource investment in improving the level of urban resilience, making their level of urban resilience relatively high. However, cities with relatively low economic and social levels have failed to invest too many resources in improving urban resilience, and their resilience levels are relatively low. This also makes the social and economic level the main driving force for the improvement of the overall resilience level of the city.

Secondly, through the analysis of the spatial differentiation characteristics of urban resilience in the study area, this study found that the level of urban resilience in the study area varies greatly, and there is an obvious siphon effect locally. This finding was also confirmed by Zhang et al. (2019) [59] and Liu et al. (2021) [35]. In the inland urban agglomeration, the scale of different cities varies greatly. Larger cities will absorb and utilize the resources of smaller cities, resulting in a siphon effect on the level of urban resilience in local areas. On this basis, this paper further explores and confirms that synergistically improving the economic and social development level of urban agglomerations can effectively reduce the gap in the resilience levels of cities in urban agglomerations and alleviate the siphon effect of urban resilience. This makes up for the lack of current scholars' research on the siphon effect of urban resilience.

Thirdly, by exploring the influencing factors of urban resilience in the study area, this paper finds that the level of openness has a negative impact on urban resilience. The study by Ma et al. (2022) [55] also confirmed this finding, arguing that the level of opening to the outside world has a negative impact on inland cities. This is mainly due to the relatively low level of opening to the outside world in most inland cities, and the relatively single and fragile economic system. The increase in the level of openness will have an impact on the urban economic system and reduce the overall resilience of the city. Meanwhile, this paper also explores and finds that influencing factors such as urbanization level, emergency facility level, and industrial structure have positive impacts on the improvement of urban resilience, which is consistent with the findings of Dong et al. (2020) [60], Khan et al. (2021) [36], and Ghouchani et al. (2021) [61]. On this basis, this paper further explores the temporal and spatial heterogeneity of influencing factors on urban resilience. It makes up for the deficiency of Chen et al.'s (2021) [54] research on the influence of influencing factors on different resilience levels, deepens the research on the influencing factors of urban resilience, and enriches the research results of the influencing factors of urban resilience.

5.2. Development Proposals

Based on the above findings, aiming at the sustainable development of cities in the area, this paper proposes the following development recommendations:

Firstly, innovate the opening-up mechanism and development mode, and promote social and economic development. The study area is located in the western inland area, and the level of social and economic is the main driving factor of urban resilience. Actively implementing the strategy of expanding opening-up, innovating the opening-up mechanism, optimizing the internal industrial structure, and vigorously developing the inland open economy are effective ways to enhance urban resilience.

Secondly, accelerate the process of urbanization and improve the level of urbanization. For the cities in the area with a relatively low level of urbanization, promoting new urbanization can strengthen urban space design and planning, rationally allocate population and natural resources, and improve infrastructure construction, which is important for improving urban resilience.

Thirdly, give play to the leading role of the government and formulate urban development plans rationally. There is a large gap in resilience levels among cities in the region, and the effects of various influencing factors also have obvious spatial heterogeneity. Each city government should actively take the lead, correctly grasp their own level of resilience, and formulate urban development plans with different focuses. Chengdu, Chongqing, and other cities with high resilience levels in the region should focus on the urbanization development and emergency facility construction that have a great impact on them, while cities with relatively low resilience levels in the region, such as Luzhou, Dazhou, and Guang'an, should focus on the optimization of industrial structure and the promotion of social and economic levels to effectively improve urban resilience.

Fourthly, strengthen regional coordinated development and solve the problem of large gaps in urban resilience between different cities. For the coordinated development of urban resilience in the area, it is necessary to comprehensively consider the demands of various cities, build a regional spatial cooperation mechanism, enhance the spatial spillover effect of talents, technology, capital and other resources in Chongqing, Chengdu, and other high-resilience cities, and overcome the siphon effect to realize the integrated improvement of urban resilience within the Chengdu–Chongqing urban agglomeration.

Finally, put emphasis on scientific and technological innovation and speed up the improvement of urban resilience. Technological innovation is a boost to the improvement of urban resilience, but the technological innovation capability of the area is relatively low and has no significant effect on the improvement of urban resilience. It is necessary to increase policy support for scientific and technological innovation and build a promotion mechanism for scientific and technological innovation to improve urban resilience, so as to make urban governance more scientific and modern and help improve the urban resilience of the area.

6. Conclusions

This paper comprehensively evaluates the urban resilience and analyzes the relevant influencing factors of urban resilience in the Chengdu–Chongqing urban agglomeration. The study is concluded as follows: first, the urban resilience of the 16 cities has improved significantly, showing an evolutionary trend from low resilience to high resilience. Second, there are obvious spatial differences in the resilience levels of cities in the study area, but with the continuous narrowing of regional social and economic gaps, the spatial differences and uneven development of urban resilience have been weakening. Third, the city's administrative level, marketization level, industrial structure, population density, urbanization level, and emergency facility level all play a significant role in promoting urban resilience, but the opening level and credit level inhibit the improvement of urban resilience in the area. Fourth, the effect of influencing factors has obvious temporal and spatial heterogeneity. The effect of influencing factors such as marketization level, industrial structure, urbanization level, and emergency facility level on urban resilience changes with time and space.

This research has a certain decision-making support for the improvement of the urban resilience level of the Chengdu–Chongqing urban agglomeration, has a certain reference significance for the resilience development of other cities in western and southwestern China, and has a certain reference value for the resilience research of inland cities. At the same time, follow-up research can explore urban resilience more deeply and comprehensively from the following aspects: first, follow-up research can further refine the research objects, locate the research objects in towns or communities, and conduct more in-depth research; second, follow-up research can fully consider the important components of the city such as policy, culture, and natural environment, and build a more comprehensive urban resilience assessment framework; and finally, follow-up research may not be limited to social and economic factors, and should further comprehensively explore the influencing factors of urban resilience and conduct more comprehensive exploratory research on effective ways to improve urban resilience.

Author Contributions: Conceptualization, B.W.; methodology, S.H.; software, S.H.; formal analysis, Y.A.; investigation, F.L.; resources, B.W.; data curation, F.L. and B.W.; writing—original draft preparation, S.H.; writing—review and editing, F.L. and B.W.; supervision, Y.A. All authors have read and agreed to the published version of the manuscript.

Funding: This research was funded by the Sichuan Science and Technology Program (2022JDR0229), National Natural Science Foundation of China (72171028), and Sichuan Mineral Resources Research Center (SCKCZY2022-YB001).

Institutional Review Board Statement: Not applicable.

Informed Consent Statement: Not applicable.

Data Availability Statement: Not applicable.

Conflicts of Interest: The authors declare no conflict of interest.

References

1. Zanotti, L.; Ma, Z.; Johnson, J.L.; Johnson, D.R.; Yu, D.J.; Burnham, M.; Carothers, C. Sustainability, resilience, adaptation, and transformation: Tensions and plural approaches. *Ecol. Soc.* **2020**, *25*, 4. [CrossRef]
2. United Nations Department of Economic and Social Affairs. World Urbanization Outlook Report: The World's Urban Population Will Increase by 2.5 Billion by 2050. Available online: https://www.un.org/development/desa/zh/news/population/world-urbanization-prospects-2014.html (accessed on 16 March 2022).
3. Guo, P.; Li, Q.; Guo, H.; Li, H.; Yang, L. A Bibliometric and Visual Analysis of Global Urban Resilience Research in 2011–2020: Development and Hotspots. *Sustainability* **2022**, *14*, 229. [CrossRef]
4. Panda, A. Foreward. In Proceedings of the 8th International Conference on Building Resilience, ICBR, Lisbon, Portugal, 14–16 November 2018.
5. Mallick, S.K. Prediction-Adaptation-Resilience (PAR) approach—A new pathway towards future resilience and sustainable development of urban landscape. *Geogr. Sustain.* **2021**, *2*, 127–133. [CrossRef]
6. Cardoso, M.A.; Brito, R.S.; Pereira, C.; Gonzalez, A.; Stevens, J.; Telhado, M.J. RAF Resilience Assessment Framework—A Tool to Support Cities' Action Planning. *Sustainability* **2020**, *12*, 2349. [CrossRef]
7. Meerow, S.; Newell, J.P.; Stults, M. Defining urban resilience: A review. *Landsc. Urban Plan.* **2016**, *147*, 38–49. [CrossRef]
8. Bruzzone, M.; Dameri, R.P.; Demartini, P. Resilience Reporting for Sustainable Development in Cities. *Sustainability* **2021**, *13*, 7824. [CrossRef]
9. China Government Net. The 14th Five-Year Plan for National Economic and Social Development of the People's Republic of China and Outline of the Vision for 2035. Available online: http://www.gov.cn/xinwen/2021-03/13/content_5592681.htm (accessed on 16 March 2022).
10. United Nations Conventions and Declarations Retrieval System. New Urban Agenda: Quito Declaration on Sustainable Cities and Human Settlements for All. Available online: https://www.un.org/zh/documents/treaty/files/A-RES-71-256.shtml (accessed on 16 March 2022).
11. PR Newswire. Rockefeller Foundation Launches 100 Cities Resilience Competition. Available online: https://www.prnasia.com/story/79454-1.shtml (accessed on 16 March 2022).
12. Brunetta, G.; Ceravolo, R.; Barbieri, C.A.; Borghini, A.; de Carlo, F.; Mela, A.; Beltramo, S.; Longhi, A.; De Lucia, G.; Ferraris, S.; et al. Territorial Resilience: Toward a Proactive Meaning for Spatial Planning. *Sustainability* **2019**, *11*, 2286. [CrossRef]
13. Jabareen, Y. Planning the resilient city:Concepts and strategies for coping with climate change and environmental risk. *Cities* **2013**, *31*, 220–229. [CrossRef]
14. Lam, N.S.-N.; Arenas, H.; Brito, P.L.; Liu, K.-B. Assessment of vulnerability and adaptive capacity to coastal hazards in the Caribbean Region. *J. Coast. Res.* **2014**, *70*, 473–478. [CrossRef]
15. Motesharrei, S.; Rivas, J.; Kalnay, E.; Asrar, G.R.; Busalacchi, A.G.; Cahalan, R.F.; Cane, M.A.; Colwell, R.R.; Feng, K.; Franklin, R.S. Modeling sustainability: Population, inequality, consumption, and bidirectional coupling of the Earth and Human Systems. *Natl. Sci. Rev.* **2016**, *3*, 470–494. [CrossRef]
16. McGill, R. Urban resilience—An urban management perspective. *Urban Manag.* **2020**, *9*, 372–381. [CrossRef]
17. Sarker, M.N.I.; Peng, Y.; Yiran, C.; Shouse, R.C. Disaster resilience through big data: Way to environmental sustainability. *Int. J. Disaster Risk Reduct.* **2020**, *51*, 101769. [CrossRef]
18. Monstadt, J.; Schmidt, M. Urban resilience in the making? The governance of critical infrastructures in German cities. *Urban Stud.* **2019**, *56*, 2353–2371. [CrossRef]
19. Bueno, S.; Bañuls, V.A.; Gallego, M.D. Is urban resilience a phenomenon on the rise? A systematic literature review for the years 2019 and 2020 using textometry. *Int. J. Disaster Risk Reduct.* **2021**, *66*, 102588. [CrossRef]
20. Sharifi, A.; Chelleri, L.; Fox-Lent, C.; Grafakos, S.; Pathak, M.; Olazabal, M.; Moloney, S.; Yumagulova, L.; Yamagata, Y. Conceptualizing Dimensions and Characteristics of Urban Resilience: Insights from a Co-Design Process. *Sustainability* **2017**, *9*, 1032. [CrossRef]
21. Serre, D.; Heinzlef, C. Assessing and mapping urban resilience to floods with respect to cascading effects through critical infrastructure networks. *Int. J. Disaster Risk Reduct.* **2018**, *30*, 235–243. [CrossRef]
22. Tong, P. Characteristics, dimensions and methods of current assessment for urban resilience to climate-related disasters: A systematic review of the literature. *Int. J. Disaster Risk Reduct.* **2021**, *60*, 102276. [CrossRef]

23. Mujuni, F.; Betts, T.; To, L.S.; Blanchard, R.E. Resilience a means to development: A resilience assessment framework and a catalogue of indicators. *Renew. Sustain. Energy Rev.* **2021**, *152*, 111684. [CrossRef]
24. Grantham, T.E.; Matthews, J.H.; Bledsoe, B.P. Shifting currents: Managing freshwater systems for ecological resilience in a changing climate. *Water Secur.* **2019**, *8*, 100049. [CrossRef]
25. Aoki, N. Adaptive governance for resilience in the wake of the 2011 great east Japan earthquake and tsunami. *Habitat Int.* **2016**, *52*, 20–25. [CrossRef]
26. Ruan, J.; Chen, Y.B.; Yang, Z.W. Assessment of temporal and spatial progress of urban resilience in Guangzhou under rainstorm scenarios. *Int. J. Disaster Risk Reduct.* **2021**, *66*, 102578. [CrossRef]
27. Hudec, O.; Reggiani, A.; Šiserová, M. Resilience capacity and vulnerability: A joint analysis with reference to Slovak urban districts. *Cities* **2018**, *73*, 24–35. [CrossRef]
28. Suárez, M.; Gómez-Baggethun, E.; Benayas, J.; Tilbury, D. Towards an urban resilience Index: A case study in 50 Spanish cities. *Sustainability* **2016**, *8*, 774. [CrossRef]
29. Joerin, J.; Shaw, R.; Takeuchi, Y.; Krishnamurthy, R. The adoption of a climate disaster resilience index in Chennai, India. *Disasters* **2014**, *38*, 540–561. [CrossRef] [PubMed]
30. Xiu, C.L.; Wei, Y.; Wang, Q. Evaluation of urban resilience of Dalian city based on the perspective of "Size-Density-Morphology". *Acta Geogr. Sin.* **2018**, *73*, 2315–2328. (In Chinese)
31. Scherzer, S.; Lujala, P.; Rød, J.K. A community resilience index for Norway: An adaptation of the Baseline Resilience Indicators for Communities (BRIC). *Int. J. Disaster Risk Reduct.* **2019**, *36*, 101107. [CrossRef]
32. Mallick, S.K.; Das, P.; Maity, B.; Rudra, S.; Pramanik, M.; Pradhan, B.; Sahana, M. Understanding future urban growth, urban resilience and sustainable development of small cities using prediction-adaptation-resilience (PAR) approach. *Sustain. Cities Soc.* **2021**, *74*, 103196. [CrossRef]
33. Zhao, R.D.; Fang, C.L.; Liu, H.M. Progress and prospect of urban resilience research. *Prog. Geogr.* **2020**, *39*, 1717–1731. [CrossRef]
34. Das, S.; Dsouza, N.M. Identifying the local factors of resilience during cyclone Hudhud and Phailin on the east coast of India, Ambio. *J. Urban Plan. Dev.* **2020**, *49*, 950–961. [CrossRef]
35. Liu, L.; Luo, Y.; Pei, J.; Wang, H.; Li, J.; Li, Y. Temporal and Spatial Differentiation in Urban Resilience and Its Influencing Factors in Henan Province. *Sustainability* **2021**, *13*, 12460. [CrossRef]
36. Khan, M.; Wu, Q.; Yan, S.Q.; Peng, J.C. Factors Affecting Urban Resilience and Sustainability: Case of Slum Dwellers in Islamabad, Pakistan. *J. Urban Plan. Dev.* **2021**, *147*, 040211053. [CrossRef]
37. Moradi, A.; Bidhendi, G.R.N.; Safavi, Y. Effective environment indicators on improving the resilience of Mashhad neighborhoods. *Int. J. Environ. Sci. Technol.* **2021**, *18*, 2441–2458. [CrossRef]
38. China Government Net. The Central Committee of the Communist Party of China and the State Council issued the "Outline of the Construction Plan for the Chengdu-Chongqing Economic Circle". Available online: http://www.gov.cn/gongbao/content/2021/content_5649727.htm (accessed on 20 March 2022).
39. Xinhua Net Sichuan. In 2021, the Chengdu-Chongqing Shuangcheng Economic Circle Will Achieve a Regional GDP of 7,391.92 Billion Yuan. Available online: http://sc.news.cn/content/2022-03/29/c_1128511978.htm (accessed on 20 March 2022).
40. China Government Net. Ministry of Emergency Management of the People's Republic of China: The Ministry of Emergency Management released the basic situation of national natural disasters in 2021. Available online: https://www.mem.gov.cn/xw/yjglbgzdt/202201/t20220123_407204.shtml (accessed on 20 March 2022).
41. Kumar, R.; Singh, S.; Bilga, P.S.; Jatin; Singh, J.; Singh, S.; Scutaru, M.-L.; Pruncu, C.I. Revealing the benefits of entropy weights method for multi-objective optimization in machining operations: A critical review. *J. Mater. Res. Technol.* **2021**, *10*, 1471–1492. [CrossRef]
42. Simmons, D.E.; Coon, J.P.; Datta, A. The von Neumann Theil index: Characterizing graph centralization using the von Neumann index. *J. Complex Netw.* **2018**, *6*, 859–876. [CrossRef]
43. Taşyürek, M.; Çelik, M. FastGTWR: Hızlı coğrafi ve zamansal ağırlıklı regresyon yaklaşımı. *Gazi Üniversitesi Mühendislik Mimar. Fakültesi Derg.* **2021**, *36*, 715–726. [CrossRef]
44. Hosseini, S.; Barker, K.; Ramirez-Marquez, J.E. A review of definitions and measures of system resilience. *Reliab. Eng. Syst. Saf.* **2016**, *145*, 47–61. [CrossRef]
45. Shen, L.Y.; Ochoa, J.J.; Shah, M.N.; Zhang, X.L. The Application of Urban Sustainability Indicators—A Comparison between Various Practices. *Habitat Int.* **2011**, *35*, 17–29. [CrossRef]
46. Xun, X.L.; Yuan, Y.B. Research on the urban resilience evaluation with hybrid multiple attribute TOPSIS method: An example in China. *Nat. Hazards* **2020**, *103*, 557–577. [CrossRef]
47. Opach, T.; Scherzer, S.; Lujala, P.; Rød, J.K. Seeking commonalities of community resilience to natural hazards: A cluster analysis approach. *Nor. Geogr. Tidsskr. Nor. J. Geogr.* **2020**, *74*, 181–199. [CrossRef]
48. Liu, X.L.; Li, S.J.; Luo, J.S. Integrated natural disasters urban resilience evaluation: The case of China. *Nat. Hazards* **2021**, *107*, 2105–2122. [CrossRef]
49. Parsons, M.; Glavac, S.; Hastings, P.; Marshall, G.; McGregor, J.; McNeill, J.; Morley, P.; Morley, I.; Stayner, R. Top-down assessment of disaster resilience: A conceptual framework using coping and adaptive capacities. *Int. J. Disaster Risk Reduction.* **2016**, *19*, 1–11. [CrossRef]

50. Javadpoor, M.; Sharifi, A.; Roosta, M. An adaptation of the Baseline Resilience Indicators for Communities (BRIC) for assessing resilience of Iranian provinces. *Int. J. Disaster Risk Reduct.* **2021**, *66*, 102609. [CrossRef]
51. Rus, K.; Kilar, V.; Koren, D. Resilience assessment of complex urban systems to natural disasters: A new literature review. *Int. J. Disaster Risk Reduct.* **2018**, *31*, 311–330. [CrossRef]
52. Fan, J.; Mo, Y.; Cai, Y.; Zhao, Y.; Su, D. Evaluation of Community Resilience in Rural China—Taking Licheng Subdistrict, Guangzhou as an Example. *Int. J. Environ. Res. Public Health* **2021**, *18*, 5827. [CrossRef] [PubMed]
53. Kammouh, O.; Noori, A.Z.; Cimellaro, G.P.; Mahin, S.A. Resilience assessment of urban communities. *ASCE-ASME J. Risk Uncertain. Eng. Syst. Part A Civ. Eng.* **2019**, *5*, 04019002. [CrossRef]
54. Chen, Y.; Zhu, M.; Zhou, Q.; Qiao, Y. Research on Spatiotemporal Differentiation and Influence Mechanism of Urban Resilience in China Based on MGWR Model. *Int. J. Environ. Res. Public Health* **2021**, *18*, 1056. [CrossRef]
55. Ma, X.; Chen, X.; Du, Y.; Zhu, X.; Dai, Y.; Li, X.; Zhang, R.; Wang, Y. Evaluation of Urban Spatial Resilience and Its Influencing Factors: Case Study of the Harbin–Changchun Urban Agglomeration in China. *Sustainability* **2022**, *14*, 2899. [CrossRef]
56. Chen, Y.; Su, X.; Zhou, Q. Study on the Spatiotemporal Evolution and Influencing Factors of Urban Resilience in the Yellow River Basin. *Int. J. Environ. Res. Public Health* **2021**, *18*, 10231. [CrossRef]
57. Zheng, Y.; Xie, X.L.; Lin, C.Z.; Wang, M.; He, X.J. Development as adaptation: Framing and measuring urban resilience in Beijing. *Adv. Clim. Change Res.* **2018**, *9*, 234–242. [CrossRef]
58. Ma, F.; Wang, Z.; Sun, Q.; Yuen, K.F.; Zhang, Y.; Xue, H.; Zhao, S. Spatial–Temporal Evolution of Urban Resilience and Its Influencing Factors: Evidence from the Guanzhong Plain Urban Agglomeration. *Sustainability* **2020**, *12*, 2593. [CrossRef]
59. Zhang, M.; Chen, W.; Cai, K.; Gao, X.; Zhang, X.; Liu, J.; Wang, Z.; Li, D. Analysis of the Spatial Distribution Characteristics of Urban Resilience and Its Influencing Factors: A Case Study of 56 Cities in China. *Int. J. Environ. Res. Public Health* **2019**, *16*, 4442. [CrossRef] [PubMed]
60. Dong, L.J.; Su, F.; Wen, Y.Q.; Wang, Y.C. Obstacle Factors and Evolution of Urban Economic Resilience of Fuxin Shrinking City and Its Obstacle Factors. *Sci. Geogr. Sin.* **2020**, *40*, 1142–1149.
61. Ghouchani, M.; Taji, M.; Roshan, A.Y.; Chehr, M.S. Identification and assessment of hidden capacities of urban resilience. *Environ. Dev. Sustain.* **2021**, *23*, 3966–3993. [CrossRef]

buildings

MDPI

Article

Identifying Critical Influencing Factors of the Value Creation of Urban Rail Transit PPP Projects in China

Xuewei Li [1], Jingfeng Yuan [1,*], Xuan Liu [2], Yongjian Ke [3] and Sijia Jia [4]

1 Department of Construction and Real Estate, School of Civil Engineering, Southeast University, Nanjing 210096, China; lxwwseu@163.com
2 Department of the Built Environment, Eindhoven University of Technology, 5600 MB Eindhoven, The Netherlands; x.liu1@tue.nl
3 School of Built Environment, University of Technology Sydney, Ultimo, NSW 2007, Australia; yongjian.ke@uts.edu.au
4 Park City Construction and Renewal Bureau of Chengdu Economic and Technological Development District, Chengdu 610100, China; 15208256930@163.com
* Correspondence: jingfeng-yuan@seu.edu.cn

Abstract: Value creation is the primary motivation for public-private cooperation. The development of urban rail transit (URT) projects requires heavy investment and abundant construction and management experience. Thus, public-private partnership (PPP) is usually adopted in URT project development to benefit the public and private sectors. However, with the high-quality development of PPP projects, the value creation of URT PPP projects is not only about achieving basic project objectives but also relying on partner synergy to achieve value-added. Based on the extended connotation of value creation, this study intends to systematically identify the influencing factors of value creation of URT PPP projects in China. The grounded theory approach was adopted to deduce the influencing factors of value creation through analyzing the various types of articles related to Chinese URT PPP projects. Resources complementarity among stakeholders, cooperation environment, and partnership synergy were identified as the main influencing factors. Meanwhile, a theoretical model that described how these influencing factors combined to promote value creation during public-private sectors cooperation of URT projects was established. This research helps broaden the understanding of how public and private sectors should cooperate and collaborate in URT projects to realize value maximization and promote the sustainable development of URT PPP projects and provides a model for further empirical examination.

Keywords: urban rail transit (URT); PPP; value creation; grounded theory

Citation: Li, X.; Yuan, J.; Liu, X.; Ke, Y.; Jia, S. Identifying Critical Influencing Factors of the Value Creation of Urban Rail Transit PPP Projects in China. *Buildings* **2022**, *12*, 1080. https://doi.org/10.3390/buildings12081080

Academic Editor: Pierfrancesco De Paola

Received: 15 June 2022
Accepted: 21 July 2022
Published: 24 July 2022

1. Introduction

Urban rail transit (URT) has formed the cornerstone of urban public transport due to its advantages of mass transportation, land saving, environment friendly, safety, and fast speed [1]. The development of URT projects requires heavy investment and abundant construction and operation experience, bringing huge financial and management pressure on governments [2]. Public-private partnership (PPP) is a long-term partnership between the public and private sectors to provide public goods or services by integrating the capacities of each sector [3]. In this context, PPP has gained popularity as a novel financing and procurement model for the delivery of URT in many countries [4].

Value creation is the primary motivation for public-private cooperation [5]. For the government, it takes advantage of the private sectors in terms of their advanced experience in investment, construction, and operation, thereby providing more URT projects with high service quality and low fare [6,7]. For the private parties, they expect to obtain profits from participating in the construction and operation of the URT project [4,8]. The opportunistic behaviors of partners caused by their heterogeneity objectives often make URT PPP projects fall into cooperation dilemmas [6]. Additionally, there are a large number of internal uncertainties and external environmental changes during the construction and operation of URT PPP projects, resulting in the loss of project value [9–11]. Therefore, it is required to identify the critical factors affecting the value creation of URT PPP projects to facilitate the realization of value for money (VFM) and promote the sustainable development of URT PPP projects.

Achieving VFM depends on high levels of performance [12]. Many scholars have conducted research on performance management (i.e., determining performance objectives and identifying corresponding critical success factors) of URT PPP projects to promote value creation [13–15]. Performance goals are the foundation of performance management. Drawing on the 3E principles (economy, efficiency, and effectiveness) of governmental funds effectiveness auditing and considering the public nature of URT PPP projects, most scholars proposed that the performance of URT PPP projects can be assessed through some basic performance objectives in compliance with contract goals, such as time, cost, quality, and public satisfaction [12,14]. Based on the defined performance objectives, different critical success factors that influence the performance of URT PPP projects have been identified from participating parties, external environment, and contracting and procurement, such as the private sector with extensive experience, policy support, public support, transit ridership, economic development level, reasonable risk allocation strategy, etc. [4,16,17].

Recently, various advanced technologies and management innovations have continuously poured into the construction industry. The PPP model is changing from high-speed to high-quality development. "Implementation Opinions on Promoting the Standardized Development of Government and Social Capital Cooperation" issued by China's Ministry of Finance in 2019 emphasizes that PPP projects should strictly perform VFM evaluation and promote PPP projects to create more value for society [18]. Therefore, achieving the basic performance management objectives in URT PPP projects can no longer meet the expectations of participants, but rather realize value-added through effective cooperation [5]. Partnership is the basic characteristic of PPP projects [19]. Kivleniece et al. [7] indicate that the stable partnership between public and private sectors based on shared resources and benefit dependence can create partner synergies, thereby promoting value-added through saving production costs, reducing transaction costs, and increasing output efficiency. Partnership value is thus proposed as an important manifestation of the value-added of PPP projects. To explore the factors affecting the partnership value of PPP projects, some scholars referring to transaction cost economics (TCE) theory proposed that effective governance strategies, including contractual and relational management, facilitate partners to share resources, and enhance partnerships, thereby increasing the efficiency of cooperation and contributing to value creation [5,20,21].

Currently, scholars have studied the connotation of value creation of PPP projects in terms of achieving basic performance management objectives and promoting partnership value and have identified corresponding influencing factors from various perspectives. However, most of the studies were conducted in a fragmented manner. Studies on the factors influencing value creation of URT PPP projects especially focused more on the critical success factors affecting basic performance management objectives, while lacking a comprehensive factor analysis that includes factors affecting partnership value. In addition, existing studies consider the impact of various factors on project value creation to be independent of each other, ignoring their interactions.

Grounded theory is an effective qualitative research method to identify core concepts of the research objective and construct the related theory model based on the relationships of these concepts [22]. The grounded theory involves the application of reasoning, which has strong application value and has been widely used in organization and management areas [23,24]. To this end, this research will adopt the grounded theory method to systematically analyze the factors influencing the value creation of URT PPP projects in China and establish a theoretical framework to maximize the joint value in public-private collaboration under the influence of complex influencing factors.

The remainder of this paper is organized as follows. Section 2 provides a literature review on the perception of the URT PPP project value creation and capture and related influencing factors. Section 3 presents the research framework. Section 4 introduces the results of data analysis based on the grounded theory method. Sections 5 and 6 present the discussions and conclusions of this study.

2. Literature Review

2.1. Value Creation of PPP Projects

Value creation is the fundamental purpose of PPP projects [5]. Kivleniece et al. [7] first proposed the concept of value creation of PPP projects and indicated that value creation of PPP projects refers to the joint realization of public and private values through the integration of the capabilities of the public and private sectors. VFM is used to evaluate whether PPP projects can create value [12]. The 3E principle including economy, efficiency, and effectiveness is widely adopted in government capital efficiency audits to evaluate whether a project achieved VFM [18]. Based on the 3E principles of VFM, various performance objectives of PPP projects are proposed to promote effective cooperation between the public and private sectors and achieve value creation. For example, Khalid et al. [25] proposed that time, cost, quality, service, profit, and variable performance are the critical performance indicators of PPP projects. Yuan et al. [12] identified 15 performance objectives through literature review and questionnaire research, mainly including making the project quality, cost, and duration more balanced, improving the quality of public services, and promoting innovation and technological progress. Specifically for URT PPP projects, Chang and Phang [9] proposed 11 performance objectives through case studies, including quality, schedule, cost, safety, environmental impact, innovativeness, operational management, service quality, public satisfaction, revenue, etc. In addition, some scholars identified the performance objectives of PPP projects as achieving reasonable public and private values [7]. Public value covers the timely delivery of high-quality public infrastructure and services to the public. The private value refers to the private sector obtaining reasonable profits and other implicit benefits (such as technology improvement, good social reputations, and more investment opportunities). Existing studies show that most scholars consistently evaluate the performance of PPP projects through cost, time, and quality. Moreover, improving the quality of public services and promoting innovation and technological progress are often used to evaluate the performance level of PPP projects. These performance objectives mainly focus on the achievement of basic project goals. With the in-depth research on the value creation of PPP projects, some scholars suggest that the value creation of PPP projects is not only to achieve the basic project goals but also to realize value-added [5,6,26].

During public-private cooperation, the public and private sectors have different resources and capabilities. Stable partnerships between public and private sectors can be established through resource sharing and effective collaboration, which promotes the realization of synergistic effects and promote value-added [5]. Zhang and Liu [27], based on TCE theory, indicated that stable partnerships between the public and private sectors are important in PPP project governance to reduce project transaction costs. Based on strategic alliance theory, Hodge et al. [28] proposed that complementary resources between the public and private sectors enable value creation through partner synergy to be greater than the sum of value created by individual sectors, which is reflected in the reduction of production costs and the increase of output efficiency. Existing studies show that the reduction of production and transaction costs and the improvement of output benefits are the value-added part of PPP projects, which are generated through stable partnerships and are defined as partnership value. Integrating studies on performance management objectives as well as the value-added of PPP projects, Matinheikki et al. [29] proposed that PPP projects should not only realize the basic project goals (e.g., cost, schedule, quality, etc.) but more importantly create partnership value. Partnership value is the value-added created by resource integration and collaboration between public and private sectors. Existing studies show that the realization of basic project objectives and the value-added based on complementary resources and synergy effective brought by the public-private cooperation and collaboration are important manifestations of value creation of PPP projects. Referring to Matinheikki et al. [29], this study divided the value creation objectives of PPP projects into the realization of project objectives and partnership value, as shown in Table 1.

Table 1. The value creation objectives of PPP projects.

Value Creation Objectives of PPP Projects	Sub-Objectives	Connotation
The realization of project objectives	The realization of quality goals	The actual engineering quality of the PPP project meets the contractual requirements.
	The realization of cost goals	The PPP project is completed within the contract budget.
	The realization of schedule goals	The PPP project completes construction and operation according to the contract schedule.
	The realization of safety and environmental goals	The development of the PPP project meets the predetermined safety standards and has no negative impact on the environment.
	The realization of stakeholder satisfaction	The development of the PPP project relieves the financial pressure on public sectors, allows the private sectors to obtain a reasonable profit, and provides good services to the public.
The realization of partnership value	Reduction of production costs	Complementary resources between the public and private sectors reduce financing costs, construction costs, and operating costs.
	Reduction of transaction costs	Partner synergies between the public and private sectors reduce opportunistic behavior and improve the efficiency of handling uncertain events, thereby reducing transaction costs.
	Improvement of output benefits	Complementary resources between the public and private sectors improve operational efficiency and thus increase output benefits.

2.2. Factors Influencing the Value Creation of URT PPP Project

Various risk factors such as stakeholder behaviors, macro-environmental risk, competition risk, and financial risk will affect the benefits of the PPP project and cause the project to fail [9,16,30]. To make PPP projects create more value and achieve VFM, many scholars have identified some critical success factors (CSFs) that affect the value creation of PPP projects based on the study of PPP project performance objectives. These CSFs can be divided into six categories: stakeholder behavior, time, public demand, public-private collaboration, cost-benefit, and environment [4,16,17]. For example, based on a review of academic literature and government reports, Henjewele et al. [31] proposed key factors affecting the achievement of performance goals of PPP projects in the UK, including information factors, task factors, decision factors, project team factors, procurement factors, macro-environmental factors, and time factors. Through case studies of PPP projects in Hong Kong, Cheung et al. [32] identified five factors that have the greatest impact on the value creation of PPP projects, including efficient risk sharing, industry competition, private sector capacity, and government regulation.

URT PPP projects have the commonality of general PPP projects, and some scholars have studied the key influencing factors for achieving the performance goals of URT PPP projects regarding the CSFs of general PPP projects. For URT PPP projects, a private sector with strong investment and financing capabilities and rich project experience could provide sustainable funds and reduce construction costs [6]. The public sector has the legitimacy to rule in URT network planning, and the division of project sovereignty can provide policy support for private sectors to engage in URT PPP projects [33]. The complementary resource advantages between public and private sectors can facilitate the achievement of intended contract objectives and create more value [5,14]. For example, the private sector can obtain loans lower than the market level with policy support from the public sector, thereby further reducing the financing costs [3,34]. The construction, operation, and maintenance costs are influenced by aspects, such as construction technology, management capacity, material/energy price, and wages in the labor market, which can be reduced by involving the private sector with extensive construction and management experience and novel management methods and tools [35,36]. Fare revenue, which is influenced by ridership and fare, is a significant revenue source for a URT project [37]. Carpintero and Petersen [15] showed that politics play an important role in the route selection of URT projects, thereby influencing passenger flow. In addition, a timely, reliable, and comfortable service could attract more commuters to ride URT [11]. The cooperation environment has an important effect on the stability and sustainability of PPP projects. The resources (e.g., material, policy and information, etc.) required for the production and delivery of public goods or services originate from the cooperative environment [5]. Some scholars explore the effects of cooperation environments on the value creation of URT PPP projects from the aspects of public participation and macro market and policy environments [17,30,38].

Current studies on the factors influencing the value creation of PPP projects are mainly related to promoting the realization of basic performance objectives (i.e., cost, quality, schedule, public satisfaction). As explained in Section 2.2, realizing value-added (i.e., partnership value) is also an important value creation objective of PPP projects. Leite and Bengtson [39] indicated that strengthening partnerships to activate consistent interests among stakeholders in PPP provides the possibility of realizing value-added. Some scholars started to explore the factors to strengthen the partnership of PPP projects. For example, Jocobson et al. [40], through interviews and qualitative research methods, proposed 10 factors that influence the partnership of PPP projects, including commitment, communication, willingness to cooperate, etc. By studying the relationship among PPP project partner subjects, cooperation environment, and public goods supply, Ye et al. [19] found that a good cooperation environment and public participation will promote the sustainability of the partnership and thus the realization of partnership value. Love et al. [41] indicated that trust among partners can also enhance partnerships, reduce transaction costs, and thus contribute to value creation. For URT PPP projects, there are relatively few studies on the influencing factors affecting its partnership value. Several scholars investigated the vertical structure of URT PPP projects and proposed that an effective vertical structure can provide a good cooperation environment for partners and thus promote partnership synergies [8]. Additionally, some scholars suggest that reasonable risk-sharing can increase the trust between partners and thus promote partner synergy [42]. Eshun et al. [43] proposed that the contract of the URT PPP project should have a high degree of completeness to guide the cooperation behavior of partners, mitigate transaction risks, and thus promote value creation.

The existing literature has illustrated that the factors influencing the value creation of URT PPP projects are complicated. However, most of the studies only explored the factors influencing the value creation of URT PPP projects on the critical success factors affecting basic performance management objectives and lack a detailed factor analysis that affects partnership value. They provided a partial understanding of the factors influencing the value creation of URT PPP projects, which left a comprehensive investigation and summarization of these factors uncovered. Thus, this study attempts to fill the gap and systematically identify critical influencing factors of the value creation of URT PPP projects.

3. Research Methodology

There are many practical cases and experience summaries of URT PPP projects in China. The qualitative research method has advantages in data information collection, data processing, and theory formation, which is suitable for exploratory research [22]. The grounded theory methodology is adopted in this study to explore the factors influencing the value creation of URT PPP projects and explain how these factors enable maximized joint value creation. The research process based on grounded theory methodology is shown in Figure 1, including data collection and data analysis parts.

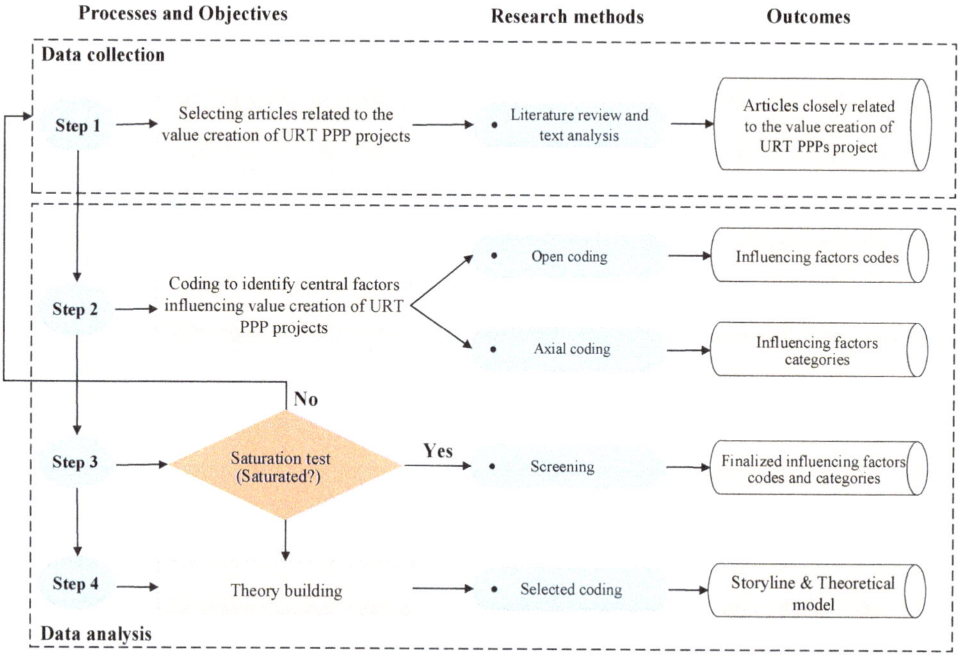

Figure 1. Research process based on grounded theory methodology.

3.1. Data Collection

Step 1: Selecting articles related to the value creation of URT PPP projects

This study adopted two ways to obtain related literature to fully identify the factors influencing the value creation of URT PPP projects.

(1) Searching academic database

To obtain literature related to the value creation of URT PPP projects, two academic databases including the Web of Science (WOS) and China National Knowledge Infrastructure (CNKI) were selected due to their widespread journal coverage [44]. After that, the keywords were determined to ensure that the selected literature is closely related to the research topic. The types of URT and their abbreviations as introduced by The World Bank [45] were presented in Keywords I of Table 2. According to PPP Knowledge Lab [46], the selected typologies of PPP and their abbreviations were presented in Keywords II of Table 2. Moreover, as explained in Section 2, studies related to the value creation of URT PPP projects include performance, critical success factors, partnerships, partner synergy, benefit, partnership value, and value-added, which were also presented in Keywords III of Table 2. The words listed in Keywords I–III were grouped; for example, the terms "urban rail transit", "public-private partnership", and "value creation" were adopted to implement a search within the WOS and CNKI database.

Table 2. List of selected keywords.

Categories	Keywords
Keywords I: Types of URT	Urban rail transit (URT)
	Rapid rail transit (RRT)
	Subway/Metro (MRT)
	Light rail transit (LRT)
	Heavy rail (HR)
	Tramways (Tram)
	Streetcar
Keywords II: Typologies of PPP	Public-private partnership (PPP)
	Build-operation-transfer (BOT)
	Build-transfer-operate (BTO)
	Design-build-finance-operate-maintain (DBFOM)
	Build-own-operate-transfer (BOOT)
	Design-build-finance-operation (DBFO)
Keywords III: Types of Value creation	Value creation
	Performance
	Critical success factors
	Partnerships
	Partner synergy
	Benefit
	Partner synergy
	Value-added

(2) Searching web-based information platform

Three web-based information platforms were selected to obtain articles related to this present study, including"China Public-Private Partnerships Centre" (CPPPC), "PPP wiki", and "PPP portal". The CPPPC is an official platform of PPP-related policies and regulations and interactive exchange sponsored and guided by the China Ministry of Finance in advancing the development of the PPP model. The platform not only provides statistics on the detailed information on all approved PPP projects in China but also reports comprehensively and objectively the new progress and new PPP project achievements. The PPP wiki and PPP portal are the most authoritative and influential platforms for knowledge-sharing of PPP in China. The platforms release various types of articles on PPP projects, including case studies, news stories, expert interviews, academic papers, and policy interpretation. In 2021, the annual reading volume in the PPP wiki and PPP portal reached 6.28 million, leading to the information aggregation of the PPP model. Thus, using CPPPC, PPP wiki, and PPP portal can capture articles in China on the value creation of the URT PPP project in a professional, timely, and comprehensive manner.

After determining the search platform, keywords that were consistent with search rules in searching academic databases were used to search on CPPPC, PPP wiki, and PPP portal. As Pettigrew [47] proposed, the most important factors to consider for raw article selection are "transparent observable", which is the same central premise adopted in this research. Thus, the following criteria were set to select the most relevant articles for the study. (1) The articles must be on the topic of the URT PPP project. (2) The articles must be related to the value creation of the PPP or URT PPP project. (3) The articles should not be out of date (within five years from the day of article collection) to represent the current characteristics of value creation.

In the first round of searching (upon updating to 10 July 2021), 1386 articles were collected through the above two ways. Second, the titles of the collected articles were browsed to refine the list of the articles and to identify whether the article is related to the research subjects. After this process, 892 items remained in the pool. In the following step, the content of the articles was read in detail to determine their relevance to the research questions. Consequently, 696 articles covering 43 academic papers, 78 case studies, 356 news stories, 166 expert interviews, and 53 policy interpretations of the URT PPP project in China were selected for coding. Corbin and Strauss [22] proposed that 25% of the obtained articles should be selected randomly for the theoretical saturation test of the model, thereby ensuring adequate validity and the credibility of the coding. Thus, 174 articles were selected randomly from 696 articles to conduct a theoretical saturation test leaving 522 articles to be coded first.

3.2. Data Analysis

Step 2: Coding to identify central factors influencing value creation of URT PPP projects

The classic grounded theory methodology includes three coding procedures: open, axial, and selective coding [22]. In this study, Nvivo12, a computer-assisted qualitative analysis software, was adopted to screen the articles and code the sentences [48]. The internal folder in Nvivo12 can include various types of sources, such as documents, web pages, and PDFs. The articles used in this study can be obtained in the web page format by using the automatic reading function (N-capture) of Nvivo12, based on which a rapid and in-depth qualitative analysis of data can be performed. First, the literature and web pages were coded according to article types, such as cases, expert interviews, academic papers, etc. The sorted web pages were then imported into Nvivo12 for standardized information management.

Open coding refers to the categorization of sentences or phrases in the texts and the procedure used to build the initial coding from the raw data by reading line-by-line or sentence-by-sentence [22]. Two principles must necessarily be complied with during the open coding process based on the data set of 522 articles to identify and depict overall constructs related to factors influencing the value creation of URT PPP projects [49]. First, the researcher needs to put aside subjective imagination and prejudice to obtain objective and rational concepts and categories. Then, a sentence-by-sentence analysis is conducted to trace continuously. "What is the relationship between the sentences and the research object?" and "What concept does this sentence provide?" One article (ID NO.2-14) is used as an example to present the open coding in Nvivo12, as shown in Figure 2. The left side of Figure 2 is the part of the NO.2-14 article, which is in Chinese. The right-side information is about the coding stripes with different colors. Two PhD graduates with a research focus on value creation of URT PPP projects undertook coding tasks separately to reduce coders' subjective influence on the work result.

Based on the results of open coding, axial coding is adopted to discover and establish relationships between subcategories and main categories [22]. The main categories of nodes are often referred to as parent nodes. The others, including subcategories and concepts, are child nodes. A child node can only have one parent node and have different relations to the parent node. The purpose of axial coding in this study is to classify the relationship between each concept and obtain the factors influencing the value creation of the URT PPP project. During the classification process, a more abstract category level can be found through the repeated comparative and cluster analysis of the relationships of concepts obtained from open coding [24]. In Nvivo12, the tree-like hierarchical structure of nodes and their relationships with each other were established to present the connections between concepts, subcategories, and main categories. Figure 3 only shows parent codes and the sub-categories level of child nodes due to the length limitations of this article. The results of open coding and axial coding are shown in Section 4.1 for details.

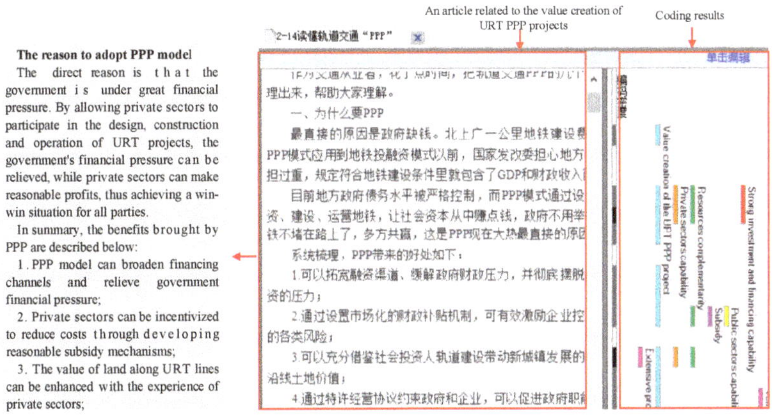

Figure 2. Open coding of one article (ID NO.2-14).

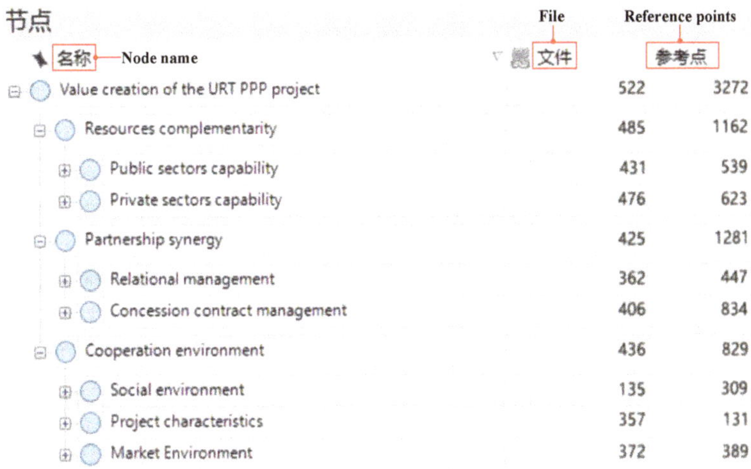

Figure 3. Axial coding process.

Step 3: Saturation test

Based on the grounded theory, all codes signed in open coding and axial coding should meet the requirements of theoretical saturation [22]. Hence, the invited two PhD graduates were invited to code the remaining 174 articles again. No new concepts, subcategories and main categories appeared during the coding process of 174 articles. This proves that the factors influencing the value creation of URT PPP projects in China were completely identified.

Step 4: Theory building

Selective coding is used to identify core categories. The objective of selective coding is to reveal a core field and systematically associate the core category with other categories by presenting a "storyline" [24]. Thus, in the last step, selective coding was adopted to integrate the identified influencing factors categories of value creation of URT PPP projects through a storyline, thereby constructing a theoretical model that described how these influencing factors combined to promote value creation during public-private sectors cooperation of URT projects. The results of selective coding are shown in Section 4.2.

4. Results

Based on open coding and axial coding, concepts and categories of the factors influencing the value creation of URT PPP projects were identified. After that, the selective coding presented a storyline and constructed the theoretical model regarding how these influencing factors combined for effective value creation of URT PPP projects. These influencing factor categories and the storyline and theoretical model are explained in detail as follows.

4.1. Categories of Factors Influencing Value Creation of URT PPP Projects

Twenty-three concepts, seven sub-categories, and three main categories were identified through open coding and axial coding, as shown in Table 3. Additionally, Table 3 also shows the connotation of each concept and its frequency of appearing in the coding process. As shown in Table 3, the top five influencing factors that occurred with frequency in the open coding process include: strong investment and financing capability (Fre. = 338), regulatory (Fre. = 312), trust (Fre. = 272), risk allocation strategy (Fre. = 225), and public participation (Fre. = 213). The occurring frequency of the influencing factor reflects the degree of concern of scholars or project participants about this factor on the value creation of URT PPP projects [24]. This study thus measures the degree of influence of the factor on the value creation of URT PPP projects by its occurring frequency. Strong investment and financing capability has the highest frequency reflecting that it has the highest degree of influence on the value creation of URT PPP projects, supporting that financing is the basic function of the PPP model and strong investment and financing capability can effectively solve the problem of insufficient funds and promote the project process [2]. Following the above factor, regulation from the public sector also has a significant impact on the value creation of URT PPP projects. Effective regulation can reduce opportunistic behavior of the private sector, allowing the private sector to deliver projects that meet public requirements, thereby reducing transaction costs and increasing revenues [9]. The impact of trust on the value creation of URT PPP projects comes in third place, reflecting that partnership is the most essential feature of PPP projects. Good trust can enhance partnership and promote partner synergy, thereby creating more value through reducing transaction costs [21]. Risk allocation strategy also has a significant influence on the value creation of URT PPP projects. A reasonable risk allocation strategy can improve the governance efficiency of risk events and reduce transaction costs [8]. Notably, the public is the end-user of URT projects. Thus, it is significant to make the public participate in the development of the projects to improve their satisfaction. Based on the coding results, the influencing factors categories are explained in detail as follows.

Table 3. Categorization of factors influencing the value creation of the URT PPP project.

Main Category	Fre.	Sub-Category	Fre.	Concept	Fre.	Connotation of the Concept
Resources complementarity	1162	Public sectors capability	539	Regulation	312	Public sectors have the legitimacy rights granted by citizens to regulate the private sectors behaviors to ensure that the services provided by URT PPP projects meet public requirements [9].
				Subsidy	125	Public sectors provide reasonable subsidies to private sectors and make them obtain reasonable revenues [10].
				Policy development and implementation	102	Supportive policies for private sector participation in URT PPP projects can increase the efficiency of project development and reduce financing costs [19].

Table 3. *Cont.*

Main Category	Fre.	Sub-Category	Fre.	Concept	Fre.	Connotation of the Concept
		Private sectors capability	623	Strong investment and financing capability	338	Strong investment and financing capability can effectively solve the problem of insufficient funds for the development of URT PPP projects and advance the process of the projects [2].
				Advanced technology	147	Advanced technologies of the private sector can effectively reduce production costs, while also increasing economic returns through improved operational efficiency [9].
				Extensive project experience	138	Extensive project experience of the private sector can reduce project sunk costs and promote project success [19].
Cooperation environment	829	Project characteristics	131	Project scale	48	Project size reflects the amount of work involved in the construction and operation of a URT PPP project, which directly affects the construction and operation costs of the project [50].
				Construction scheme	36	The construction scheme reflects the level of difficulty of the project construction, which directly affects the construction costs of the project [10].
				Geological conditions and surrounding environment	47	Adverse geological conditions can increase construction difficulties and thus increase construction costs [16].
		Social environment	309	Public participation	216	The public is the end-user of URT projects. Public participation makes URT PPP projects meet public requirements and thus improve public satisfaction and increase ridership [18].
				Media reports	93	Media reports are the main channel for the public to obtain project information. Unfavorable media reports can cause public dissatisfaction [6].
		Market environment	389	Business environment	152	The business environment reflects daily average transit ridership, carrying capacity, and property rents at stations [51].
				Economic development level	123	A lower economic level can increase the financing cost and discourage the positive externality benefits of a URT project [52].
				Industry environment	114	The industry environment reflects the number of buses and other URT lines, which can threaten the ridership of the developed URT PPP projects [53].

Table 3. *Cont.*

Main Category	Fre.	Sub-Category	Fre.	Concept	Fre.	Connotation of the Concept
Partnership synergy	1281	Concession contract management	834	Risk allocation strategy	225	A reasonable risk allocation strategy can improve the governance efficiency of risk events and reduce transaction costs [8].
				Revenue sharing strategy	213	A reasonable revenue sharing strategy can enable partners to obtain reasonable benefits, thus stimulating partners' motivation and reducing their opportunistic behavior [8].
				Vehicle structure	93	The vertical structure of URT PPP contracts reflects the responsibilities and the possible benefits of each partner [51].
				Subsidy strategy	87	A reasonable subsidy strategy can reduce public sector pressure, allow private sectors to receive reasonable benefits, and thus promote partner synergy and realize project sustainability [54].
				Pricing mechanism	82	The pricing mechanism directly affects the revenue of the URT PPP project and public satisfaction [6].
				Duration	33	Duration refers to the time that the private sector can participate in the construction and operation of URT PPP projects [54].
				Contract flexibility	101	Contractual flexibility reflects the ability to protect stakeholders' interests through contract renegotiation when uncertain events arise [6].
		Relational management	447	Trust	272	Trust means that a party believes that its partner can cooperate fairly and actively fulfill their commitments [21].
				Communication and coordination	175	Communication and cooperation mean that partners can proactively share their experiences and information [43].

Note: Fre. refers to Frequency.

4.1.1. Resource Complementarity

Resource complementarity between partners is a critical factor in the value creation of the URT PPP project [5,6]. The coding results show that the integration of the unique capabilities of the public and private sectors can provide sufficient financial, technical, and policy support for the development of URT PPP projects that cannot be realized by just one party and thus facilitate the achievement of contractual objectives. In addition, the complementarity of different types of capabilities can enhance operational efficiency and enable projects to cope with more risks, thereby realizing value-added, such as minimizing cost, reducing the duration, and improving the functional structure. Public sector capability and private sector capability are the two sub-categories of resource complementarity. The occurring frequency of private sector capability and public sector capability is 623 and 539, respectively. It is thus inferred that the private sector capability has a greater impact on the value creation of URT PPP projects than the public sector has on it.

Public sector capability: The public sector is ultimately responsible for providing URT projects and has the legitimacy rights granted by the general public, such as regulation, policy development, providing subsidies, etc. Government regulation (Fre. = 312) is the most important factor in public sector capability. Effective government regulation can ensure that URT projects meet public demand, thereby inducing more public ridership on URT and creating value in terms of providing high-quality public goods and services and increasing economic benefits [9].

During the coding process, some articles indicated that public sector incentives to the private sector can increase the private sector's motivation to enhance management and innovation, which has a positive effect on reducing production costs and increasing economic benefits [33]. For example, URT projects generally require considerable investment and public welfare characteristics, leading to difficulties in recovering costs. Chiara and Kokkaew [55] showed that the discrepancies between URT PPP projects' operational expenditure and fare revenue could reach 29–89%. Thus, government subsidies can mitigate passenger flow risk and motivate private sectors to provide better projects and services [10].

Policy support from the public sector for the development of URT PPP projects is a key factor in attracting private sector participation and enhancing the efficiency of project collaboration [19]. Some articles show that excessive subsidies would bring financial burden to the government and decrease the opportunities for other infrastructure investments, which then affects social benefits. URT investment can lead to higher land and property values along the route to bridging the gap between affordable fares and business feasibility [56]. Thus, land value capture (LVC) has been promoted as an alternative financing policy to bridge the gap between affordable fares and the business feasibility of URT PPP projects. Some LVC policies, such as tax instruments and joint development of PPP have been adopted to capture the increased value of the land along the route [14]. For example, Mass Transit Railway Corporation Limited (MTRCL) of Hong Kong applies the developed-based LVC policy and creates the synergy between LVC and URT operation: MTRCL convert the loss status in the 1980s into profit worth 16 billion yuan in 2015 by adopting the develop-based LVC policy [52].

Private sector capability: The private sector is directly involved in the design, construction, and operation of URT PPP projects. Private sector capabilities, such as investment and financing capability, advanced technology, extensive project experience, etc., have a significant effect on value creation (i.e., cost, revenue, and delivery of a project) [19]. The construction and operation of the URT project require significant investment. In China, the cost per kilometer of URT is up to 600 to 900 million yuan [2]. Strong financing and management capability (Fre. = 338) can provide sufficient financial support for the successful delivery of URT projects and advance the project process, which is the most important factor in private sector capability.

The construction and operation of URTs require advanced technology and management levels. Some articles propose that the private sector with advanced technology and extensive project experience can reduce trial-and-error costs and sunk costs to realize the successful implementation of URT projects [9]. Additionally, the patents, efficient management, and innovative business models of private sectors can effectively reduce the production costs of a project [19], while also increasing economic benefits through improved operational efficiency.

4.1.2. Cooperation Environment

Chung and Hensher [6] confirmed that transport project benefits are highly exposed and strongly influenced by the cooperation environment. Cooperation environment factors such as project characteristics, market environment, and social environment can directly influence the project's cost and revenues, which the affects URT projects' value creation. The market environment (Fre. = 389) is the most important cooperation environment factor. Besides, the public is the end-user of URT PPP projects. The coding results indicated that the social environment (Fre. = 309) is also a critical cooperation environment factor that influences the value creation of URT PPP projects.

Project characteristics: Project characteristics, which include project scale, construction scheme, geological conditions, and surrounding environments, are the fundamental factors affecting the project cost [50]. For example, an article proposes that "the adverse geological conditions will increase the construction difficulty, thereby increasing construction costs." Therefore, ecological and geological surveys are necessary to design a reasonable construction plan and reduce the project construction cost.

Market environment: A stable market environment can provide good resources for the development of URT PPP projects [29]. An article indicated that economic development level can affect the operating policies of URT projects, financial environment, and urban GDP. A lower economic level can increase the financing cost and discourage the positive externality benefits of a URT project, which can affect the project's operating revenues. In addition, some articles proposed that the business environment including daily average transit ridership, carrying capacity, and property rents at stations affect the revenue of a URT project. The business environment (Fre. = 152) is the most important factor in the market environment. The deterioration of the business environment can lead directly to lower revenues and even project failure. Furthermore, industrial environments, such as the number of buses and other URT lines and their route plans can threaten the ridership of the developed URT PPP projects, which would also affect project revenues.

Social environment: URT is a public good and has a profound effect on social welfare. Enhanced public participation can enable decisions on URT PPP projects to meet public requirements, thereby reducing project rework and increasing public satisfaction [50]. In addition, public supervision can encourage the public and private sectors to provide more resources and generate more social benefits. The rapid development of the Internet has enabled the media to play an important role in guiding social opinion [6]. Some articles indicated that adverse media reports on URT PPP projects are likely to stimulate public discontent and lead to social risks that affect the reputation of the government and the profits of the private sectors.

4.1.3. Partnership Synergy

The public and private sectors have different expectations to participate in URT PPP projects and aim to obtain more benefits through resource complementarity [7]. The heterogeneity of goals often leads to conflicts in public-private cooperation [39]. Therefore, the success of URT PPP projects not only depends on resource complementarity but also balances the conflicting interests of partners. Partner synergy is a critical factor in ensuring the smooth construction and operations of the URT PPP project. Partner synergy manifested as a close trusting relationship and active contract compliance attitude between the public and private sectors can effectively reduce opportunistic behavior of partners and enhance the ability to deal with problems, thereby reducing the transaction costs of the project and realizing value-added [41]. Notably, the occurring frequency of concession contract management (Fre. = 834) is much more than relational management (Fre. = 447). It can be concluded that contract management is thought to be a more effective governance strategy to promote partnership synergy. Relational management mainly depends on ethics to bind partners' behavior, while contract management guarantee partners' behavior through contract clauses. Contract management can thus better maintain a good partnership between public and private partners and promote partnership synergy.

Concession contract management: Concession contractual management of URT PPP projects aims to regulate the rights and obligations of public and private sectors through formal agreements [20]. Some articles show that the vertical structure, duration, pricing mechanism, revenue sharing strategy, and risk allocation strategy of the URT PPP project should be defined clearly in the concession agreement to reduce the occurrence of uncertainties and reduce transaction costs. Coding results show that risk allocation strategy (Fre. = 225), revenue sharing strategy (Fre. = 213), and Contract flexibility (Fre. = 101) are the most important concession contract management factor. Specifically, the vertical structure of PPP contracts, which is determined by considering the characteristics of the project and the resource advantages of the government and private sectors, can specify the responsibilities and benefits of each partner [51]. The coding results show that various vertical structures in bundled or unbundled models were adopted in URT PPP projects. The bundled model enables the public sector to transfer all the responsibilities and risks related to the lifecycle of the URT project to the private sector and capture more cost-effectiveness because it can motivate private sectors to minimize costs and maximize revenues. The unbundled model refers to the public sector involved in the private sector in the design, construction, operation, maintenance, and management of URT projects through various separated PPP contracts [15]. There is no standard answer to choosing between bundled and unbundled models of URT PPP contracts, and instead requires a combined consideration of the government's financial capacity, revenue sources, project characteristics, etc.

Concession duration length influences the private sector's opportunities to accumulate operational experience and capability-building and obtain fare revenues to resist uncertainties [54]. Some articles indicate that "the shorter concession durations enable the public sector to achieve early control of the URT PPP project with a good asset state, but negatively affect private sectors to increase investment for construction and operation; Conversely, the longer concession durations are conducive to improving the return on investment of private sectors, but making the public sectors take over the URT project of lower asset state after the concession durations." Thus, the public and private sectors need to determine a reasonable concession duration by considering various uncertainties to balance the different expectations of the public and private sectors.

Fare revenue is an important aspect of maintaining the financial sustainability of URT projects [8]. Reasonable pricing mechanisms that can balance the benefits of government, passengers, and the private sector are essential. A pricing mechanism that combines government regulations and market mechanisms may allow dynamic fare adjustment according to the market environments [6]. The complementary government regulations and market mechanisms can balance multiple interests and promote value creation [57].

Profit-seeking often causes the private sector to pursue profit maximization with less consideration for the social benefits, usually leading to a value level achieved lower than the optimal value level [54]. Thus, the public sector provides subsidies to improve the performance of the URT project. However, some articles show that the public sector is likely to suffer from financial losses because the private sector may deliberately present deficits in their revenues to obtain a minimum revenue guarantee from the public sector. Hence, combining performance evaluation and reasonable subsidies would motivate private sectors to improve project performance.

Some selected articles explain that the private sector obtaining excessive profits without re-investment to improve the URT performance will damage the social benefits. A reasonable revenue-sharing strategy can facilitate the formation of aligned goals between the public and private sectors that allows the private sector to earn profits rather than windfall profits while providing extra funds to the public sector for URT improvement and other infrastructure development, thereby realizing the maximization of value creation [8].

Many uncertainties, such as adverse natural environment, and market environment exist in the URT PPP projects investment; these uncertainties affect the costs and revenues of the project [42]. Some articles indicate that "risks of PPP projects should be allocated to the most suitable stakeholders to minimize risk management costs" [8]. Based on these principles, the government should take risks of political factors and the lowest operating revenues. The private sector should be responsible for risks in aspects such as financing, organization management, and construction and operating costs. For other types of risks, the dominant stakeholder should take the corresponding risks.

For URT PPP project concession contracts, anticipating all uncertainties (e.g., changes in public demand, policy changes, organizational changes, etc.) is impossible, and thus, there is a need to develop a sound mechanism to manage conflicts and risks. Some articles indicated that the concession contract of the URT PPP project should be flexible enough to provide partners with negotiating opportunities to adjust terms and ensure that partners receive rational returns when suffering various risks and promote partnership synergy [6].

Relational management: Effective relationship governance, including building trust and increasing communication between partners, can drive partners to proactively share technology, resources, and experience, thereby facilitating the realization of value-added [39].

A good trust between public and private sectors can increase the willingness to cooperate between partners and motivate them to solve various risks actively and promptly [21], thereby improving mutual satisfaction, reducing project costs, accelerating project progress, and providing a guarantee for the realization of value creation. Additionally, some articles indicated that active communication and collaboration between partners can enhance partnerships and make partners sincerely share technology and experience [43], thereby providing more complete construction solutions for URT project development, improving project construction efficiency, and creating more value for the project.

4.2. Selective Coding

The aforementioned categories of influencing factors are critical for the value creation of the URT PPP project. The open and axial coding process showed that those influencing factors categories are interrelated. For example, "public and private sectors with advanced project experience and management capabilities" has been posited by several studies to be the prerequisite to realizing value creation while a "good social environment" would significantly increase the performance of resources complementarity by providing a stable cooperation environment. "A good communication and coordination between partners" motivate partners to share knowledge and experience openly and promote partnership synergy and create more values. Therefore, the selective coding helped explicitly link the three influencing factors categories through the following storyline.

(1) Resource complementarity between public and private can directly influence the value creation of URT PPP projects.

As explained in Section 4.1.1, the distinct resources and capabilities of the public and private sectors are the starting point for the value creation of URT PPP projects. The integration of complementary resources ensures the smooth construction and operation of URT projects following the basic contract goals (e.g., quality, schedule, and cost objectives). In addition, the complementarity of different types of resources can enhance the partners' ability to cope with risks, thereby improving operational efficiency, reducing production costs, and realizing value-added.

(2) Partnership synergy can directly influence the value creation of URT PPP projects.

As explained in Section 4.1.3, appropriate governance strategies belonging to "concession contract management" and "relational management" need to be implemented to control the heterogeneous goals and opportunistic behavior of partners and thus realize "partnership synergy". Effective partnership synergy can reduce transaction costs by reducing opportunistic behaviors of partners and improving efficiency in dealing with problems, thereby creating more partnership value.

(3) Resource complementarity has a mediating effect on the relationship between partnership synergy and value creation of URT PPP projects.

The coding results show that higher partnership synergy implies a stable partnership between the public and private sectors. This makes partners show a strong willingness to cooperate and adopt cooperative behaviors, such as devoting more dedicated resources and sharing more information. Thus, partner synergy can promote resource complementarity and thus create more value.

(4) Cooperation environment has a moderating effect on the relationship between resource complementarity and value creation of URT PPP projects.

The coding results show that the cooperation environment is also a critical factor that influences the value creation of URT PPP projects. Influencing factors belonging to the "cooperation environment" provides the basic resource foundation of public-private cooperation and influence the resource complementarity performance by affecting project cost and revenues. Therefore, a theoretical model was built based on the storyline, illustrating how the various influencing interacts to realize the maximization of value creation of the URT PPP projects, as shown in Figure 4.

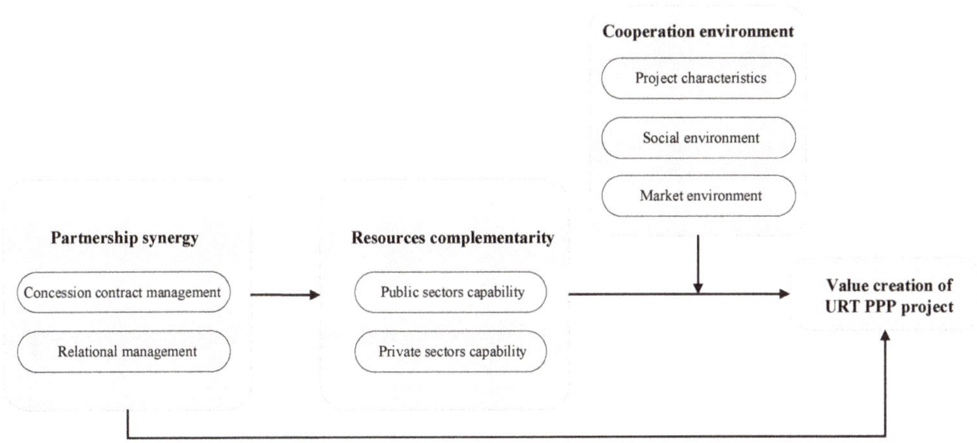

Figure 4. The generation mechanism of the value creation of the URT PPP projects under the influence of various factors.

5. Discussion

5.1. Theoretical Contribution

Previous studies on the value creation of URT PPP projects mainly focused on the achievement of basic performance objectives (e.g., time, quality, cost, and public satisfaction) [12,14]. However, with the high-quality development of PPP projects, the value creation of URT PPP projects is not only about achieving basic project objectives but relying on partner synergy to achieve value-added [5]. This study thus defines the objectives of value creation of URT PPP projects as the achievement of project basic goals and the realization of partnership value (value-added). Based on the extended connotation of value creation, this study explores what and how the factors influence the value creation of URT PPP projects. The study proposes that public-private cooperation is a generator to make URT projects bring more value and develops some contributions.

First, this study proposed that resource complementarity between the public and private sectors is a source of value creation. The public and private sectors that offer more complementary resources or capabilities can provide products or services that meet the public requirements more easily and create extra partnership values through production cost savings and reduced transaction costs, which many researchers emphasized as the primary driving factor of value creation of URT PPP projects [5,6,26]. Notably, the coding results show that private sector capabilities are considered to have a greater impact on value creation than public sector capabilities. This supports that the private sector is responsible for the entire design, construction, and operation of the URT PPP project, and its capabilities and resources directly affect the project′s cost and efficiency [19]. Additionally, to create more extra value for URT PPP projects, especially the development-based LVC policy, prior studies argued that the public sector should consider implementing an LVC policy, which can not only bring steady long-term revenues through leasing or rental of retail as well as commercial and residential spaces for private sectors, but also provide better accessibility for the public through integrating the property and commercial developments into the URT investment [11,52].

Second, this study proposed that the cooperation environment has a moderating effect on the relationship between resource complementarity and value creation of URT PPP projects. Various uncertainties risks, such as demand risk, operation risk, competition risk, and financial risk, from a cooperation environment, can affect the project′s financing costs, production costs, operating revenues, and thus the resources complementarity performance between partners. The public is the end-user of URT PPP projects. However, existing studies focused more on the impact of the public and private sectors on the value creation of URT PPP projects and neglected the role of the public. This study finds that public participation will monitor the behavior of the public and private sectors and motivate them to invest more resources, thus contributing to value creation. Moreover, public satisfaction directly influences the costs and revenues of the project.

Partnership is the basic feature of PPP projects [41]. However, there is little research on the impact of partnership synergy on the value creation of URT PPP projects. This study finds that partnership synergy is in activating the consistent interests between public and private sectors and providing the possibility of creating joint value maximization. Both concession contract management and relational management are critical factors to promote partnership synergy. The coding results show that contract management is considered to have a greater impact on value creation than relational management. Relational management mainly depends on ethics to bind partners' behavior, while contract management guarantees partners' behavior through contract clauses [18]. Contract management can thus better maintain a good partnership between public and private partners and promote partnership synergy. As for concession contract management of the URT PPP project, the vertical structure of the URT PPP project should be first determined, determining the responsibilities and the possible benefits of each partner. In addition, to align the interests of each partner with the overall value creation, the public and private sectors need to play the game through an integrated consideration of concession duration, pricing mechanism, revenue sharing strategy, and risk allocation strategy, and explicitly indicate them in the contract. Existing studies also validated the importance of contract flexibility to improve partnership synergy and promote value creation. Alvanchi et al. [20] found that flexible terms in contracts allow partners to deal with uncertainty risks more efficiently and ensure that they obtain reasonable benefits. As for the relational management of the URT PPP project, trust and communication between partners can help motivate partners to share their resources and technologies and elevate their willingness to be involved in joint working and decision making, thereby improving cooperation efficiency and promoting value creation.

Finally, the study proposed that resource complementarity, partnership synergy, and a cooperation environment are the decisive elements for bringing the maximized value creation of URT PPP projects. Resources complementarity incentivizes the public and private sectors to become involved in cooperation. The cooperation environment has a moderate effect on resource complementarity. During the cooperation, partners' interests become interdependent through the effective contract and relational management, thereby activating the alignment in the interests of partnerships. This finding indicates that resource complementarity among partners together with the cooperation environment and partnership synergy generates the proper conditions to realize the joint value maximization in public-private collaboration.

5.2. Implications for Practice

This study provides a comprehensive framework for public and private sectors to better understand value creation in the cross-sector cooperation of URT projects. Based on the constructed theory model, the study proposes that identifying the advantages of each partner, fully considering the influence of the cooperation environment, and activating the commonality from partners' heterogeneous motives would promote mutual support among the cross-sector in achieving the maximization of the joint value of public, private and partnership values.

Public sectors should cooperate with private sectors with advanced technology and management experience in the construction and operation of the URT PPP project to improve cost-revenue efficiency. As an example, the public sector can select private sectors with advanced technology and experience by adopting a prequalification system. In addition, the public sector should enact favorable policies to support the URT project to obtain more benefits. For example, LVC bridges the gap between affordable fares and the business feasibility of URT PPP projects [11]. The government could adopt a development strategy that combines LVC and transit-oriented development (TOD). TOD improves the traffic network and business environment along the URT lines, thereby incentivizing the public to take the URT and indirectly increasing the land values along the route [53].

To facilitate partnership synergy, governments could consider formulating a framework of disclosure to increase information transparency among stakeholders during the lifecycle of URT PPP projects. Increasing information transparency during cooperation has been advocated to improve trust among partners and reduce public misgivings, thereby enhancing the performance of resource complementarity among partners [43]. However, finding a balance between providing critical information to inform and obtain the trust and support of stakeholders and guaranteeing business confidentiality, and complying with the legal provisions can be difficult [50]. Thus, the public sector should better provide the information to satisfy the stakeholders′ curiosity and concerns and simultaneously maintain business confidentiality. Additionally, the government should thoroughly consider adopting some effective strategies and identifying them in the contract to strengthen the cohesiveness of motives among partners. The vertical structure of URT PPP projects with the bundled model is recommended to ensure project feasibility. The bundled model enables the public sector to transfer the responsibility for the design, construction, operation, maintenance, and management of URT projects to the private sector [15]. Therefore, the private sector can optimize costs and improve revenues, thereby obtaining the expected profits. At the same time, the public sector can devote more energy and funds to other infrastructure investments and management. It is worth noting that the government should conduct continuous monitoring of the construction and operational performance of the private sector to avoid focusing on short-term interests at the expense of project sustainability.

The findings also indicate that public involvement is a critical cooperation environment factor that influences resource complementarity performance. Thus, the public sector can build more information communication channels for the public to obtain their suggestions in time.

6. Conclusions

The significance of public-private cooperation in the success of URT projects has been recognized in some previous studies. However, in-depth studies on the influencing factors and the mechanism of value creation beyond self-interest maximization in cross-sector cooperation of URT projects have been limited. The study obtains concepts from selected articles, explores relationships between concepts, and finally constructs a theoretical model on the generation mechanism of the value creation of URT PPP projects. The findings suggest that value creation comes from the combination of resources complementarity, cooperation environment, and partnership synergy. URT PPP projects can create more values that are difficult to achieve depending on any partner on their own by accessing and integrating the legitimacy advantages of the public sector and the competence in the construction and operation of private sectors. The influence of project characteristics and market environment on project cost and revenues should be considered, and more focus should be given to the public and media attitudes towards the project to strengthen the performance of resource complementarity. However, the heterogeneity of expectations between the public and private sectors often leads to the expectation of maximizing self-interest. Therefore, the interaction partner's in PPP need to explore the balance criteria to satisfy heterogeneous expectations through effective contract management and relational management, thereby promoting joint value maximization.

In conclusion, the study assists the public and private sectors in better understanding the factors and relationships that influence the value creation in public-private cooperation of URT projects, leading them to make more reasonable benefit adjustments, sharing and governance strategies in the URT PPP project's lifecycle. The finding enables stakeholders to become more aware of the resource complementarity, cooperation environment and cohesiveness of motives among partners to realize the value creation of URT PPP projects.

Moreover, the study can serve as a research foundation for further analyzing the value creation of the URT PPP project. Future studies can use detailed quantitative analysis to explore the action mechanism of different factors in the value creation of URT PPP projects. A simulation analysis would also be beneficial in generating strategies for the dynamic adjustment of value creation.

This study has some limitations, and further research needs to be conducted to obtain a more detailed and practical perspective on value creation. First, the data collected in this study came from China. Due to differences in institutions and cultural norms across countries, it is possible to extend the scope of data collection to other countries in a future study to demonstrate the generality of the results. Next, the object of this present study focused on URT PPP projects. For other types of inter-sector cooperation projects, factors influencing the realization of value creation should be further identified. Nonetheless, the findings in this study can provide a reference for future research on value creation.

Author Contributions: Conceptualization, formal analysis, visualization, writing—original draft preparation, X.L. (Xuewei Li); Methodology, validation, writing—review & editing, funding acquisition, J.Y.; Data curation, software, writing—original draft preparation, X.L. (Xuan Liu); Resources, supervision, project administration, writing—review & editing, Y.K.; Conceptualization, resources, investigation, writing—original draft preparation, S.J. All authors have read and agreed to the published version of the manuscript.

Funding: This research was funded by "Jiangsu Graduate Innovative Research Program, grant number KYCX20_0161", "Fundamental Research Funds for the Central Universities, grant number 3205002104D", "National Natural Science Foundation of China, grant number 71671042 and 72072031".

Institutional Review Board Statement: No applicable.

Informed Consent Statement: No applicable.

Data Availability Statement: The data generated or analyzed during the study are available from the corresponding author on request.

Conflicts of Interest: The authors declare no conflict of interest.

References

1. Graham, D.J.; Carbo, J.M.; Anderson, R.J.; Bansal, P. Understanding the costs of urban rail transport operations. *Transp. Res. Part B Methodol.* **2020**, *138*, 292–316.
2. Yang, L.; Chen, Y.; Xu, N.; Zhao, R.; Chau, K.W.; Hong, S. Place-varying impacts of urban rail transit on property prices in Shenzhen, China: Insights for value capture. *Sustain. Cities Soc.* **2020**, *58*, 102140. [CrossRef]
3. DeCorla-Souza, P.; Lee, D.; Timothy, D.; Mayer, J. Comparing Public-Private Partnerships with Conventional Procurement: Incorporating Considerations from Benefit-Cost Analysis. *Transp. Res. Rec.* **2013**, *2346*, 32–39. [CrossRef]
4. Taecharungroj, V. An analysis of tripadvisor reviews of 127 urban rail transit networks worldwide. *Travel Behav. Soc.* **2022**, *26*, 193–205. [CrossRef]
5. Villani, E.; Greco, L.; Phillips, N. Understanding value creation in public-private partnerships: A comparative case study. *J. Manag. Stud.* **2017**, *54*, 876–905. [CrossRef]
6. Chung, D.M.; Hensher, D.A. Public private partnerships in the provision of tolled roads: Shared value creation, trust and control. *Transp. Res. Part A Policy Pract.* **2018**, *118*, 341–359. [CrossRef]
7. Kivleniece, I.; Quelin, B.V. Creating and capturing value in public-private ties: A private actor's perspective. *Acad. Manag. Rev.* **2012**, *37*, 272–299. [CrossRef]
8. Roumboutsos, A.; Pantelias, A. Allocating Revenue Risk in Transport Infrastructure Public Private Partnership Projects: How it Matters. *Transp. Rev.* **2015**, *35*, 183–203. [CrossRef]
9. Chang, Z.; Phang, S.Y. Urban rail transit PPPs: Lessons from East Asian cities. *Transp. Res. Part A Policy Pract.* **2017**, *46*, 35–46. [CrossRef]
10. Hu, Y.P.; Wang, J.P.; Sun, H.L. Optimisation of pricing and subsidies for urban rail transit PPP projects based on satisfactions of main stakeholders. *J. Environ. Prot. Ecol.* **2018**, *19*, 435–449.
11. Zhao, J.B.; Li, C.S.; Zhang, R.H.; Palmer, M. Cost of an urban rail ride: A nation-level analysis of ridership, capital costs and cost-effectiveness performance of urban rail transit projects in China. *J. Transp. Land Use* **2018**, *11*, 1173–1191. [CrossRef]
12. Yuan, J.; Zeng, A.Y.; Skibniewski, M.J.; Li, Q. Selection of performance objectives and key performance indicators in public-private partnership projects to achieve value for money. *Constr. Manag. Econ.* **2009**, *27*, 253–270. [CrossRef]

13. Yuan, J.; Wang, C.; Skibniewski, M.J.; Li, Q. Developing key performance indicators for public-private partnership projects: Questionnaire survey and analysis. *J. Manag. Eng.* **2012**, *28*, 252–264. [CrossRef]
14. Li, X.; Love, P.E.D. State-of-the-Art Review of Urban Rail Transit Public-Private Partnerships. *J. Infrastruct. Syst.* **2020**, *26*, 03120002. [CrossRef]
15. Carpintero, S.; Petersen, O.H. Bundling and Unbundling in Public-Private Partnerships: Implications for Risk Sharing in Urban Transport Projects. *Proj. Manag. J.* **2015**, *46*, 35–46. [CrossRef]
16. Ke, Y.; Hao, W.; Ding, H.; Wang, Y. Factors influencing the private involvement in urban rail public-private partnership projects in China. *Constr. Econ. Build.* **2017**, *17*, 90–106. [CrossRef]
17. Xiahou, X.; Tang, L.; Yuan, J.; Zuo, J.; Li, Q. Exploring social impacts of urban rail transit PPP projects: Towards dynamic social change from the stakeholder perspective. *Environ. Impact Assess. Rev.* **2022**, *93*, 106700. [CrossRef]
18. Tian, B.; Wang, Z.; Li, C.; Fu, J. Can relational governance improve sustainability in public-private partnership infrastructure projects? An empirical study based on structural equation modeling. *Eng. Constr. Archit. Manag.* **2021**. *ahead-of-print*. [CrossRef]
19. Ye, X.; Shi, S.; Chong, H.Y.; Fu, X.; Liu, L.; He, Q. Empirical analysis of firms' willingness to participate in infrastructure PPP projects. *J. Constr. Eng. Manag.* **2018**, *144*, 04017092. [CrossRef]
20. Alvanchi, A.; Hosseini, S.M.T.; Nili-Ahmadabad, M.H.; AmiriDiba, A. Improving public-private partnership project procurement, addressing major shortfalls in the standard-form contract. *Int. J. Procure. Manag.* **2020**, *13*, 482–506. [CrossRef]
21. Benitez-Avila, C.; Hartmann, A.; Dewulf, G.; Henseler, J. Interplay of relational and contractual governance in public-private partnerships: The mediating role of relational norms, trust and partners' contribution. *Int. J. Proj. Manag.* **2018**, *36*, 429–443. [CrossRef]
22. Corbin, J.; Strauss, A. Grounded theory research—Procedures, canons and evaluative criteria. *Z. Fur Soziologie* **1990**, *19*, 418–427. [CrossRef]
23. Tetteh, M.O.; Chan, A.P.; Darko, A.; Yevu, S.K.; Boateng, E.B.; Nwaogu, J.M. Key drivers for implementing international construction joint ventures (ICJVs): Global insights for sustainable growth. *Eng. Constr. Archit. Manag.* **2021**. *ahead-of-print*. [CrossRef]
24. Walker, D.; Myrick, F. Grounded theory: An exploration of process and procedure. *Qual. Health Res.* **2006**, *16*, 547–559. [CrossRef]
25. Almarri, K.; Boussabaine, H. Interdependency of the critical success factors and ex-post performance indicators of PPP projects. *Built Environ. Proj. Asset Manag.* **2017**, *7*, 546–556. [CrossRef]
26. Crane, A.; Palazzo, G.; Spence, L.J.; Matten, D. Contesting the Value of "Creating Shared Value". *Calif. Manag. Rev.* **2014**, *56*, 130–149. [CrossRef]
27. Zhang, X.; Liu, J. Incentive Mechanism and Value-Added in PPP Projects Considering Financial Institutions' Early Intervention. *J. Constr. Eng. Manag.* **2022**, *148*, 04022001. [CrossRef]
28. Hodge, G.A.; Greve, C. Public-private partnerships: An international performance review. *Public Adm. Rev.* **2007**, *67*, 545–558. [CrossRef]
29. Matinheikki, J.; Rajala, R.; Peltokorpi, A. From the profit of one toward benefitting many—Crafting a vision of shared value creation. *J. Clean. Prod.* **2017**, *162*, S83–S93. [CrossRef]
30. Liu, S.; Yao, E.; Li, B. Exploring urban rail transit station-level ridership growth with network expansion. *Transp. Res. Part D Transp. Environ.* **2019**, *73*, 391–402. [CrossRef]
31. Henjewele, C.; Sun, M.; Fewings, P. Analysis of factors affecting value for money in UK PFI projects. *J. Financ. Manag. Prop. Constr.* **2012**, *17*, 9–28. [CrossRef]
32. Cheung, E.; Chan, A.P.; Kajewski, S. Factors contributing to successful public private partnership projects: Comparing Hong Kong with Australia and the United Kingdom. *J. Facil. Manag.* **2012**, *10*, 45–58. [CrossRef]
33. Parrado, S.; Reynaers, A.M. Managing Public Values in Public-Private Partnerships: Do Public Authorities Succeed? *Gestión Política Pública* **2021**, *30*, 163–196. [CrossRef]
34. Liu, F.R.; Liu, J.; Yan, X.D. Quantifying the Decision-Making of PPPs in China by the Entropy-Weighted Pareto Front: A URT Case from Guizhou. *Sustainability* **2018**, *10*, 1753. [CrossRef]
35. Soliño, A.S.; Vassallo, J.M. Using public-private partnerships to expand subways: Madrid-Barajas international airport case study. *J. Manag. Eng.* **2009**, *25*, 21–28. [CrossRef]
36. Babatunde, S.O.; Perera, S. Analysis of traffic revenue risk factors in BOT road projects in developing countries. *Transp. Policy* **2017**, *56*, 41–49. [CrossRef]
37. Lesley, L. Public and private funding in new urban public transport. *Public Money Manag.* **1995**, *15*, 61–64. [CrossRef]
38. Ma, L.; Fu, H. A Governance Framework for the Sustainable Delivery of Megaprojects: The Interaction of Megaproject Citizenship Behavior and Contracts. *J. Constr. Eng. Manag.* **2022**, *148*, 04022004. [CrossRef]
39. Leite, E.; Bengtson, A. A business network view on value creation and capture in public-private cooperation. *Ind. Mark. Manag.* **2018**, *73*, 181–192. [CrossRef]
40. Jacobson, C.; Choi, S.O. Success factors: Public works and public-private partnerships. *Int. J. Public Sect. Manag.* **2008**, *21*, 637–657. [CrossRef]
41. Love, P.E.; Ika, L.; Matthews, J.; Fang, W. Shared leadership, value and risks in large scale transport projects: Re-calibrating procurement policy for post COVID-19. *Res. Transp. Econ.* **2021**, *90*, 100999.
42. Phang, S.Y. Urban rail transit PPPs: Survey and risk assessment of recent strategies. *Transp. Policy* **2007**, *14*, 214–231. [CrossRef]

43. Eshun, B.T.B.; Chan, A.P.C.; Osei-Kyei, R. Conceptualizing a win-win scenario in public-private partnerships: Evidence from a systematic literature review. *Eng. Constr. Archit. Manag.* **2021**, *28*, 2712–2735. [CrossRef]
44. Chadegani, A.A.; Salehi, H.; Yunus, M.M.; Farhadi, H.; Fooladi, M.; Farhadi, M.; Ebrahim, N.A. A comparison between two main academic literature collections: Web of Science and Scopus databases. *Asian Soc. Sci.* **2013**, *9*, 18–26. [CrossRef]
45. The World Bank. Railway Reform: A Toolkit for Improving Rail Sector Performance. 2017. Available online: https://ppiaf.org/ppiaf/sites/ppiaf.org/files/documents/toolkits/railways_toolkit/index.html (accessed on 6 July 2022).
46. PPP Knowledge Lab. PPP Reference Guide. 2017. Available online: https://pppknowledgelab.org/guide (accessed on 6 July 2022).
47. Pettigrew, A.M. Longitudinal field research on change: Theory and practice. *Organ. Sci.* **1990**, *1*, 267–292. [CrossRef]
48. Liu, X.M.; Zhou, J.Y.; Xue, Y.T.; Qian, S.Y. Analysis of property management ecological behavior in China based on the grounded theory: The influencing factors and the behavior model. *J. Clean. Prod.* **2019**, *235*, 44–56. [CrossRef]
49. Strauss, A.; Corbin, J. Grounded theory methodology. *Handb. Qual. Res.* **1994**, *17*, 273–285.
50. Ho, S.P.; Levitt, R.; Tsui, C.W.; Hsu, Y.W. Opportunism-focused transaction cost analysis of public-private partnerships. *J. Manag. Eng.* **2015**, *31*, 04015007.
51. Yuan, J.; Ding, H.; Huang, Z.; Deng, B.; Li, S.; Huang, W. Influence of market structures on concession pricing in Public-Private-Partnership utilities with asymmetric information. *Util. Policy* **2021**, *69*, 101162. [CrossRef]
52. Li, X.; Love, P.E. Procuring urban rail transit infrastructure by integrating land value capture and public-private partnerships: Learning from the cities of Delhi and Hong Kong. *Cities* **2022**, *122*, 103545. [CrossRef]
53. Cervero, R.; Murakami, J. Rail and property development in Hong Kong: Experiences and extensions. *Urban Stud.* **2009**, *46*, 2019–2043. [CrossRef]
54. Chung, D. Risks, Challenges and Value for Money of Public-Private Partnerships. *Financ. Account. Manag.* **2016**, *32*, 448–468. [CrossRef]
55. Chiara, N.; Kokkaew, N. Alternative to Government Revenue Guarantees: Dynamic Revenue Insurance Contracts. *J. Infrastruct. Syst.* **2013**, *19*, 287–296. [CrossRef]
56. Xu, H.; Yan, Y. Integrated Planning Model of Land-Use Layout and Transportation Network Design for Regional Urbanization in China Based on TOD Theory. *J. Urban Plan. Dev.* **2021**, *147*, 04021013. [CrossRef]
57. Jin, H.; Liu, S.; Li, J.; Liu, C. Imperfect information bargaining model for determining concession period of PPPs under revenue uncertainty. *J. Leg. Aff. Disput. Resolut. Eng. Constr.* **2020**, *12*, 04520012. [CrossRef]

buildings

Article

A Classification-Based Blockchain Architecture for Smart Home with Hierarchical PoW Mechanism

Weilu Lv [1,2,†], Ning Wang [3,*,†], Xianwang Xie [4] and Zhen Hong [5,*]

1 School of Art and Archaeology, Zhejiang University City College, Hangzhou 310015, China
2 School of Architecture, Tsinghua University, Beijing 100084, China
3 School of Spatial Planning and Design, Zhejiang University City College, Hangzhou 310015, China
4 School of Cyber Security, University of Chinese Academy of Sciences, Beijing 101408, China
5 Institute of Cyberspace Security, Zhejiang University of Technology, Hangzhou 310023, China
* Correspondence: wangning@zucc.edu.cn (N.W.); zhong1983@zjut.edu.cn (Z.H.)
† These authors contributed equally to this work.

Abstract: Smart home, as a typical Internet of Things (IoT) application, provides people with a variety of conveniences. Unfortunately, it may suffer from security and privacy issues. Currently, blockchain theory is considered as one of the potential solutions to the IoT security problem. However, according to the rules of blockchain, it requires large storage to store distributed ledgers and undertakes long latency caused by proof of work (PoW), which cannot be performed by resource-constrained IoT devices. To address the issue, we propose a classification-based blockchain architecture with a hierarchical PoW mechanism, which can reduce the storage consumption and decrease the latency. In our architecture, we divide IoT devices into several child nodes by data classification and convert the data storage into partial network storage. Furthermore, we try to set the moderate-cost security grades (SG) to adjust the difficulty of PoW for reduction of latency. Finally, comparing the performance of our scheme with the traditional method and current technology, the proposed architecture not only takes up less storage (i.e., almost 90% reduction) but also increases efficiency (i.e., almost 50% running time saving) while ensuring safety.

Keywords: smart home; secure architecture; blockchain; storage efficiency; IoT

Citation: Lv, W.; Wang, N.; Xie, X.; Hong, Z. A Classification-Based Blockchain Architecture for Smart Home with Hierarchical PoW Mechanism. *Buildings* **2022**, *12*, 1321. https://doi.org/10.3390/buildings12091321

Academic Editors: Liyin Shen, Jorge Ochoa and Haijun Bao

Received: 30 June 2022
Accepted: 24 August 2022
Published: 29 August 2022

1. Introduction

The smart city refers to the use of various information technologies or innovative ideas to build and optimize the urban management framework [1,2]. It usually integrates the systems and services of the city to improve the efficiency of resource utilization and the quality of citizens' lives. In a sense, a smart city is the product of the rapid development of information technology, the high-quality and sustainable development of modern cities. As an important part of the smart city, the smart home, which is one of the applications filed on the Internet of Things (IoT), has brought a new modern concept of people living in recent years [3–5]. It integrates with a series of digital techniques that influence the daily life of individuals [6]. As millions of devices are continuously being linked to the IoT networks, how to keep IoT systems secure and avoid various kinds of malicious attacks is an open issue and a matter of great concern [7–9]. Currently, a highly centralized security framework is widely used for IoT due to its easy control. However, it is incompletely suitable for IoT since a single central control node may be vulnerable by attackers [10].

One effective solution to protect the IoT network is to employ blockchain technology [11–16]. Usually, blockchain is an open distributed digital ledger that maintains a growing list of blocks one after another within a chain. Each block is added to the ledger after mining, which is verified by the participating nodes. To mine a block, some specific nodes called miners try to solve a time-consuming cryptographic problem known as proof of work (PoW) [17]. This is how blockchain eliminates the need for trusted third parties through the distributed record preservation and verification system. Currently, blockchain-based technology is widely used in various fields, such as smart education [18], smart healthcare [19], smart home [12], etc.

Recently, there has been much research regarding secure IoT systems [20–23]. Dorri et al. [24] propose a blockchain-based architecture for IoT devices that supports security and privacy. However, it is not fully built on a distributed architecture due to the use of a central cloud storage. Furthermore, they try to reduce the latency by removing the PoW consensus mechanism, but cannot prove whether it would withstand attacks performed by compromised nodes [25]. Similarly, to eliminate the PoW mechanism, a blockchain-enabled architecture of software-defined networking (SDN) controllers using a cluster structure with a new routing protocol is proposed for resource-constrained IoT device scenarios [26]. It actually uses public and private blockchains for peer to peer (P2P) communication between IoT devices and SDN controllers. In order to improve the architecture (or features, e.g., structure, verification, storage) of the original blockchain, as shown in Table 1, Qu et al. [27] propose a hypergraph-based blockchain model to reduce data storage, but cannot deal with the long latency caused by PoW. Mohanty et al. [28] develop an integrated blockchain model that includes a lightweight consensus algorithm, certificateless cryptography, and distributed throughput management scheme. It generates an overlay network to assign higher resources to a public blockchain to guarantee the dedicated security and privacy. But this scheme seems a bit complex for smart home scenarios. We can see the existing blockchain-based architecture for smart home devices face the challenge of imbalanced security and efficiency [29]. It exposes the traditional highly centralized architecture to huge security risks and vulnerabilities. Therefore, it is necessary to design a decentralized, safe, and efficient blockchain-based smart home architecture for human living.

Table 1. Comparison of blockchain models.

Features	Description	
	Original Blockchain	**Hypergraph-Based Blockchain**
Structure	One chain	Several subchains
Verification	By node itself	By other nodes
Storage	One node one copy	Partial nodes have a copy
Miners' function	PoW	PoW and linear independence matrix

In this paper, we propose a classification-based blockchain architecture for smart homes with a hierarchy-based PoW mechanism. In our architecture, we focus on reducing storage for IoT devices while decreasing the latency caused by PoW in the condition of acceptable security risks. The major contributions of this paper can be summarized as follows.

- To replace the high-risk centralized frameworks, we propose a classification-based blockchain architecture for smart homes that stores data in a fully decentralized way. In the architecture, we divide IoT devices into several child nodes by data classification and convert the data storage into the partial network storage. It not only helps decrease risks such as single point failure but also reduces almost 90% storage for resource-constrained IoT devices.
- We design a moderate-cost hierarchical PoW mechanism, i.e., set different security grades according to the security requirements, which can reduce the latency and the security risks to an acceptable level. By experimenting, the proposed architecture can help reduce running time by almost 50%.

The rest of this paper is organized as follows. Section 2 discusses the current problem associated with centralized blockchain-based architectures. In Section 3, we design and propose a new improved blockchain-based architecture that is a typically distributed mode. Furthermore, we propose a hierarchical PoW mechanism to balance the performance of security and computational complexity in Section 4. Experiments are conducted to further analyze the proposed scheme on storage, security, and latency in Section 5. Finally, we conclude this paper in Section 6.

2. Problem Statement

In the traditional smart home, as shown in Figure 1, the architecture is so highly centralized that the key node (i.e., control center) is located at the center of the IoT network to control all the devices. However, it cannot always guarantee services availability because it is vulnerable to a single point of failure and malicious attacks such as Sybil and DDoS attacks [30]. Furthermore, the control center acts as the data switching station and the interactive information is prone to eavesdropping under the transmission process. In order to protect user privacy, we try to design a blockchain-based decentralized architecture for the smart home.

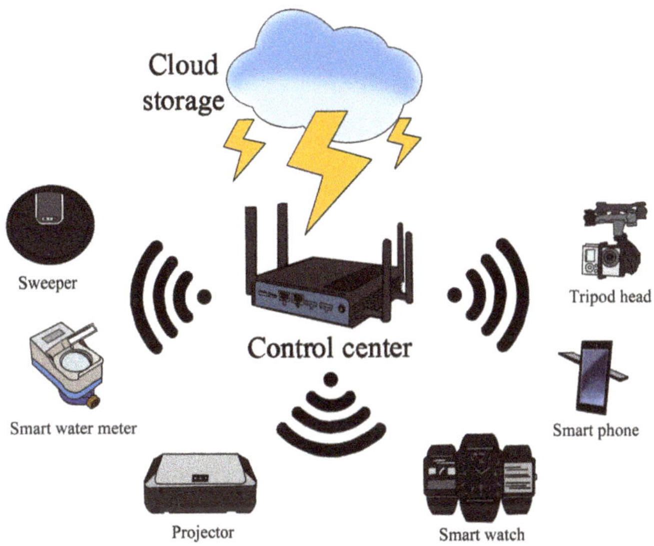

Figure 1. The traditional highly centralized smart home architecture.

The distributed ledger of the blockchain requires a full network accounting model. All nodes in the blockchain retain a ledger that contains all transaction data, and update it to maintain integrity if a new transaction is available. When a transaction occurs, all of the participant nodes would verify it during the mining process which may cause long latency according to the PoW mechanism. The higher the difficulty of the PoW mechanism, the more secure the transaction data, and the greater the latency. Once the transaction is verified and added to the blockchain, it will be stored in all nodes and cannot be tampered unless the attacker can simultaneously control more than 51% of the nodes in the system.

Consequently, it is not always necessary for all nodes to store all of the transaction records in the blockchain network. Actually, there is no need to set the same high level of security for all categories of transaction data. For one transaction record, it is enough to guarantee that it is stored by a sufficient number of nodes and it only needs to ensure that each kind of transaction is at an acceptable security level. When a new transaction occurs, only the associated nodes will verify and store the transaction record.

3. System Architecture

3.1. Architecture Overview

To address the above problem, we design an improved blockchain-based architecture. Firstly, we introduce the main objects within the architecture that are described as follows.

- **Node**: a device with storage in a blockchain. Each node contains several child nodes (CNs), and it belongs to at least one vertex set.
- **Miners**: are devices used to calculate encryption block hash keys in the blockchain.
- **Vertex set (VS)**: contains a number of CNs that are involved in different devices and store the same category of transaction data. Each VS maintains a sub-blockchain.

Figure 2 shows an example of the proposed blockchain-based architecture. In Figure 2, our blockchain network contains 7 devices ($Node_1$ to $Node_7$), 19 CNs (CN_1 to CN_{19}), 2 miners ($Miner_1$ and $Miner_2$), and 2 local networks (LN_1 and LN_2). Moreover,we classify CNs which record the same category of data to the same VS, and they are divided into five sets (VS_1 to VS_5) that are represented as connected blocks of the same color. Here, a device can be involved in two or more VSs at the same time. For example, $Node_4$ belongs to VS_1 and also belongs to VS_5. In addition, devices belonging to the same VSs may or may not be in the same local network.

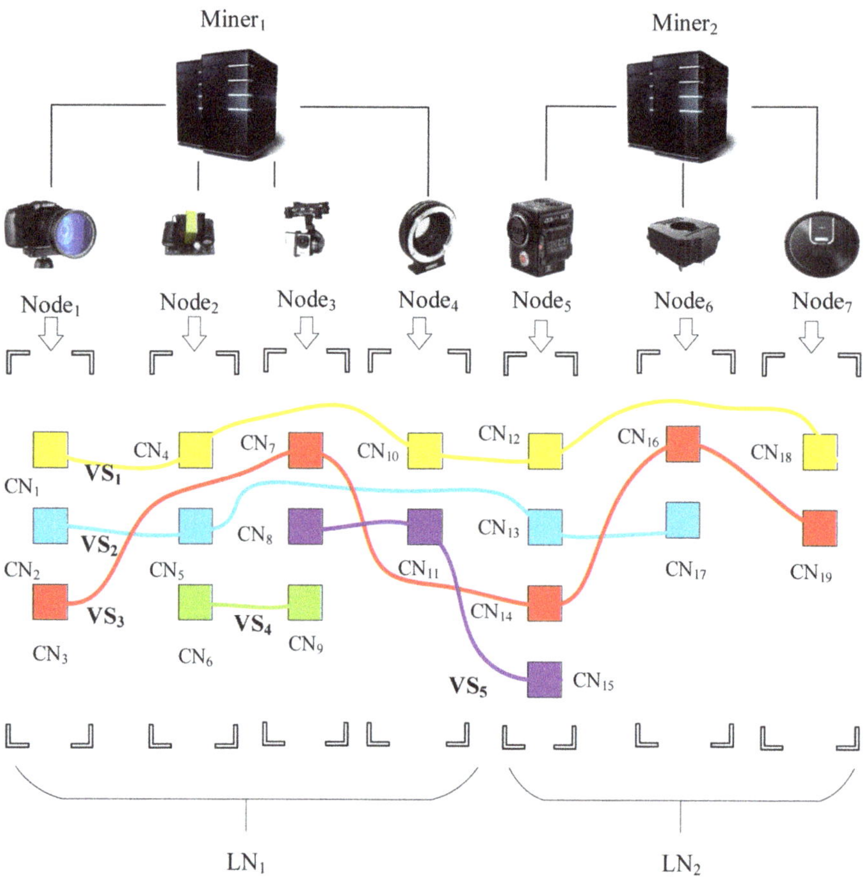

Figure 2. A classification-based blockchain decentralized architecture.

In the proposed architecture, a CN can only belong to one VS. The CNs in the same VS must be synchronized in the storage process. In order to balance the storage distribution and avoid the phenomenon that some CNs in the largest VS store too much data, we define the maximum and minimum size of a VS as $maxn$, $minn$, respectively, where $minn = maxn/4$.

3.2. The Data Structure of Nodes

Since a node in the blockchain must contain all transaction data related to the device, it involves the categories of transaction data generated from both itself and other devices. Meanwhile, the node must store the synchronized transaction data in different VSs. However, the original working mechanism of blockchain cannot reach the requirements due to its structure. Therefore, we designed a data structure for each node.

As shown in Figure 3, the storage structure designed for each node includes three parts: the blockchain-list, sub-blockchain, and relation vector. The blockchain-list involves several indexes of sub-blockchains that store synchronous transaction data related to the device, which means each VS maintains a sub-blockchain. Specifically, the total number of indexes is equal to the number of categories of data associated with the device in the whole blockchain. Each sub-blockchain is stored in the CNs of the device, and the data category between sub-blockchains are different from each other. The relation vector is a vector that records all the indexes of CNs related to this device, where r_k represents the indexes of CNs related to CN_k.

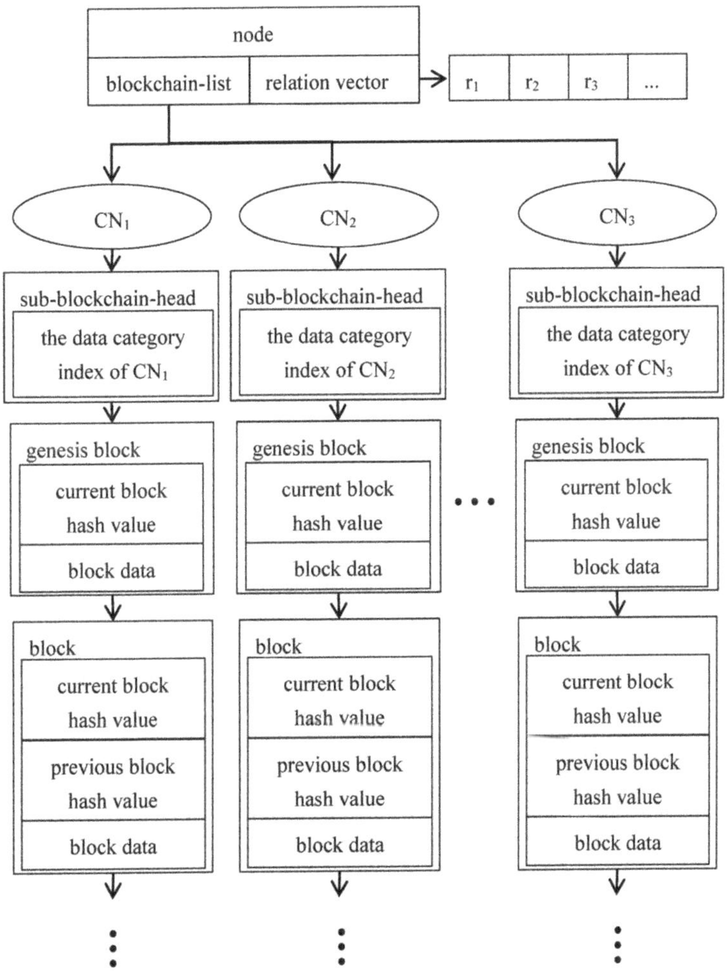

Figure 3. The data structure of nodes.

4. Hierarchical PoW Mechanism

As far as we know, PoW is the most widely used consensus algorithm in the blockchain which can effectively defend against various malicious attacks [17,22]. However, it is overloaded for power-constrained IoT devices. We cannot eliminate PoW since it may cause system vulnerabilities and threats. To address the above problem, we propose a moderate-cost hierarchical PoW mechanism for such power-constrained IoT devices to make the trade-off between efficiency and security.

In our architecture, we use small-scale private blockchain and each sub-blockchain only records the same category of data. According to the security requirements, we define that a data category has a security grade (SG), i.e., the SG of each data category must be positively related to its security requirement and cannot be much higher to make the IoT device overload. On the other hand, each CN also has the same security grade as a data category. The difficulty of PoW is self-adaptive according to the SG of each CN. The higher the SG, the longer it takes to run the PoW mechanism. Thus, this mechanism allows the CNs that store the data category with low-security requirements to consume fewer resources. However, letting the miners know the SG of the transaction data and run a PoW of corresponding difficulty when a transaction is released is a key problem.

We built a blockchain between miners to record the mapping of all the categories of data in the blockchain system to SGs that have been initialized. When a transaction occurs, the source CN constructs a record that includes information such as timestamp, the index of the category of transaction data, transaction content. The miners read the index from the constructed records and obtain the security grade through the mapping. Then, they run the PoW with corresponding difficulty for verification. If the transaction is verified to be legal, the record is added to the current block of the sub-blockchain with the same index of transaction data category.

When the current block in a sub-blockchain of a CN is full, according to the working principle of blockchain, the data in the current full block, the hash value of previous block and other information will be published to the whole sub-blockchain network. Miners receive this data and competitively calculate the cryptographic hash value. Once a miner settles down the puzzle, it will publish to the sub-blockchain for verification. If the verified result is acceptable, the block will be encrypted and stored, otherwise, it will be discarded and the above process will be repeated.

In addition to setting the security grade, the number of CNs in each VS must be sufficient to reach the security requirements. To avoid the construction of a VS with only a few CNs (e.g., some CNs are deleted from the blockchain), we designed a series of algorithms to manage the process of node joining (i.e., connect to network) and deletion (disconnection).

When a new node is connected to the network, each of its CNs is added to the VS that contains its other associated CNs and stores the same data category. If there is no VS associated with the new node in the network, its CNs will be randomly added to a VS in which the stored data category is the same as the corresponding CNs. On the other hand, if the number of CNs in a VS is greater than $maxn$, then the VS is split into two sets, one of which has a number of $minn$ CNs and the other is $(maxn\text{-}minn)$. Specifically, there is no association for CNs in these two VSs. Here we can assume that the number of interconnected devices is less than $minn$ since there are not many associated devices in the context of the smart home. The process for node addition is shown in Algorithm 1. In contrast, when a node is deleted from the network, i.e., disconnected from the network, it may cause the number of CNs in a VS to be less than $minn$. At this time, we merge this VS and the other VS whose number of child nodes does not exceed $(maxn\text{-}minn)$. The process of node deletion is given in Algorithm 2.

Algorithm 1 Node Addition

```
for each CN in NewAddSet do
    k ← index(NewAddSet, CN)
    if RelationVector[k] ≠ null then
        r_k ← RelationVector[k]
    else
        r_k ← random()
    end if
    j ← index(VS, r_k)
    VS[j] ← VS[j] ∪ CN
    if size(VS[j]) > maxn then
        split minn CNs in VS[j] to a new VS
    end if
end for
```

Algorithm 2 Node Deletion

```
for each CN in deletedSet do
    i ← index(VS, CN)
    VS[i] ← VS[i] − CN
    if size(VS[i]) < minn then
        select VS[j] whose size < (maxn − minn)
        VS[j] ← VS[i] ∪ VS[j]
    end if
end for
```

5. Performance Evaluations

To evaluate the proposed architecture, in this paper, one real smart home scenario ($maxn$ = 5, the number of categories is 100) is conducted for emulation and verification. Specifically, as shown in Figure 4, we designed a small testbed with the self-design IoT devices (nodes) to emulate the scenario of the smart home. In our testbed, we used PCs as miners and used Raspberry Pi Model 3B with 1 GB memory as a normal node which is integrated with various physical sensors.

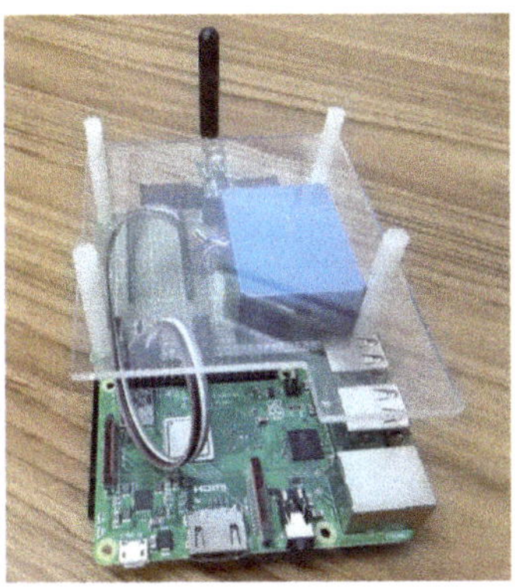

Figure 4. The IoT device.

For a given N IoT nodes in the network, we try to calculate the average storage of each node and the running time of generating a certain amount of blocks. Furthermore, we try to find the relationship among the $maxn$ of VS, the average storage of each node, and the security. Here we define the safety factor for security evaluation as the maximum number of malicious CNs that the system can tolerate. In order to prove the advantage of our classification-based blockchain architecture, we compare with original blockchain and hypergraph-based blockchain [27] on the performance of total used memory capacity and running time of generating a certain amount of blocks, respectively. All the analysis is verified under the average results of multiple experiments, since the evaluation may have random factors.

5.1. Storage Used Analysis

Figure 5 shows the used memory comparison between three architectures in a real smart home scenario. As shown in Figure 5, we can easily find each node in an original blockchain architecture consumes more memory than that in the other two architectures. This is because every node stores a copy of all records (all transaction data), and the used memory capacity of the entire network is proportional to the number of categories of data in each node. In contrast, our architecture and the hypergraph-based blockchain architecture require much smaller storage consumption because both schemes use multiple blockchains to store data. On the other hand, our architecture has almost the same result as the hypergraph-based blockchain architecture in memory consumption but is a little better in some scenarios. Specifically, the number of CNs in each VS which maintains a sub-blockchain is limited in our architecture, thus the average storage of each node and the transaction data for synchronization are also limited to a certain range. In our experiments, it can save up to 90% of storage space when the network is large with many nodes/devices. Thus, our scheme needs less storage through experiments analysis while comparing with the same type of methods.

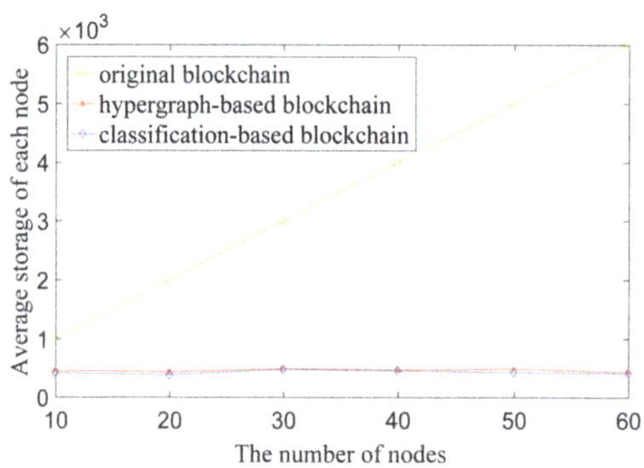

Figure 5. The used memory comparison among three architectures in real smart home scenario.

5.2. Latency and Security Evaluation

In this section, we evaluate the performance of the hierarchical PoW mechanism while comparing it with the traditional PoW. Generally, the running time of PoW is a linear positive correlation with the difficulty. Both the original and hypergraph-based blockchain architecture use traditional PoW so that they can only set one kind of difficulty for all data categories. In order to ensure safety, they have to set all categories of data to the highest difficulty. However, our architecture with hierarchical PoW mechanism can set the appropriate difficulty to each data category. As shown in Table 2, we compare the running time of generating a certain amount of blocks among three architectures. The results reflect the running time of ours is almost 50% less than other architectures, due to our proposed hierarchical PoW mechanism. That means our scheme has less latency than the others. Moreover, in our experimental test, the difficulty of each security grade is not high, and the average block time of all security grades is only about 3 s.

Table 2. Comparison of the running time of generating certain number of blocks among three architectures.

Number of Blocks	Running Time(s)		
	Original Blockchain	**Hypergraph-Based Blockchain**	**Classification-Based Blockchain**
1	5.7	5.1	2.8
2	10.8	10.4	5.6
3	16.9	16.2	7.9
4	21.5	21.2	10.6
5	27.5	27.1	14.1
6	32.9	32.5	17.4
7	37.2	36.8	19.8
8	44.3	43.9	22.7

To further evaluate our safety performance, we conducted several attacks on the system, tampering with data with malicious nodes to affect integrity. As shown in Figure 6, in our experiment, both the safety factor and average storage of each node are proportional to the $maxn$ of a VS (i.e., the maximum number of participated devices in a sub-network). Obviously, the security level is determined by the maximum size of the VS. The greater the $maxn$ of a VS is, the higher the security, and vice versa. In other words, the specific number of participating devices determines the safety factor of the system. Since smart homes usually contain dozens of devices, the systems have a high safety factor, and the cost of hacking is quite high. Consequently, the safety factor can be improved by increasing the number of participating devices depending on the specific scenarios. In summary, our scheme has a good integrity performance.

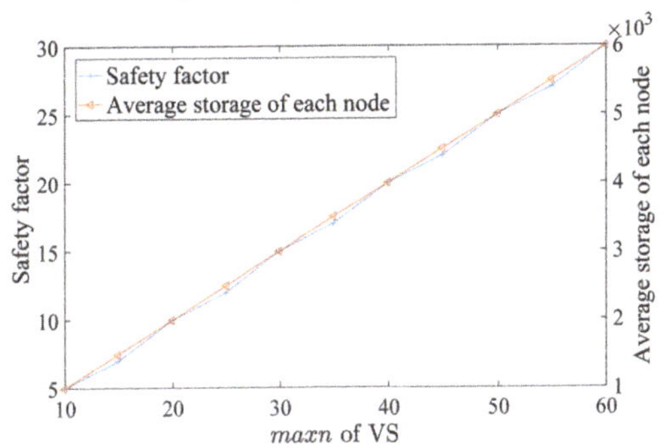

Figure 6. The relationship among the $maxn$ of VS, the average storage of each node, and the security.

6. Conclusions

In this paper, we propose a classification-based blockchain architecture with hierarchical PoW mechanism in the smart home to address security challenges for resource-constrained IoT. With the proposed scheme, the experimental results show that it decreases risks to a certain degree, and reduces storage by almost 90%. Meanwhile, our moderate-cost hierarchical PoW mechanism balances the security and performance to an acceptable level so that it can reduce the running time by almost 50%.

As we know, the PoW-based mechanism always needs to consume a lot of device resources for the blockchain calculation. Although we use a moderate-cost strategy to reduce the resource consumption in our proposed architecture, unfortunately, the efficiency of the system is still not enough. Consequently, our next work will focus on further improving the efficiency of the system. The possible research direction may use a more lightweight approach to replace the PoW-based scheme.

Author Contributions: Conceptualization, W.L., N.W., X.X. and Z.H.; methodology, N.W. and Z.H.; software, X.X.; validation, W.L. and X.X.; formal analysis, W.L., N.W. and X.X.; investigation, W.L. and N.W.; writing—original draft preparation, W.L., N.W. and X.X.; writing—review and editing, Z.H.; visualization, X.X.; funding acquisition, Z.H. All authors have read and agreed to the published version of the manuscript.

Funding: This research was funded by the National Natural Science Foundation of China under Grant No. 62072408, Zhejiang Provincial Natural Science Foundation of China under Grant No. LY20F020030, and New Century 151 Talent Project of Zhejiang Province.

Institutional Review Board Statement: Not applicable.

Informed Consent Statement: Not applicable.

Data Availability Statement: Not applicable.

Acknowledgments: We would like to thank all of the anonymous reviewers who spent their own time to review this article and provide suggestions.

Conflicts of Interest: The authors declare no conflict of interest.

References

1. Camero, A.; Alba, E. Smart city and information technology: A review. *Cities* **2019**, *93*, 84–94. [CrossRef]
2. Laufs, J.; Borrion, H.; Bradford, B. Security and the smart city: A systematic review. *Sustain. Cities Soc.* **2020**, *55*, 102023. [CrossRef]
3. Dattana, V.; Kumar, A.; Kush, A.; Kazmi, S.I.A. Manet for Stable Data flow in Smart home and Smart city. In Proceedings of the 2019 4th MEC International Conference on Big Data and Smart City (ICBDSC), Muscat, Oman, 15–16 January 2019; pp. 1–4.
4. Almusaylim, Z.A.; Zaman, N. A review on smart home present state and challenges: Linked to context-awareness internet of things (IoT). *Wirel. Netw.* **2019**, *25*, 3193–3204. [CrossRef]
5. Sovacool, B.K.; Del Rio, D.D.F. Smart home technologies in Europe: A critical review of concepts, benefits, risks and policies. *Renew. Sustain. Energy Rev.* **2020**, *120*, 109663. [CrossRef]
6. Scuotto, V.; Ferraris, A.; Bresciani, S. Internet of Things: Applications and challenges in smart cities: A case study of IBM smart city projects. *Bus. Process Manag. J.* **2016**, *22*, 357–367. [CrossRef]
7. Hoque, M.A.; Davidson, C. Design and Implementation of an IoT-Based Smart Home Security System. *Int. J. Netw. Distrib. Comput.* **2019**, *7*, 85–92. [CrossRef]
8. Touqeer, H.; Zaman, S.; Amin, R.; Hussain, M.; Al-Turjman, F.; Bilal, M. Smart home security: Challenges, issues and solutions at different IoT layers. *J. Supercomput.* **2021**, *77*, 14053–14089. [CrossRef]
9. Yu, R.; Zhang, X.; Zhang, M. Smart home security analysis system based on the internet of things. In Proceedings of the IEEE 2nd International Conference on Big Data, Artificial Intelligence and Internet of Things Engineering (ICBAIE), Nanchang, China, 26–28 March 2021; pp. 596–599.
10. Roman, R.; Zhou, J.; Lopez, J. On the features and challenges of security and privacy in distributed internet of things. *Comput. Netw.* **2013**, *57*, 2266–2279. [CrossRef]
11. Song, J.C.; Demir, M.A.; Prevost, J.J.; Rad, P. Blockchain Design for Trusted Decentralized IoT Networks. In Proceedings of the 2018 13th Annual Conference on System of Systems Engineering (SoSE), Paris, France, 19–22 June 2018; pp. 169–174.
12. Moniruzzaman, M.; Khezr, S.; Yassine, A.; Benlamri, R. Blockchain for smart homes: Review of current trends and research challenges. *Comput. Electr. Eng.* **2020**, *83*, 106585. [CrossRef]
13. Arif, S.; Khan, M.A.; Rehman, S.U.; Kabir, M.A.; Imran, M. Investigating smart home security: Is blockchain the answer? *IEEE Access* **2020**, *8*, 117802–117816. [CrossRef]
14. Khan, M.A.; Abbas, S.; Rehman, A.; Saeed, Y.; Zeb, A.; Uddin, M.I.; Ali, A. A machine learning approach for blockchain-based smart home networks security. *IEEE Netw.* **2020**, *35*, 223–229. [CrossRef]
15. Baucas, M.J.; Gadsden, S.A.; Spachos, P. IoT-based smart home device monitor using private blockchain technology and localization. *IEEE Netw. Lett.* **2021**, *3*, 52–55. [CrossRef]
16. Giannoutakis, K.M.; Spathoulas, G.; Filelis-Papadopoulos, C.K.; Collen, A.; Anagnostopoulos, M.; Votis, K.; Nijdam, N.A. A blockchain solution for enhancing cybersecurity defence of IoT. In Proceedings of the 2020 IEEE International Conference on Blockchain (Blockchain), Rhodes, Greece, 2–6 November 2020; pp. 490–495.
17. King, S. Primecoin: Cryptocurrency with Prime Number Proof-of-Work. 2013. Available online: http://primecoin.io/bin/primecoin-paper.png (accessed on 7 July 2013).
18. Khan, A.A.; Laghari, A.A.; Shaikh, A.A.; Bourouis, S.; Mamlouk, A.M.; Alshazly, H. Educational blockchain: A secure degree attestation and verification traceability architecture for higher education commission. *Appl. Sci.* **2021**, *11*, 10917. [CrossRef]
19. Khan, A.A.; Shaikh, Z.A.; Baitenova, L.; Mutaliyeva, L.; Moiseev, N.; Mikhaylov, A.; Laghari, A.A.; Idris, S.A.; Alshazly, H. QoS-ledger: Smart contracts and metaheuristic for secure quality-of-service and cost-efficient scheduling of medical-data processing. *Electronics* **2021**, *10*, 3083. [CrossRef]

20. Suchaad, S.A.L.; Mashiko, K.; Ismail, N.B.; Abidin, M.H.Z. Blockchain use in home automation for children incentives in parental control. In Proceedings of the 2018 International Conference on Machine Learning and Machine Intelligence, Hanoi, Vietnam, 28–30 September 2018; pp. 50–53.
21. Tantidham, T.; Aung, Y.N. Emergency service for smart home system using ethereum blockchain: System and architecture. In Proceedings of the 2019 IEEE international conference on pervasive computing and communications workshops (PerCom Workshops), Kyoto, Japan, 11–15 March 2019; pp. 888–893.
22. Saxena, U.; Sodhi, J.S.; Tanwar, R. Augmenting smart home network security using blockchain technology. *Int. J. Electron. Secur. Digit. Forensics* **2020**, *12*, 99–117. [CrossRef]
23. Qashlan, A.; Nanda, P.; He, X. Security and privacy implementation in smart home: Attributes based access control and smart contracts. 2020 IEEE 19th International Conference on Trust, Security and Privacy in Computing and Communications (TrustCom), Guangzhou, China, 29 December–1 January 2021; pp. 951–958.
24. Dorri, A.; Kanhere, S.S.; Jurdak, R. Blockchain in internet of things: Challenges and Solutions. *arXiv* **2016**, arXiv:1608.05187.
25. Dorri, A.; Kanhere, S.S.; Jurdak, R. Towards an Optimized BlockChain for IoT. In Proceedings of the 2017 IEEE/ACM Second International Conference on Internet-of-Things Design and Implementation (IoTDI), Pittsburgh, PA, USA, 18–21 April 2017; pp. 173–178.
26. Yazdinejad, A.; Parizi, R.M.; Dehghantanha, A.; Zhang, Q.; Choo, K.K.R. An energy-efficient SDN controller architecture for IoT networks with blockchain-based security. *IEEE Trans. Serv. Comput.* **2020**, *13*, 625–638. [CrossRef]
27. Qu, C.; Tao, M.; Yuan, R. A Hypergraph-Based Blockchain Model and Application in Internet of Things-Enabled Smart Homes. *Sensors* **2018**, *18*, 2784. [CrossRef] [PubMed]
28. Mohanty, S.N.; Ramya, K.C.; Rani, S.S.; Gupta, D.; Shankar, K.; Lakshmanaprabu, S.K.; Khanna, A. An efficient Lightweight integrated blockchain (ELIB) model for IoT security and privacy. *Future Gener. Comput. Syst.* **2020**, *102*, 1027–1037. [CrossRef]
29. Yazdinejad, A.; Srivastava, G.; Parizi, R.M.; Dehghantanha, A.; Karimipour, H.; Karizno, S.R. SLPoW: Secure and low latency proof of work protocol for blockchain in green IoT networks. In Proceedings of the 2020 IEEE 91st Vehicular Technology Conference (VTC2020-Spring), Antwerp, Belgium, 25–28 May 2020; pp. 1–5.
30. Yu, H.; Gibbons, P.B.; Kaminsky, M.; Xiao, F. SybilLimit: A Near-Optimal Social Network Defense against Sybil Attacks. In Proceedings of the 2008 IEEE Symposium on Security and Privacy (S&P 2008), Oakland, CA, USA, 18–22 May 2008; pp. 3–17.

buildings

MDPI

Article

Decarbonization of the Colombian Building Sector: Social Network Analysis of Enabling Stakeholders

John Salazar [1,*], Jose Guevara [1], Monica Espinosa [2], Felipe Rivera [2] and Juan F. Franco [2]

[1] Department of Civil and Environmental Engineering, Universidad de los Andes, Bogota 111711, Colombia
[2] Hill Consulting, Bogota 111711, Colombia
* Correspondence: js.salazarf@uniandes.edu.co

Abstract: Reducing greenhouse gas (GHG) emissions is one of the main challenges to stopping climate change; in particular, the building sector acts as one of the main emitters. In response, governments have been developing nationally determined contributions (NDCs) and roadmaps to establish measures to achieve net-zero emissions. One of the main barriers to implementing these measures, particularly in the building sector, underlays in stakeholder integration. Through social network analysis (SNA) concepts, this research explores the roles of the actors whose participation is required in decarbonizing the Colombian building sector. These stakeholders engage in enabling categories (e.g., policy, finance, technology, and capacity development) required to achieve net-zero emissions, according to the goals proposed by the Colombian Green Building Council (CGBC). For the network analysis, we employ the results of semi-structured interviews led by the CGBC within the framework of the Zero Carbon Building Accelerator (ZCBA) project. Findings show highly interconnected networks characterized by redundant connections among actors. Three types of actors are identified within each enabler network: prominent actors with high centrality values, in charge of coordinating most of the actions required to achieve net-zero emissions; second-level actors limited to specific roles in policy-making processes; and perimeter actors focused on a few particular actions.

Keywords: climate change; GHG mitigation; public policy; enabler networks; net-zero roadmap; developing countries; social network analysis

Citation: Salazar, J.; Guevara, J.; Espinosa, M.; Rivera, F.; Franco, J.F. Decarbonization of the Colombian Building Sector: Social Network Analysis of Enabling Stakeholders. *Buildings* **2022**, *12*, 1531. https://doi.org/10.3390/buildings12101531

Academic Editor: Francesco Asdrubali

Received: 28 August 2022
Accepted: 14 September 2022
Published: 26 September 2022

1. Introduction

According to the Intergovernmental Panel on Climate Change (IPCC), in 2019, the building sector emitted 19% of global greenhouse gases (GHGs) and 31% of carbon dioxide (CO_2) emissions [1]. Under the current policy scenario, GHGs associated with the construction sector will increase by 2.2% yearly [2]. Developing countries are one of the main drivers of global emissions because these economies are growing in population and economy, with increasing floor areas per capita, while employing non-efficient construction methods as a standard practice [1,3]. Building-related emissions, particularly CO_2, are closely linked to energy production and use. Energy is responsible for 67% of the emissions from buildings [4,5]. Future energy–building consumption growth is a major concern because emerging economies hold a large portion of the world's housing demand potential [6], and more than 80% of the nations with the highest projected population growth through 2030 lack any kind of obligatory energy code [5].

Although carbon emissions per capita in high- and upper-middle-income countries are more elevated than those in low- and lower-middle-income countries, most industrialized economies have implemented programs to reduce energy consumption and mitigate GHG emissions [7], in particular, in the building sector [5]. In contrast, many developing nations have chosen to expand their investment in fossil fuel energy and keep their tendencies in the construction and operation of buildings instead of migrating to cleaner options [8,9]. The development of programs to reduce energy consumption and mitigate GHG emissions remains one of the main challenges for all sectors and regions, including the building sector in developing countries.

Within the Paris Agreement, 196 participants presented their updated nationally determined contributions (NDCs) in COP26 in 2020 to reiterate their commitment to reducing GHG emissions [10]. The two most common GHG mitigation measures in international pledges are to increase renewable energy use and enhance building energy efficiency [5]. However, many nations have struggled to address GHG mitigation in the life cycle of buildings and continue to use inefficient construction and building operation methods [5,11]. Scholars, industry practitioners, and government officials have proposed ambitious measures to reduce buildings' energy consumption and GHG emissions in buildings throughout their life cycle. There are different alternatives to reduce emissions at the product stage, construction phase, usage stage, and end-of-life stage [12]. Among others, the options include changes in the steel [13] and cement production [14] processes; optimization of building designs and alternative construction systems in the construction stage [15]; passive design and service systems in the operational stage [16]; and circularity of materials at the end of life stage [17].

Despite extensive research on GHG emission reduction strategies for the building industry, these strategies are only just beginning to be implemented globally [5]. A lack of integration among stakeholders is one of the key obstacles to GHG emissions mitigation actions in the building sector [18]. The reasons for this are multiple. First, the plurality of participants throughout all life cycle phases creates complicated relationships in the building sector [19]. There are different actors intervening in building design, construction, financing, operation, and maintenance processes [20]. Second, actors have different interests, affecting decision-making procedures [20–22]. Third, different players are impacted in very diverse ways by the adoption of GHG mitigation strategies. Some actors win, and some actors lose, depending on the type of interventions used to minimize GHG emissions [23]. These factors generate differences and conflicts between actors. One of the main goals established during COP26 to develop mitigation actions to face climate change is mutual work among all stakeholders [24]. This includes governments, businesses, academia, and civil society. In order to understand the role and importance of different stakeholders inside specific contexts, social network analysis (SNA) has been widely applied [25,26]. In the building sector, SNA has been used to understand the relationships between stakeholders of the biomass industry [25], comprehend the influence of the actors impacting building energy efficiency [27], and understand stakeholders' influence on green retrofit projects' success [28], among other analyzes.

Therefore, even though SNA has been applied in the building field, and the absence of integration among stakeholders has been recognized as one of the main barriers to achieving GHG emissions mitigation, most studies have focused on specific problems rather than the overall characterization of the sector [29]. In particular, building sector stakeholders' characterization via SNA strives to improve engagement and knowledge transfer [30], align internal collaboration [29], and identify potential problems [31]. Thus, due to the necessity of lining up stakeholders toward common goals to achieve GHG emissions mitigation, this study analyzes the network of key actors and stakeholders involved in the design and implementation of the Colombian Net-Zero Carbon Buildings Roadmap.

This study aimed to identify the key players within the major enablers of the roadmap (policy, technology, finance, and capacity development) and to identify the critical links and relationships among stakeholders. The results of this analysis are useful for the implementation phase of the Colombian Net-Zero Carbon Buildings Roadmap. Policymakers can take advantage of the findings in multiple ways. First, they can identify fundamental actors per category and their tasks. Second, they also can recognize potential challenges, such as the lack of integration among crucial stakeholders in certain links within the networks. Third, SNA helps identify potential opportunities for collaboration. Due to the complexity of relations among actors in the different enablers to achieving GHG emissions mitigation, SNA is a suitable tool for supporting the subsequent phases of the roadmap.

2. Background

2.1. Zero Carbon Building Accelerator Project in Colombia

There are different international initiatives to support compliance with the long-term mitigation goals established in the Paris Agreement. An example of these initiatives is the Zero Carbon Building Accelerator (ZCBA) project carried out by the World Resources Institute (WRI) with the support of global partners such as the Global Environment Facility (GEF), the United Nations Environment Program (UNEP), and the World Green Building Council (WGBC) [32]. In the first stage, the program supports Colombia in mitigating buildings' GHG emissions. The project led by the CGBC consisted in designing the Colombian Net-Zero Carbon Buildings Roadmap. Between 2021 and 2022, different stakeholders from the national government, local governments, building industry, and academia participated in formulating the roadmap. The CGBC performed nine workshops between May 2021 and February 2022. Each month, nine groups of experts met to elaborate and define the roadmap by discussing multiple points of view. The CBGC employed a snowball technique [33,34] to gather as many experts as possible during the workshops [35]. This technique involved beginning the initial workshops with a group of experts and gradually approaching new experts through the initial group. In total, 357 actors participated in the workshops, representing universities, private companies, construction guilds, the Colombian government, NGOs, and international organizations, among others [35]. Information about the participants is shown in Table 1.

Table 1. Workshop participants.

Organization Role	Number of Participants	Roles of Participants
Universities	35	Professors, graduate students, legal representatives, and program directors.
Construction guilds	33	Technical experts, consultants, technical directors, project directors, and coordinators.
Private companies	191	Analysts, architects, CEOs, consultants, coordinators, directors, technical experts, engineers, researchers, builders, and contractors.
Colombian government	79	Advisors, contractors, coordinators, directors, and technical specialists.
Non-governmental organizations	11	Managers, consultants, coordinators, directors, and technical experts.
International organizations	8	Consultants, directors, and CEOs.

In the process conducted by the CGBC, an exhaustive literature review to define the transformative actions required to achieve net-zero emissions in the Colombian building industry [35] was developed. These actions were established in concordance with the national policy of sustainable buildings [36] and classified according to their strategic importance in first-, second-, and third-level action categories. Additionally, actions were examined through the lens of four enablers (i.e., policy, technology, finance, and capacity development) (Table 2), as defined by the Global ABC Roadmap for Latin America [37]. Transformative first-level measures were defined (i.e., life cycle assessment, energy efficiency, green labeling, promotion of sustainable materials and systems, decarbonization of energy sources, sustainability standards, sustainability practices in the industry sector, information management, integrated urban planning, resilience, ecosystemic services, construction processes, and cross-cutting actions). Based on that, second-level actions were established for every first-level category within each enabler (i.e., 54 for policy, 43 for technology, 15 for capacity development, and 50 for finance). Subsequently, every second-level action was associated with a set of third-level action categories (or subgroups). Table 3 displays a graphical representation of a typical enabler associated with first level-measures, second-level actions, and third-level action categories.

Table 2. Definition of enablers in the Colombian Net-Zero Carbon Buildings Roadmap.

Enabler	Definition
Policy	Includes processes to be developed through regulation and other public policy instruments.
Technology	Includes processes of technological improvement.
Capacity development	Includes processes to improve the capabilities of the actors in the supply chain of the building sector.
Finance	Includes processes to create financial mechanisms to make possible the actions required.

Table 3. Example of a typical enabler.

First-Level Measures	Second-Level Actions	Action Categories or Subgroups						
		Group 1	Group 2	Group 3	Group 4	Group 5	Group 6	Group 7
	1.1		x	x	x			
	1.2				x			
1	1.3		x				x	
	...				...			
	1.n	x				x		
...	...				...			
	12.1	x			x		x	x
	12.2		x		x		x	
12	12.3		x	x		x		
	12.4		x					x
	...				...			
	12.m	x		x			x	

The working groups, one per action category, responded to a questionnaire (Appendix A) [35] to evaluate second-level actions within the enabling groups. The results of this process were the base for the network analysis presented in this manuscript.

2.2. SNA in Construction and Sustainability

SNA has been implemented in a great variety of research fields for more than 80 years [34,38]. Grounded on graph theory, SNA takes advantage of its notation to represent sets of actors (nodes) and their relationships (links or edges) [39]. Therefore, it is frequently considered a relational model focused mainly on the stakeholders' connections instead of their individual attributes [40]. Accordingly, SNA grants information about social structures, recognizing that each stakeholder is embedded in multiple systems defined by its connections [34]. To grasp information and construct SNA models, researchers usually rely on qualitative (e.g., semi-structured interviews) and quantitative (e.g., SNA metrics) methods [41].

Those qualitative and quantitative methods have been widely applied in the construction and sustainability fields. Schröpfer et al. (2017) evaluated, via questionnaires, the flow of knowledge of sustainable construction project teams in the UK and Germany [42]. Alexandrescu et al. (2016) studied the social network of brownfield regeneration actors through semi-structured interviews, evaluating their embeddedness across regeneration goals [43]. Xu et al. (2021) investigated the stakeholders' power in cutting emissions and energy savings in building energy performance; this was achieved through literature review and semi-structured interviews [27]. More recently, Jin et al. (2021) proposed qualitative and quantitative methods to create an SNA model to evaluate construction industrialization in the Hong Kong building sector, focusing on industrial performance and sustainability [44]. These studies collected qualitative information through surveys, which subsequently were processed to build social networks and compute network- and actor-based metrics to understand underlying information about network structures and stakeholders [21,45,46].

Furthermore, similar studies within specific contexts have found network structures for green building projects prone to be dominated by consultant enterprises rather than universities [1], highlighting the importance of studying network structures rather than assuming main actors. Moreover, SNA studies focused on timber structure building observed that a lack of collaboration and understanding of network structures could jeopardize a project's quality [4]. Indeed, researchers have identified major project concerns to achieve common goals through the position of stakeholders in networks, prioritizing the main concerns according to the actor's centrality indexes [2]. In line with this, this study strived to identify the potential network structures of the four major action categories (policy, technology, finance, and capacity development) of the Colombian net-zero roadmap for the building sector, finding the prominent actors and underlying network structures of each category.

3. Methodology

This study sought to analyze the network of key actors and stakeholders involved in the design and implementation of the Colombian Net-Zero Carbon Buildings Roadmap. We conducted an SNA to characterize and examine prominent actors and critical relationships associated with achieving a net-zero carbon transition in the Colombian building sector. We followed a three-step methodological approach, as shown in Figure 1. Stage 1 involved collecting data from the results of the questionnaires conducted by the CGBC. The data referred to information that regarded stakeholders that had to participate in the main goals established to achieve net-zero emissions. These data were represented initially within reference matrices. In the matrix, if actor *i* participated in the second-level action j, the value of this cell was 1. With the expert answers, we filled out one reference matrix per each enabler, following the rule: a cell filled with the number "one" represented the situation when, according to the experts' answers, there was a common ground of the necessity of an actor to participate in an SLA (Figure 2). In the second stage, we processed the collected data and developed four two-mode networks following the methodology proposed in previous studies [21,34]. For each enabler, we built a two-mode network. In step three, the two-mode networks were transformed into one-mode networks by multiplying each enabler matrix by their transpose matrix. We developed four actor networks per enabler and finally computed the SNA metrics. These networks were drawn and computed with UCINET 6 [47].

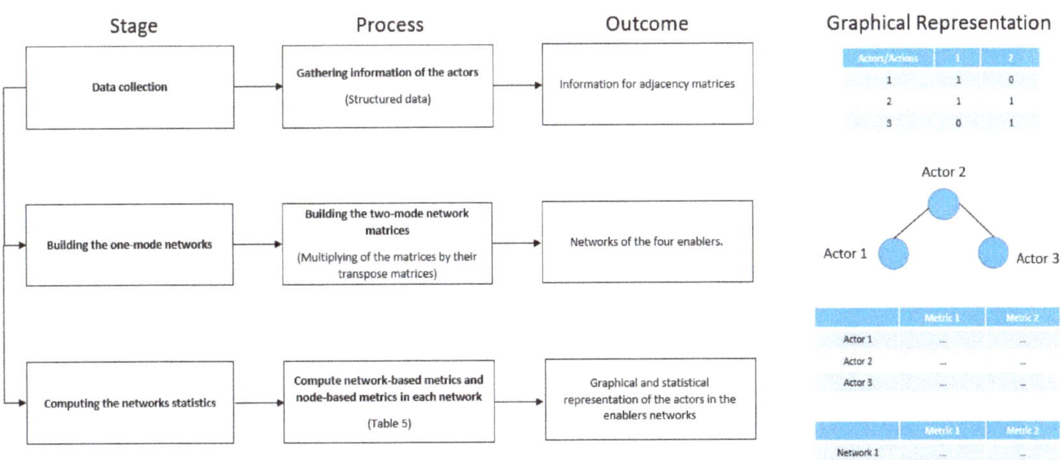

Figure 1. Methodology.

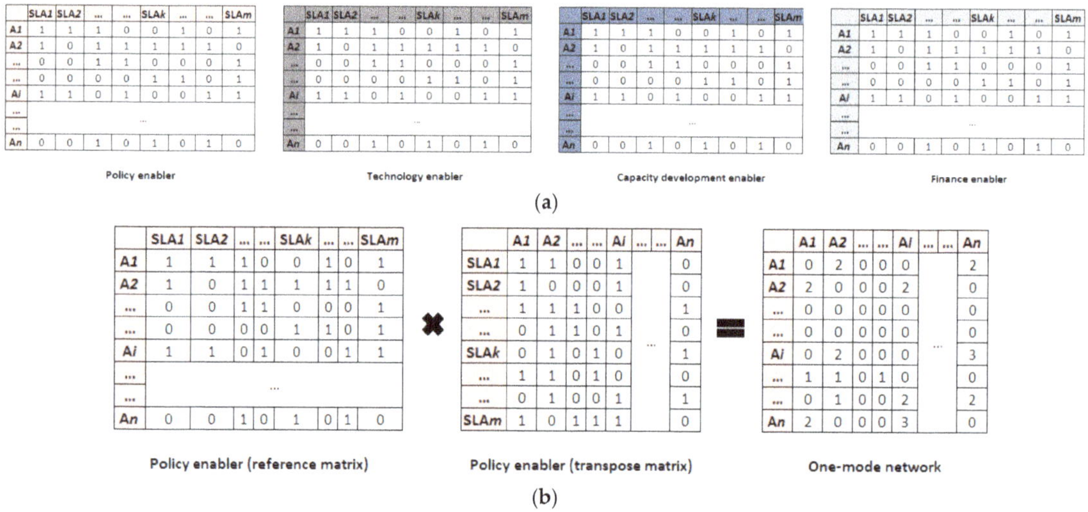

Figure 2. Reference matrices (**a**). Multiplication of the reference matrix by its transpose matrix (**b**).

3.1. Stage 1: Data Collection

We employed the information collected by the CGBC, supplementary information (https://www.cccs.org.co/wp/download/reporte-de-recomendaciones-proyecto-acelerador-de-edificaciones-neto-cero-carbono/, accessed on 28 August 2022), across the workshops (Appendix A) and analyzed the responses to the questionnaires to develop network diagrams and indicators. We identified participants and actor categories within the Colombian building sector (see Table 4) and their corresponding links with second-level actions (SLAs) in each one of the four enablers (e.g., policy, technology, finance, and capacity development actions). We considered actors' and SLAs' complexity, nature, and specific properties.

Table 4. Actor categories identified by the workshop participants.

Actors	Role
National government	Official entities with jurisdiction at the national level.
Local governments	Official entities with jurisdiction at the local level.
Guilds and professional associations	Different groups of affiliated companies participating in the operation, construction, and maintenance of buildings.
Public utility companies	Entities in charge of providing public services across Colombia.
Standards organizations	Technical standardization entities.
Private sector	Private companies participating in the life cycle of buildings.
Financial institutions	Banks, pension funds, insurance companies, and brokerage commission companies related to the building sector.
Academia	Universities and research entities working in Colombia in related areas to buildings, sustainability, and carbon markets.
Civil society	Different groups representing civil society working in Colombia in related areas to buildings, sustainability, and low-carbon projects.

Relationships between actors and SLAs were organized into four reference matrices (one per enabler) (Figure 2a). We followed the methodology proposed in similar analyzes [21]. For each enabler, the rows corresponded to actors, and the columns represented the second-level actions. In each cell in this matrix, A_{ik} was assigned a value of 1 if actor i participated in the SLA k; or 0 otherwise.

3.2. *Stage 2: One-Mode Networks*

Once the reference matrices (two-mode arrays) were developed, we calculated the adjacency matrix (one-mode array) associated with each enabler. To obtain the one-mode network adjacency matrix per enabler, it was required to multiply the reference matrices obtained in Figure 2a by each one of their transpose matrices. This step followed the projection method for transforming two-mode networks to one-mode networks presented in previous studies [48]. Figure 2b represents this process for the policy enabler network. This process allowed for obtaining the arrangements representing one-mode networks, which related to all the participants in any given enabler [21]. The cells A_{ik} and A_{ki} in Figure 2b represented the number of SLAs in which actor *i* (A*i*) needed to participate with actor j to develop the established actions per enabler.

3.3. *Stage 3: Computing Network Statistics*

After developing the four one-mode matrices, the authors input them into UCINET 6 in order to produce network metrics and diagrams. Table 5 describes the two types of network metrics employed in this study. Network-based metrics helped to understand each network globally [21]. Actor-based metrics provided information on the role of each individual stakeholder within their specific network. The selection of these metrics was consistent with previous studies in the fields of construction and sustainability [21,34,41–45,49], which have proven to provide valuable information about network configuration [21,50]. For each one of the four enablers (e.g., policy, technology, finance, and capacity development), using the matrices obtained in stage 2, this last stage consisted of drawing one-mode networks with UCINET 6 [47] and computing network statistics according to the metrics presented in Table 5.

Table 5. Network-based metrics and Actor-based metrics.

(a)		
	SNA Metric	**Definition in Construction and Sustainability**
Network-based metrics	Network size	The number of stakeholders in each category of enablers [21,50–52].
	Short average path length	The average minimum number of links separating two actors [45,53].
	Density	The ratio between the total number of links and the theoretical maximum number of relationships [21,41,54].
	Average weighted degree	The mean number of relationships of an actor in a network [21,45].
	Degree centralization	The measure of the concentration of the degree of centrality in a few actors [45,55].
	Average stakeholders	The average number of stakeholders participating per second-level action in each enabler.
Actor-based metrics	Degree centrality (D)	The number of links of each stakeholder within each enabler network [21,53,56].
	Betweenness centrality (B)	The propensity of each stakeholder to be a bridge that communicates multiple actors [21,49,50].
	Closeness centrality (C)	The propensity of each stakeholder to be close to all the other actors in a given network [21,49,50].
	Eigenvector centrality (E)	The propensity of each stakeholder to communicate with the most important actors in each network [21,49,50].

4. Results

The networks developed for each enabler are shown in Figure 3. These networks showed the ties established between actors and the way each actor was integrated into the set of SLAs per enabler. This reflected the way the roadmap of the Colombian Net-Zero Carbon Building Roadmap was intended to be implemented. In each network, the size of the node representing each of the actors was proportional to the number of relationships of each stakeholder.

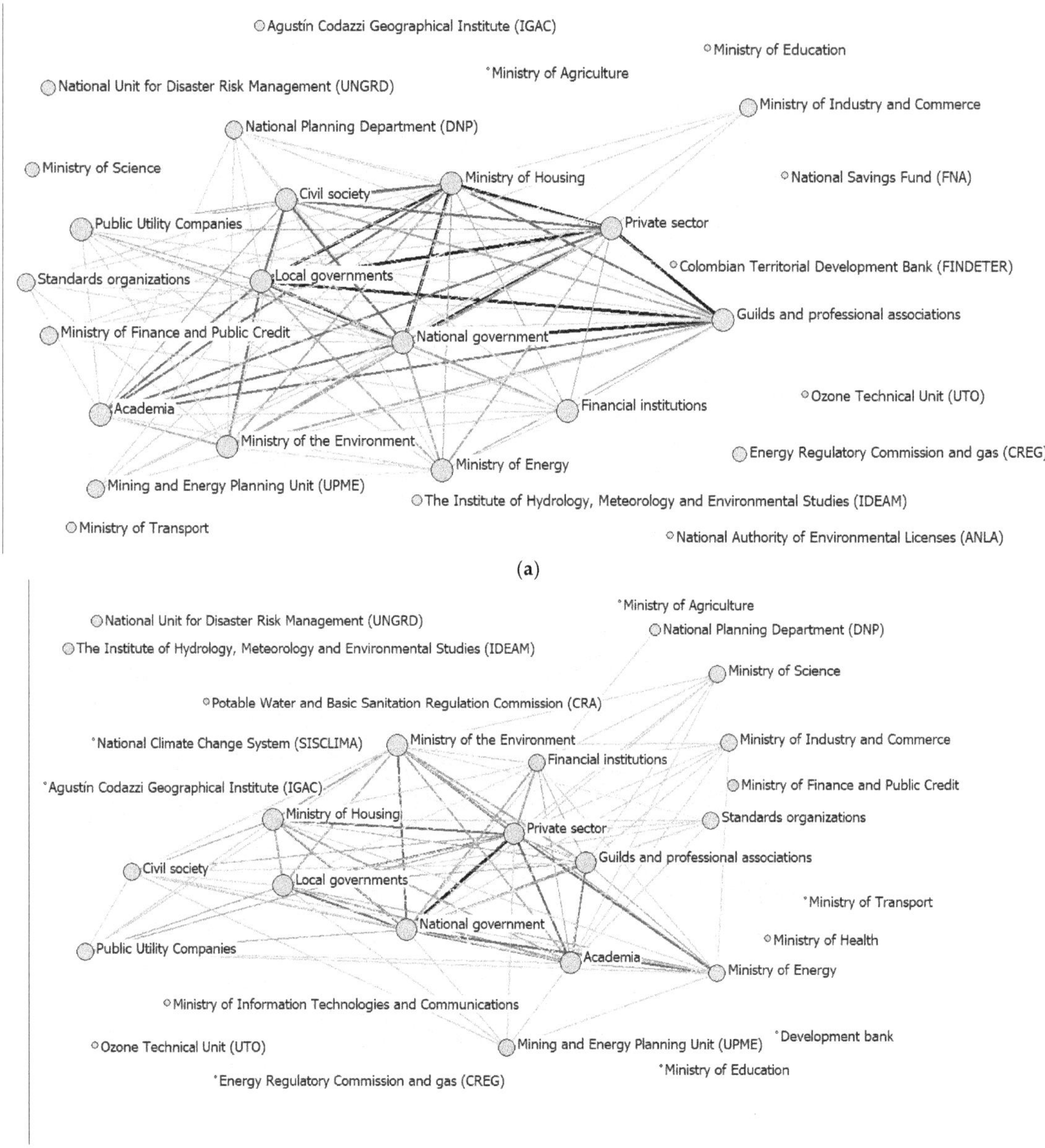

Figure 3. *Cont.*

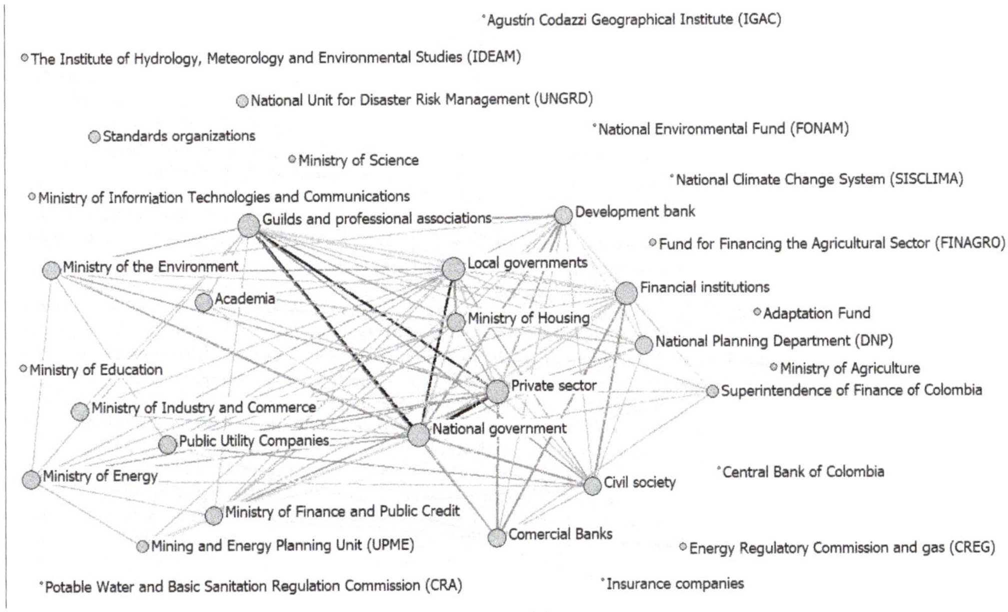

(c)

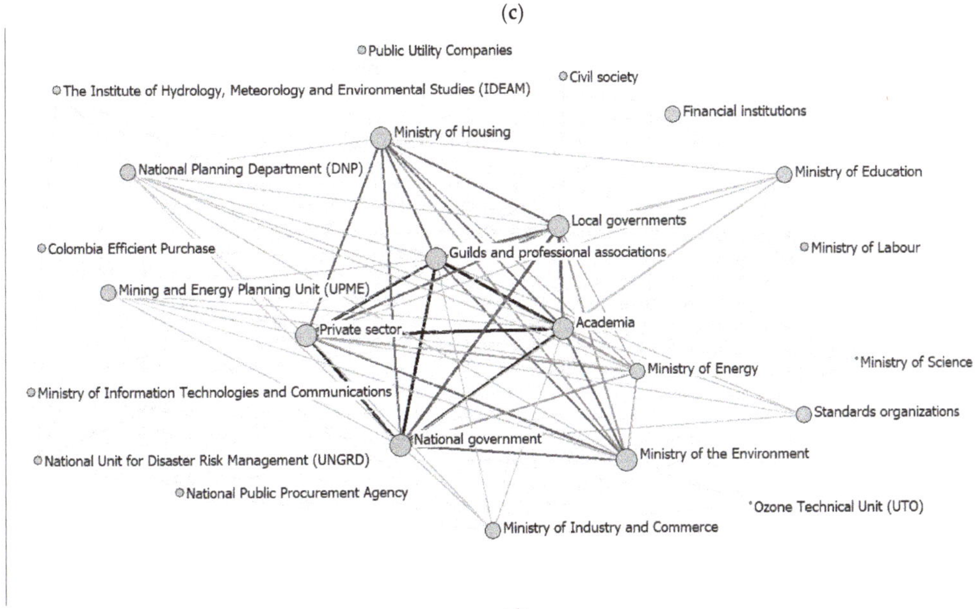

(d)

Figure 3. (**a**) Public policy network; (**b**) technology network; (**c**) finance network; and (**d**) capacity development network.

For each link in any network, the thickness and darkness of color were proportional to the number of times the pair of actors needed to participate together per enabler. The darker and thicker the link, the stronger the relationship between stakeholders because they had to participate more times together in second-level actions per enabler. To provide a quantitative interpretation of Figure 3, Tables 6 and 7 show the results of the network-based metrics and actor-based metrics per network, respectively. These results allowed comparing the networks and actors participating in each enabler.

Table 6. Network-based metrics per enabler.

Network of Enablers	Network Size	Short Average Path Length	Density	Average Weighted Degree	Degree Centralization	Average Stakeholders
Policy	28	1.36	0.64	17.36	0.37	10.40
Technology	30	1.39	0.61	17.73	0.42	9.56
Finance	35	1.43	0.57	18.94	0.45	8.82
Capacity development	23	1.23	0.77	17.04	0.25	9.23

Table 7. Network-based metrics per actor.

Policy	D	C	E	B	Technology	D	C	E	B
National government	18.15	1.00	0.51	0.07	National government	12.79	1.00	0.54	0.06
Local governments	18.07	0.90	0.51	0.02	Private sector	12.41	1.00	0.53	0.06
Private sector	17.44	0.96	0.50	0.04	Ministry of the Environment	10.24	0.94	0.44	0.04
Ministry of Housing	16.48	0.96	0.47	0.06	Academia	10.03	0.91	0.44	0.04
Guilds and professional associations	16.26	0.93	0.47	0.04	Local governments	9.86	0.97	0.43	0.05
Academia	13.33	0.87	0.39	0.02	Guilds and professional associations	9.07	0.85	0.41	0.03
Civil society	12.44	0.90	0.37	0.03	Ministry of Housing	8.83	0.91	0.39	0.04
Ministry of the Environment	11.07	0.87	0.33	0.02	Ministry of Energy	7.90	0.81	0.36	0.02
Ministry of Energy	10.70	0.84	0.31	0.01	Financial institutions	7.00	0.88	0.32	0.03
Financial institutions	9.33	0.90	0.27	0.03	Civil society	6.52	0.85	0.29	0.02
Public utility companies	9.30	0.87	0.28	0.02	Public utility companies	5.52	0.81	0.25	0.02
Standards organizations	6.59	0.75	0.21	0.00	Ministry of Industry and Commerce	4.72	0.69	0.22	0.00
National Planning Department (DNP)	5.44	0.79	0.17	0.02	Standards organizations	4.21	0.78	0.19	0.01
Ministry of Finance and Public Credit	5.44	0.75	0.17	0.00	Mining and Energy Planning Unit (UPME)	3.79	0.73	0.18	0.01
Mining and Energy Planning Unit (UPME)	5.04	0.77	0.15	0.00	Ministry of Science	3.48	0.67	0.16	0.00
Finance	**D**	**C**	**E**	**B**	**Capacity Development**	**D**	**C**	**E**	**B**
National government	10.82	1.00	0.54	0.07	Guilds and professional associations	5.55	1.00	0.52	0.03
Private sector	10.30	0.94	0.52	0.05	National government	5.46	1.00	0.51	0.03
Guilds and professional associations	8.70	0.87	0.45	0.03	Academia	5.46	1.00	0.51	0.03
Local governments	8.24	0.94	0.42	0.05	Private sector	5.27	1.00	0.50	0.03
Financial institutions	7.94	0.89	0.42	0.04	Local governments	4.82	0.98	0.46	0.02
Development Bank	6.58	0.87	0.35	0.03	Ministry of Housing	4.59	0.98	0.44	0.02
Civil society	6.42	0.77	0.35	0.02	Ministry of the Environment	4.41	1.00	0.41	0.03
Ministry of Housing	6.09	0.92	0.33	0.04	Ministry of Energy	3.86	1.00	0.35	0.03
Ministry of the Environment	5.27	0.83	0.28	0.02	National Planning Department (DNP)	2.50	0.93	0.23	0.01
National Planning Department (DNP)	4.94	0.85	0.27	0.03	Mining and Energy Planning Unit (UPME)	2.09	0.93	0.19	0.02
Commercial bank	4.85	0.73	0.28	0.01	Standards organizations	1.86	0.84	0.19	0.01
Ministry of Energy	4.82	0.77	0.26	0.01	Ministry of Industry and Commerce	1.82	0.88	0.16	0.02
Ministry of Finance and Public Credit	4.64	0.81	0.25	0.02	Ministry of Education	1.82	0.88	0.20	0.00
Public utility companies	4.58	0.81	0.25	0.02	Financial institutions	1.59	0.78	0.15	0.00
Ministry of Industry and Commerce	3.33	0.73	0.18	0.00	Ministry of Labour	1.05	0.76	0.10	0.00

Degree centrality (D), betweenness centrality (B), closeness centrality (C), and eigenvector centrality (E).

According to the network-based metrics (Table 6), all networks showed at least 23 stakeholders and exhibited density values higher than 0.5. The density values obtained meant that more than 50% of the possible relationships between actors took place within the proposed structures. Such density values also indicated that the actors participating in achieving net-zero emissions in the Colombian building sector needed to keep redundant relationships among them. The density values obtained showed a difference from previous studies, in which similar networks exhibited density values lower than 0.5 [21,41,45]. The redundancy in network relationships could also be examined by exploring indicators such as average distance and degree. While many studies in the extant literature exhibited short average path lengths higher than 1.5 [45,50], the four structures presented in this study exhibited values lower than those. This denoted that Colombian stakeholders required fewer links to communicate with each other, suggesting that all actors in the enabling networks remained highly interconnected. Furthermore, regarding the average degree, most stakeholders revealed multiple relationships, supporting the idea of a vastly interconnected network.

Even though the above-mentioned network-based metrics (e.g., density and short average path length) suggested the idea of highly interrelated networks with well-connected actors in each enabler, the degree of centralization indicated that the studied networks seemed to be dominated by central actors. In particular, the degree centralization exhibited its highest value in the finance network, in which the degree centralization for the national government showed a value of 0.45 (see Table 7). Overall, degree centralization values were higher than 0.25 in all networks, indicating the dominance of well-connected players across all arrangements.

Table 7 identifies the main actors whose efforts are necessary to achieve net-zero emissions in the Colombian building sector. This table shows the 15 most prominent actors in each network by considering multiple actor-based metrics (i.e., D—degree centrality, C—closeness centrality, B—betweenness centrality, and E—eigenvector centrality). It is important to highlight that the national government, local governments, guilds and professional associations, financial institutions, the Ministry of Environment, the Ministry of Housing, and the private sector were cross-sectional participants in all enabling networks within the building sector. This means that they all should participate as leading actors in supporting the proposed SLAs.

4.1. *Characterization of Enabling Networks: Similarities and Differences*

All the enabling networks shared some common structures. Figure 3 and Table 6 show that the short average path length in all networks exhibited low values, varying between 1.23 and 1.36, thus, indicating efficiency and few intermediaries in the communication among stakeholders [50,53]. In respect of the average stakeholders per network, it is worth appreciating that the average number of actors in charge of each second-level action varied between 8.82 and 10.4, exhibiting high levels of participation per SLA in each enabler. In this sense, the density values varied between 0.57 and 0.77, and the average weighted degree indicated very interrelated networks, strengthening the idea of highly cohesive networks with redundant components and connectivity [41,50,57]. Even though there were common attributes across the enabling networks and relative homogeneity in their network-based metrics, there were also some singular attributes. Specifically, in terms of network sizes, it is important to highlight that despite differences in the number of SLAs assigned to each network, the number of participants in every structure remained very similar across the four studied structures. For instance, while the capacity development network incorporated three times fewer SLAs than the policy network (i.e., 15 vs. 54 SLAs), the number of actors in each one was 23 and 28, respectively. Similarly, the technology and finance networks had associated 43 and 50 SLAs and 30 and 35 participants, respectively. This indicated that the number of actors was not related to the number of second-level actions but to the complexity and synergies of each specific enabling network. Consequently, the set of actors in charge of developing the proposed enablers varied according to the priorities, value chains, and skillsets [58].

On the other hand, the degree centralization metric displayed in Table 6 highlighted differences among enablers. Even though all the degree centralization values were low (less than 0.5) compared to some values found in the literature [59,60], the enabling networks denoted important variations in this metric. In particular, the values of the finance (0.45) and technology (0.42) networks were close to 0.5, indicating the presence of intertwined structures prone to be controlled by a few main actors (i.e., the national government). This tendency was smaller in the policy and capacity development networks due to these exhibiting less centralized structures. In general, while high centralization values were associated with the degree of power of an actor in the decision-making process, low centralization figures indicated plurality in such a process [61,62]. Thus, and according to Tables 6 and 7, the national government seemed to act to coordinate and avoid conflicts among actors, mainly in the policy, technology, and finance enabling networks, as it was the most dominant player in these structures. In contrast, in the capacity development network, in which there was not a clear, prominent player, the guilds and professional associations, national government, and academia seemed to be responsible for playing a crucial function in coordinating their roles to develop innovation [61].

This proposed set of network-based metrics allowed for understanding the overall structure of the networks' actors in charge of decarbonizing the Colombian building sector. This analysis exhibited the strengths and weaknesses of each enabler network in terms of connectivity, participation, and centralization by finding similarities and distinctions between the networks of stakeholders. A deeper analysis of the main actors participating in each of the four enabling networks is presented below.

4.2. *Characterization of ZCBA Actors across the Enabling Networks*

Table 7 displays the 15 most important stakeholders in each enabling network according to their degree centrality (D), closeness centrality (C), betweenness centrality (B), and eigenvector centrality (E). Most of these actors were public entities (Colombian ministries, national government, and local governments). Still, many actors belonged to non-public sectors (private companies, guilds, standards organizations, and civil society), showing the need for joint work and coordination among different actors in achieving net-zero emissions goals in the Colombian building sector.

4.2.1. Public Policy Enabling Network

According to Figure 3a and Table 6, the public policy enabling network allowed for visualizing a highly interconnected structure within one single cluster. In this network, the five most prominent actors were the national government, local governments, the private sector, the Ministry of Housing, and guilds and professional associations. These players participated in at least 47 (87%) of the 54 SLAs proposed for this network. They held the highest values in all the actor-based metrics, showing the need to achieve a balance between the public sector and other actors to reach the net-zero emissions targets. Specifically, while the public sector seemed to be in charge of defining technical specifications, determining environmentally friendly procurement methods, and establishing mandatory energy codes, the non-public sector seemed to require working on procurement processes focused on the mitigation of CO_2 emissions [63].

In addition to the five main actors in this network, four additional stakeholders appeared as second-tier actors, participating in more than 50% of the SLAs. In particular, academia, civil society, the Ministry of Environment, and the Ministry of Energy were seemingly important in implementing 29 of the 54 second-level actions within this network. According to the connection exhibited in Figure 3a and the metrics shown in Table 6, these second-tier actors seemed to focus on objectives associated with social inclusion and structural changes within the public policy realm [64].

4.2.2. Technology Enabling Network

According to Figure 3b and Table 7, the technology-enabling network showed two prominent actors, the national government and the private sector. These two participants were involved in 42 second-level actions within this structure (i.e., 98% of all SLAs in this network). Both of these actors had the highest values in all actor-based metrics, showing their importance in developing the technology actions required to achieve net-zero emissions in the Colombian building sector. As proposed in previous studies [65], the government seemed fundamental in supporting research and development for environmental sustainability, while the private sector had a role in supporting innovation by investing in cleaner productive processes [65].

Apart from the two most prominent actors, eight stakeholders also exhibited essential values in their actor-based metrics (i.e., the Ministry of the Environment, academia, local governments, guilds and professional associations, the Ministry of Housing, the Ministry of Energy, financial institutions, and civil society). All these actors were influential in at least 21 second-level actions (i.e., 49% of all SLAs in this network). These stakeholders are prone to pursue multiple goals: improving sustainability, research, and development by establishing frameworks and supporting innovation, supporting the technological transformation financially, and veiling up for societal welfare.

4.2.3. Finance Enabling Network

Although highly interconnected, the finance enabling network was the least dense network within the four studied structures (Figure 3c and Table 7). This can be partially explained by the roles of the leading, prominent actors in this arrangement. In particular, the finance enabling network had the same two prominent actors as the technology enabling network (i.e., the national government and the private sector). However, and in contrast to the policy enabler network and the technology enabler network, the national government and the private sector participated in at least 42 SLAs (i.e., 84% of all SLAs within the network). This percentage was marginally smaller than the share of participation of the main actors in the policy and technology networks, even though the network-based metric values were in line with the values of the previously analyzed structures.

In this sense, the role of the government in this network seemed to be providing financial incentives and resources to make the transition towards net-zero emissions in the building sector economically viable. On the other hand, as suggested by previous studies, the private sector seemed to be involved in continuous collaboration with all stakeholders by mobilizing capital and capabilities [66].

Along with the leading actors in the finance enabler network, participants such as guilds and professional associations, local governments, financial institutions, the Development Bank, and civil society also stood out as important players in this structure. All these actors participated in at least 24 SLAs (i.e., 48% of all SLAs within the network). Interestingly, this set of actors contained mainly stakeholders belonging to the non-public sector. This group of participants seemed to focus on developing financial mechanisms to achieve net-zero emissions and guarantee coordination among government actors and other players.

4.2.4. Capacity Development Enabling Network

The capacity development enabling network exhibited four main stakeholders, namely, guilds and professional associations, the national government, academia, and the private sector (Figure 3d and Table 7). In general, these leading actors had the highest actor-based metrics and dominated the flow of information within the network, as they participated in at least 14 SLAs (i.e., 63% of all SLAs in the structure). However, compared to the other three enabling networks, these actors exhibited slightly less centralized behaviors, which made relationship patterns less dependent on the national government and private sector. Instead, relationships seemed to focus on the roles of guilds and professional associations, and academia, as these players seemed to be centered on disseminating the knowledge and establishing the technical bases required to achieve net-zero emissions.

In addition to the leading actors mentioned before, the local governments, the Ministry of Housing, the Ministry of Environment, and the Ministry of Energy exhibited an important role within this network, as each one of these stakeholders participated in at least eight SLAs (i.e., 53% of all SLAs within the structure). While local governments seemed to be focused on coordinating the dissemination of information and knowledge at local scales, the ministries of housing, environment, and energy showed behaviors associated with developing standards and defining regulations for establishing common ground regarding the knowledge and capacity required to reach net-zero emissions.

5. Discussion

There were common actors leading the four enablers (policy, technology, finance, and capacity development) to achieve GHG emissions reduction in the building sector. Three of these actors, the national government, local governments, and the private sector, appeared as one of the main five leaders in all the categories, suggesting common main actors of all networks. These similitudes were strengthened with the network-based metrics, presenting high values compared to previous literature analyzes [21,41,45]. Despite this, the action category networks also had distinct features. For instance, while in the policy network, the Ministry of Housing was the main actor, in the technology network, this role was occupied by the Ministry of Environment. The guilds and professional associations became the leaders in the finance and capacity development networks.

The results suggest multiple ways to take advantage of each enabler's network structures and show options to anticipate the best strategies. Regarding the policy networks, the two main actors were the national government and local governments. The experts recognized the role of the national government in leading the decision-making process to implement the roadmap to net-zero buildings. However, according to the results, this is only possible with the intervention of local governments implementing the policies in a differentiated way according to each region's context. Therefore, it is essential to consider decentralization mechanisms [67] for a successful low-carbon roadmap application. Additional to this, other actors such as the private sector, the guilds and professional associations, academia, and civil society exhibit the importance of coordinating public policies articulated by the interest of all the actors in the Colombian building sector.

Concerning the technology network, in addition to the national government and the local governments, the private sector, the Ministry of Environment, and academia were the following three main actors. It is possible to visualize the role of the private sector in supporting the adoption of new technology via the Ministry of Environment's regulations and the academia's innovation [65].

The two main actors in the finance network corresponded to the national government and the private sector. The private sector plays a role in funding sustainable infrastructure jointly with the national government [68] and simultaneously opened the debate on the feasibility of exploring alternative financial methods such as public–private partnerships [69].

In contrast to the other networks, the guilds and professional associations played the primary role in the capacity development network. They are vital in adopting new technologies and in promoting new capacities. The national and local governments, academia, and the private sector are essential in supporting the new capacity formation in the entire Colombian building sector.

Lastly, it is necessary to depict potential problems associated with the enablers' network structure. Even though it has been widely assumed that high cohesion values, associated with density, lead to improving team performance, some studies have shown that excessive density values can exhibit underperformance issues [70]. The four major categories of the roadmap presented network-based metrics higher than previous studies [21,41], potentially leading to stagnation, poor team performance, and lack of coordination [70]. For this reason, the Colombian government should constantly evaluate the role of the main actors and define their tasks specifically. Additionally, future studies based on improving team performance can be carried out to the extent of the execution of the Colombian roadmap.

6. Limitations and Future Research

This research had several limitations. Even though the sample size corresponded to 357 participants from diverse sectors, the inclusion of participants in the building sector from rural and other areas, rather than main cities, might add vital information to further studies.

Regarding how the CGBC classified actors in the survey, it would be better to have more specific categories of actors for future analysis. For instance, within the private sector would be valuable information to know the types of companies they represent.

This study adopted many metrics from the literature [45,50]; however, other methodologies, such as community analysis, might allow obtaining more specific results for the different groups of participants. Future investigations could also explore metrics at different points in time; one option is to use temporal social network analysis [71].

7. Conclusions

We analyzed the networks of actors involved in designing and implementing the Colombian Net-Zero Carbon Buildings Roadmap. Through SNA, we identified the key players within the major categories of the roadmap (policy, technology, finance, and capacity development) and the critical links and relationships among actors. Compact and dense structures characterized the four enabling networks (e.g., public policy, finance, technology, and capacity development) required to achieve net-zero emissions in the Colombian building sector. Small short average path lengths and a high degree of collaboration defined these network structures. Three types of players composed the networks:

- Leading stakeholders participated in more than two-thirds of the SLAs. They exhibited high centrality values and dominated most network connections and information flows.
- Second-tier actors participated in approximately one-half of the SLAs and coordinated specific objectives and information flows.
- Perimeter actors had low centrality values and participated in less than one-half of the SLAs. They were in charge of developing punctual actions of the roadmap and worked together with the leading and second-tier actors.

The studied networks had singularities, most of them regarding their leading actors and roles. While the national government and the private sector participated as leading actors in all enabling fields, other main actors changed according to the attributes of each network. For example, while academia was one of the five most prominent actors in the technology and capacity development networks, its role was less pronounced in the policy network and very limited in the finance network.

Overall, this research supports the field of sustainability and management in several ways. Even though the academic literature provides examples of social networks for sustainability in specific contexts, there is little evidence of using this methodology to analyze a whole economic sector. Social network analyzes allow identifying the actors, their interactions, and their roles in implementing net-zero roadmaps in the building sector. The diversity of actors intervening in the building sector and the complexity of the relations are vital factors in implementing effective GHG mitigation strategies.

This study provides a novel approach to studying decarbonization roadmaps by using SNA. Developing a social network through the actions required to achieve net-zero emissions allows a better definition of responsible actors at different levels and is an alternative for changing the focus from traditional actor maps to relational structures incorporating communication flows between multiple stakeholders. Governments and policymakers can take advantage of the shape of the enabling networks to achieve strategic goals within their roadmaps toward net-zero emissions.

Author Contributions: Conceptualization, J.S., J.G., M.E., F.R. and J.F.F.; Data curation, J.S.; Formal analysis, J.S., J.G., M.E., F.R. and J.F.F.; Investigation, J.S., J.G., M.E., F.R. and J.F.F.; Methodology, J.S. and J.G.; Project administration, J.G. and J.F.F.; Resources, J.F.F.; Supervision, J.G., M.E. and J.F.F.; Validation, J.S., J.G., M.E., F.R. and J.F.F.; Visualization, J.S.; Writing—original draft, J.S., M.E. and F.R.; Writing—review & editing, J.G., M.E., F.R. and J.F.F. All authors have read and agreed to the published version of the manuscript.

Funding: This research was funded by Hill Consulting and Universidad de los Andes.

Data Availability Statement: Data, models, and codes that support the findings of this study are available from the corresponding author upon reasonable request.

Acknowledgments: We thank the Colombian Green Building Council (CGBC), especially its director Angelica Ospina, and the World Resource Institute (WRI) for supporting this research and providing the required information.

Conflicts of Interest: The authors declare no conflict of interest.

Appendix A

Semi-structured interview for the group of experts in the ZCBA project.

Question 1.
Please provide a score from zero to one for each cross-cutting issue (e.g., equity, resilience, consumption habits, and habitability) within the second-level action you are analyzing.
Question 2.
In your opinion, what should happen at the national level to implement this second-level action?
Question 3.
What are the current barriers at the national level to implementing this second-level action?
Question 4.
In which subsectors of the third or residential sectors should this action be prioritized first?
Question 5.
What is the gradual time (dates) where this action should occur?
Question 6.
What actors should participate in this second-level action?
Question 7.
In your opinion, are there additional enablers required for this second-level action to be effective?
Question 8.
Do you have any comments regarding the four cross-cutting issues identified (e.g., equity, resilience, consumption habits, and habitability)?

References

1. IPCC. *AR6 Climate Change 2022: Mitigation of Climate Change*; IPCC: Geneva, Switzerland, 2022.
2. IEA. World Energy Outlook 2019–Analysis—IEA. Available online: https://www.iea.org/reports/world-energy-outlook-2019 (accessed on 25 April 2022).
3. Patiño, L.I.; Padilla, E.; Alcántara, V.; Raymond, J.L. The relationship of energy and CO_2 emissions with GDP per capita in Colombia. *Atmosphere* **2020**, *11*, 778. [CrossRef]
4. Patiño, L.I.; Alcántara, V.; Padilla, E. Driving forces of CO_2 emissions and energy intensity in Colombia. *Energy Policy* **2021**, *151*, 112130. [CrossRef]
5. United Nations Environment Programme. *2021 Global Status Report for Buildings and Construction: Towards a Zero-Emission, Efficient and Resilient Buildings and Construction Sector*; United Nations: Nairobi, Kenya, 2021.
6. Escamilla, E.Z.; Habert, G.; Daza, J.F.C.; Archilla, H.F.; Echeverry Fernández, J.S.; Trujillo, D. Industrial or Traditional Bamboo Construction? Comparative Life Cycle Assessment (LCA) of Bamboo-Based Buildings. *Sustainability* **2018**, *10*, 3096. [CrossRef]
7. Wu, Y.; Zhu, Q.; Zhu, B. Decoupling analysis of world economic growth and CO2 emissions: A study comparing developed and developing countries. *J. Clean. Prod.* **2018**, *190*, 94–103. [CrossRef]
8. Mehmood Mirza, F.; Sinha, A.; Rehman Khan, J.; Kalugina, O.A.; Wasif Zafar, M. Impact of energy efficiency on CO2 Emissions: Empirical evidence from developing countries. *Gondwana Res.* **2022**, *106*, 64–77. [CrossRef]
9. United Nations. *The Sustainable Development Goals Report 2022*; United Nations: New York, NY, USA, 2022.
10. Arora, N.K.; Mishra, I. COP26: More challenges than achievements. *Environ. Sustain.* **2021**, *4*, 585–588. [CrossRef]
11. Di Placido, A.M.; Pressnail, K.D.; Touchie, M.F. Exceeding the Ontario Building Code for low-rise residential buildings: Economic and environmental implications. *Build. Environ.* **2014**, *77*, 40–49. [CrossRef]

12. Ruiz, A.; Guevara, J. Energy Efficiency Strategies in the Social Housing Sector: Dynamic Considerations and Policies. *J. Manag. Eng.* **2021**, *37*, 04021040. [CrossRef]
13. International Energy Agency. *Iron and Steel Technology roadmap: Towards more sustainable steelmaking*; International Energy Agency: Paris, France, 2020; Volume 3.
14. Cement Sustainability Initiative. *Existing and Potential Technologies for Carbon Emissions Reductions in the Indian Cement Industry*; International Finance Corporation: Delhi, India, 2013.
15. Basbagill, J.; Flager, F.; Lepech, M.; Fischer, M. Application of life-cycle assessment to early stage building design for reduced embodied environmental impacts. *Build. Environ.* **2013**, *60*, 81–92. [CrossRef]
16. Cao, X.; Dai, X.; Liu, J. Building energy-consumption status worldwide and the state-of-the-art technologies for zero-energy buildings during the past decade. *Energy Build.* **2016**, *128*, 198–213. [CrossRef]
17. Zhang, N.; Han, Q.; de Vries, B. Building circularity assessment in the architecture, engineering, and construction industry: A new framework. *Sustainability* **2021**, *13*, 12466. [CrossRef]
18. Feige, A.; Wallbaum, H.; Krank, S. Harnessing stakeholder motivation: Towards a Swiss sustainable building sector. *Build. Res. Inf.* **2011**, *39*, 504–517. [CrossRef]
19. Yang, J.; Shen, Q.; Ho, M. An overview of previous studies in stakeholder management and its implications for the construction industry. *J. Facil. Manag.* **2009**, *7*, 159–175. [CrossRef]
20. Salazar, J.; Guevara, J.; Verhoest, K. Inferential Analysis of Road Infrastructure PPP Sponsor Networks. *J. Manag. Eng.* **2021**, *37*, 04021069. [CrossRef]
21. Guevara, J.; Salazar, J.; Garvin, M.J. Social Network Analysis of Road PPP Equity Markets in Canada, Chile, and the United States. *J. Manag. Eng.* **2020**, *36*, 04020058. [CrossRef]
22. Matinheikki, J.; Naderpajouh, N.; Aranda-Mena, G.; Jayasuriya, S.; Teo, P. Befriending Aliens: Institutional Complexity and Organizational Responses in Infrastructure Public–Private Partnerships. *Proj. Manag. J.* **2021**, *52*, 453–470. [CrossRef]
23. Karunathilake, H.; Hewage, K.; Brinkerhoff, J.; Sadiq, R. Optimal renewable energy supply choices for net-zero ready buildings: A life cycle thinking approach under uncertainty. *Energy Build.* **2019**, *201*, 70–89. [CrossRef]
24. COP26 COP26 Goals—UN Climate Change Conference (COP26) at the SEC–Glasgow 2021. Available online: https://ukcop26.org/cop26-goals/ (accessed on 13 February 2022).
25. Zhu, J.; Lin, H.; Yang, X.; Yang, X.; Jiang, P.; Del Valle, T.M. Social Network Relationships between Biomass Industry Stakeholders in the Agricultural Waste Power Generation Industry—A Case of Northern Jiangsu, China. *Sustainability* **2022**, *14*, 571. [CrossRef]
26. Matous, P.; Pollack, J.; Helm, J. Reprint of: Collecting experimental network data from interventions on critical links in workplace networks. *Soc. Netw.* **2022**, *69*, 274–292. [CrossRef]
27. Xu, X.; Xiao, B.; Li, C.Z. Stakeholders' power over the impact issues of building energy performance gap: A two-mode social network analysis. *J. Clean. Prod.* **2021**, *289*, 125623. [CrossRef]
28. Liang, X.; Yu, T.; Guo, L. Understanding stakeholders' influence on project success with a new sna method: A case study of the green retrofit in china. *Sustainability* **2017**, *9*, 1927. [CrossRef]
29. Wang, G.; Li, Y.; Zuo, J.; Hu, W.; Nie, Q.; Lei, H. Who drives green innovations? Characteristics and policy implications for green building collaborative innovation networks in China. *Renew. Sustain. Energy Rev.* **2021**, *143*, 110875. [CrossRef]
30. Mok, K.Y.; Shen, G.Q.; Yang, R. Stakeholder complexity in large scale green building projects: A holistic analysis towards a better understanding. *Eng. Constr. Archit. Manag.* **2018**, *25*, 1454–1474. [CrossRef]
31. Goforth, E.; Yosri, A.; El-Dakhakhni, W.; Wiebe, L. Infrastructure Asset Management System Optimized Configuration: A Genetic Algorithm–Complex Network Theoretic Metamanagement Approach. *J. Infrastruct. Syst.* **2022**, *28*, 04022029. [CrossRef]
32. World Resource Institute Global Launch: Zero Carbon Building Accelerator. Available online: https://www.wri.org/events/2021/6/global-launch-zero-carbon-building-accelerator (accessed on 15 September 2022).
33. Ghaljaie, F.; Naderifar, M.; Goli, H. Snowball Sampling: A Purposeful Method of Sampling in Qualitative Research. *Strides Dev. Med. Educ.* **2017**, *14*, e67670. [CrossRef]
34. Castelblanco, G.; Guevara, J.; Salazar, J. Remedies to the PPP Crisis in the Covid-19 Pandemic: Lessons from the 2008 Global Financial Crisis. *J. Manag. Eng.* **2022**, *38*, 04022017. [CrossRef]
35. Consejo Colombiano de la Construcción Sostenible. *Reporte de Recomendaciones Proyecto Acelerador de Edificaciones Neto Cero Carbono*; Consejo Colombiano de la Construcción Sostenible: Bogotá, Colombia, 2022.
36. Manuel Santos Calderón, J.; Abel Rivera Flórez, G.; Cárdenas Santamaría, M.; Carlos Villegas Echeverri, L.; Guillermo Zuluaga Cardona, J.; Gaviria Uribe, A.; Janeth Restrepo Gallego, G.; Arce Zapata, G.; Lorena Gutiérrez Botero, M.; Giha Tovar, Y.; et al. *Documento Conpes 3919*; Departamento Nacional de Planeación: Cartagena, Colombia, 2018.
37. GlobalABC (Global Alliance for Buildings and Construction); IEA; UNEP (Nations Environment Programme). *GlobalABC Regional Roadmap for Buildings and Construction in Latin America: Towards a Zero-Emission, Efficient and Resilient Buildings and Construction Sector*; United Nations: Paris, France, 2020.
38. Moreno, J.L. Sociometry in Relation to Other Social Sciences. *Sociometry* **1937**, *1*, 206. [CrossRef]
39. Eissa, R.; Eid, M.S.; Elbeltagi, E. Current Applications of Game Theory in Construction Engineering and Management Research: A Social Network Analysis Approach. *J. Constr. Eng. Manag.* **2021**, *147*, 04021066. [CrossRef]
40. Lusher, D.; Koskinen, J.; Robins, G. *Exponential Random Graph Models for Social Networks: Theory, Methods, and Applications*; Cambridge University Press: Cambridge, UK, 2013; Volume 123, ISBN 9780521193566.

41. Karali, E.; Bojovic, D.; Michalek, G.; Giupponi, C.; Schwarze, R. Who is connected with whom? *A Social network analysis of institutional interactions in the European CCA and DRR landscape. Sustainability* **2020**, *12*, 1275. [CrossRef]
42. Schröpfer, V.L.M.; Tah, J.; Kurul, E. Mapping the knowledge flow in sustainable construction project teams using social network analysis. *Eng. Constr. Archit. Manag.* **2017**, *24*, 229–259. [CrossRef]
43. Alexandrescu, F.M.; Rizzo, E.; Pizzol, L.; Critto, A.; Marcomini, A. The social embeddedness of brownfield regeneration actors: Insights from social network analysis. *J. Clean. Prod.* **2016**, *139*, 1539–1550. [CrossRef]
44. Jin, X.; Shen, G.Q.P.; Ekanayake, E.M.A.C. Improving construction industrialization practices from a socio-technical system perspective: A hong kong case. *Int. J. Environ. Res. Public Health* **2021**, *18*, 9017. [CrossRef] [PubMed]
45. Guevara, J.; Herrera, L.; Salazar, J. Interorganizational Sponsor Networks in Road and Social Infrastructure PPP Equity Markets. *J. Constr. Eng. Manag.* **2022**, *148*, 04022009. [CrossRef]
46. Salazar, J.; Guevara, J.; Herrera, L. Transferal of responsibilities of PPP European Equity Markets: Dependency Analysis. In Proceedings of the Construction Research Congress 2022, Arlington, VA, USA, 9–12 March 2022.
47. Borgatti, S.P.; Everett, M.G.; Freeman, L.C. UCINET 6 for Windows: Software for social network analysis (Version 6.102). *Harvard MA Anal. Technol.* **2002**, *6*, 12–15.
48. Malik, H.A.M.; Mahesar, A.W.; Abid, F.; Waqas, A.; Wahiddin, M.R. Two-mode network modeling and analysis of dengue epidemic behavior in Gombak, Malaysia. *Appl. Math. Model.* **2017**, *43*, 207–220. [CrossRef]
49. Eteifa, S.O.; El-adaway, I.H. Using Social Network Analysis to Model the Interaction between Root Causes of Fatalities in the Construction Industry. *J. Manag. Eng.* **2018**, *34*, 04017045. [CrossRef]
50. Pryke, S.; Badi, S.; Almadhoob, H.; Soundararaj, B.; Addyman, S. Self-Organizing Networks in Complex Infrastructure Projects. *Proj. Manag. J.* **2018**, *49*, 18–41. [CrossRef]
51. Borgatti, S.P.; Everett, M.G.; Johnson, J.C. *Analyzing Social Networks*; Sage: Newcastle upon Tyne, UK, 2018.
52. Newman, M.E.J. The structure of scientific collaboration networks. *Proc. Natl. Acad. Sci. USA* **2001**, *98*, 404–409. [CrossRef]
53. Borgatti, S.P.; Mehra, A.; Brass, D.J.; Labianca, G. Network analysis in the social sciences. *Science* **2009**, *323*, 892–895. [CrossRef]
54. Wasserman, S.; Faust, K. *Social Network Analysis: Methods and Applications*; Structural Analysis in the Social Sciences; Cambridge University Press: Cambridge, UK, 1994.
55. Freeman, L.C.; Roeder, D.; Mulholland, R.R. Centrality in social networks: Ii. *experimental results. Soc. Netw.* **1979**, *2*, 119–141. [CrossRef]
56. Freeman, L.C. Centrality in social networks conceptual clarification. *Soc. Netw.* **1978**, *1*, 215–239. [CrossRef]
57. Wu, G.; Qiang, G.; Zuo, J.; Zhao, X.; Chang, R. What are the key indicators of mega sustainable construction projects?-A stakeholder-network perspective. *Sustainability* **2018**, *10*, 2939. [CrossRef]
58. Global Alliance for Buildings and Construction; OID. *Buildings and Climate Change Adaptation: A Call for Action*; United Nations: Paris, France, 2021.
59. Gui, Q.; Liu, C.; Du, D. Bin Globalization of science and international scientific collaboration: A network perspective. *Geoforum* **2019**, *105*, 1–12. [CrossRef]
60. Gui, Q.; Liu, C.; Du, D. Bin The structure and dynamic of scientific collaboration network among countries along the belt and road. *Sustainability* **2019**, *11*, 5187. [CrossRef]
61. Giannoccaro, I. Centralized vs. decentralized supply chains: The importance of decision maker's cognitive ability and resistance to change. *Ind. Mark. Manag.* **2018**, *73*, 59–69. [CrossRef]
62. Fu, D.; Ionescu, C.M.; Aghezzaf, E.H.; De Keyser, R. Decentralized and centralized model predictive control to reduce the bullwhip effect in supply chain management. *Comput. Ind. Eng.* **2014**, *73*, 21–31. [CrossRef]
63. Roelich, K.; Giesekam, J. Decision making under uncertainty in climate change mitigation: Introducing multiple actor motivations, agency and influence. *Clim. Policy* **2019**, *19*, 175–188. [CrossRef]
64. Jakob, M.; Flachsland, C.; Christoph Steckel, J.; Urpelainen, J. Actors, objectives, context: A framework of the political economy of energy and climate policy applied to India, Indonesia, and Vietnam. *Energy Res. Soc. Sci.* **2020**, *70*, 101775. [CrossRef]
65. Ganda, F. The impact of innovation and technology investments on carbon emissions in selected organisation for economic Co-operation and development countries. *J. Clean. Prod.* **2019**, *217*, 469–483. [CrossRef]
66. Alkhani, R. Understanding private-sector engagement in sustainable urban development and delivering the climate agenda in northwestern europe—A case study of london and copenhagen. *Sustainability* **2020**, *12*, 8431. [CrossRef]
67. Lowatcharin, G.; Stallmann, J.I. The differential effects of decentralization on police intensity: A cross-national comparison. *Soc. Sci. J.* **2019**, *56*, 196–207. [CrossRef]
68. Azhgaliyeva, D.; Kapoor, A.; Liu, Y. Green bonds for financing renewable energy and energy efficiency in South-East Asia: A review of policies. *J. Sustain. Financ. Investig.* **2020**, *10*, 113–140. [CrossRef]
69. Koppenjan, J.F. Public-private partnerships for green infrastructures: Tensions and challenges. *Curr. Opin. Environ. Sustain.* **2015**, *12*, 30–34. [CrossRef]
70. Wise, S. Can a team have too much cohesion? *The dark side to network density. Eur. Manag. J.* **2014**, *32*, 703–711. [CrossRef]
71. Kim, H.; Anderson, R. Temporal node centrality in complex networks. *Phys. Rev. E-Stat. Nonlinear Soft Matter Phys.* **2012**, *85*, 026107. [CrossRef] [PubMed]

buildings

MDPI

Article

Structural Relationship between COVID-19, Night-Time Economic Vitality, and Credit-Card Sales: The Application of a Formative Measurement Model in PLS-SEM

Seong-a Kim and Heungsoon Kim *

Department of Urban Planning and Engineering, Hanyang University, Wangsimri-ro 222, Seongdong-gu, Seoul 04763, Korea
* Correspondence: soon@hanyang.ac.kr

Abstract: Cities worldwide are actively promoting their Night-Time Economies (NTEs) to recover from the economic crisis caused by COVID-19. However, in the case of Seoul, Korea, the interest in the NTE from an urban perspective remains insufficient. Therefore, this study was performed with the following two objectives: (1) To empirically identify the characteristics of Korea's NTE and derive an indicator of the nighttime economic vitality (NTEV) by considering the NTE in urban regions; (2) to explore the structural relationship between NTEV, COVID-19, and credit-card sales in Seoul, to which operational restrictions were stringently applied according to the COVID-19 policy of Korea. The NTEV was evaluated using indicators of the nightly floating population, night-lighting value, and number of entertainment facilities. Moreover, to identify the structural relationship between COVID-19, NTEV, and credit-card sales based on abnormal analysis data, a formative measurement model of the partial least squares structural equipment modeling framework was used. The results highlighted that the effect of COVID-19 differed depending on the density of facilities to which the "social distancing policy" was applied, and the NTEV boosted the consumption economy of the entire city. Moreover, we empirically confirmed that an increase in the number of confirmed COVID-19 patients directly or indirectly decreased credit-card sales, which deteriorated the urban economy.

Keywords: COVID-19; COVID-19 response policy; operational restrictions on facilities; Night-Time Economy (NTE); Night-Time Economic Vitality (NTEV); credit-card sales; PLS-SEM (partial least square structural equation modeling); formative measurement model

Citation: Kim, S.-a.; Kim, H. Structural Relationship between COVID-19, Night-Time Economic Vitality, and Credit-Card Sales: The Application of a Formative Measurement Model in PLS-SEM. *Buildings* **2022**, *12*, 1606. https://doi.org/10.3390/buildings12101606

Academic Editors: Liyin Shen, Jorge Ochoa and Haijun Bao

Received: 5 September 2022
Accepted: 28 September 2022
Published: 4 October 2022

1. Introduction

COVID-19 has affected various sectors of the society, culture, economy, and environment worldwide. In particular, the pandemic has led to massive losses in economic fields such as trade, domestic demand, stock, and labor markets [1]. Consumer spending, which supports 70% of the economy, has declined with people avoiding visiting restaurants, cinemas, offices, and other public places [2]. In other words, the pandemic has directly shrunk the floating population, the card-transaction volume, and sales at both the national and urban levels [3,4].

As the pandemic continues, cities in various countries are pursuing diverse night policy projects in an attempt to recover from the pandemic-induced economic crisis. Night-Time Economy (NTE) is considered an important aspect to revitalize the urban economy, and thus, cities are encouraging people to engage in various activities and boost consumption by promoting night tours, night markets, and night festivals [5]. In China, NTE is rapidly emerging as an urban trend given that the country has mobilized various support policies to revitalize the NTE, which has boosted the sluggish economies of various cities such as Shanghai, Beijing, and Guangzhou [6]. In contrast, in the case of Seoul, Korea, the Korea Tourism Organization organized only one forum in 2020 based on the theme of revitalizing the NTE through night tourism, and interest in restoring and revitalizing the NTE from an urban perspective remains limited.

Seoul is known as "a city that does not sleep", "a city that is awake 24 h", and "a city with active economic activities in the nighttime" [7]. However, from the beginning of the pandemic, Seoul has strictly limited the operating hours of all industries to 9 p.m. or 10 p.m. as part of "social distancing", a COVID-19 response policy. Consequently, the appearance of Seoul's night streets after COVID-19 has changed rapidly. The COVID-19 response policy of limiting operating hours has led to a decline in family outings, work dinners, and restaurant sales, and people are returning home earlier. Consequently, 20,000 commercial entities in Seoul closed down in the first quarter of 2020 alone [8]. This economic impact highlights the significance of the NTE as a key factor supporting the vitality of Seoul's urban economy.

Against the background of the perception that the NTE is important for urban vitality, this study is aimed at empirically verifying whether COVID-19 actually affected Seoul's self-employment sales and whether the policy of restriction on operating hours to limit the spread of COVID-19 influenced the vitality of Seoul's NTE.

The objectives of this study can be summarized as follows: First, although Korea is one of the countries in which most commercial facilities such as restaurants, cafes, and shopping centers operate until late, there are no positive indicators pertaining to the NTE. Moreover, although the NTE theory mainly focuses on tourism and economics, the number of NTE indicators that can be used in diverse urban studies remains insufficient. Therefore, we refer to the NTE theory applicable to urban studies as Night-Time Economic Vitality (NTEV) and attempt to construct the NTEV indicators that reflect the characteristics of Korea. Second, to determine whether the pandemic actually had an adverse effect on the urban economy, we investigate the structural relationship between COVID-19, NTEV, and credit-card sales and compare the differences in the structural relationships by industry. To these ends, partial least square structural equation modeling (PLS-SEM) is performed to clarify the structural relationships among multiple variables. The spatial scope of the study is Seoul, where social distancing and operating restriction policies have been most strictly applied in Korea. The temporal scope of the study is 2021, when the level of social distancing and number of confirmed COVID-19 cases in Seoul were higher than those in 2020, which is the year of the COVID-19 outbreak.

Figure 1 shows the process flow of this study. The remaining paper is organized as follows: Section 2 describes the concepts related to the design of the NTEV indicators and presents a literature review to highlight the novelty of this study. Section 3 describes the variable selection and establishment of hypotheses. After collecting and processing the data suitable for selected variables and reviewing the data through exploratory analysis, the analysis method and model were identified. Section 4 describes the PLS-SEM analysis performed to compose the NTEV indicators and identify the structural relationship between COVID-19, NTEV, and credit-card sales. Moreover, the differences in the structural relationships across industries were examined. Section 5 presents the concluding remarks and discusses the significance and implications of our results.

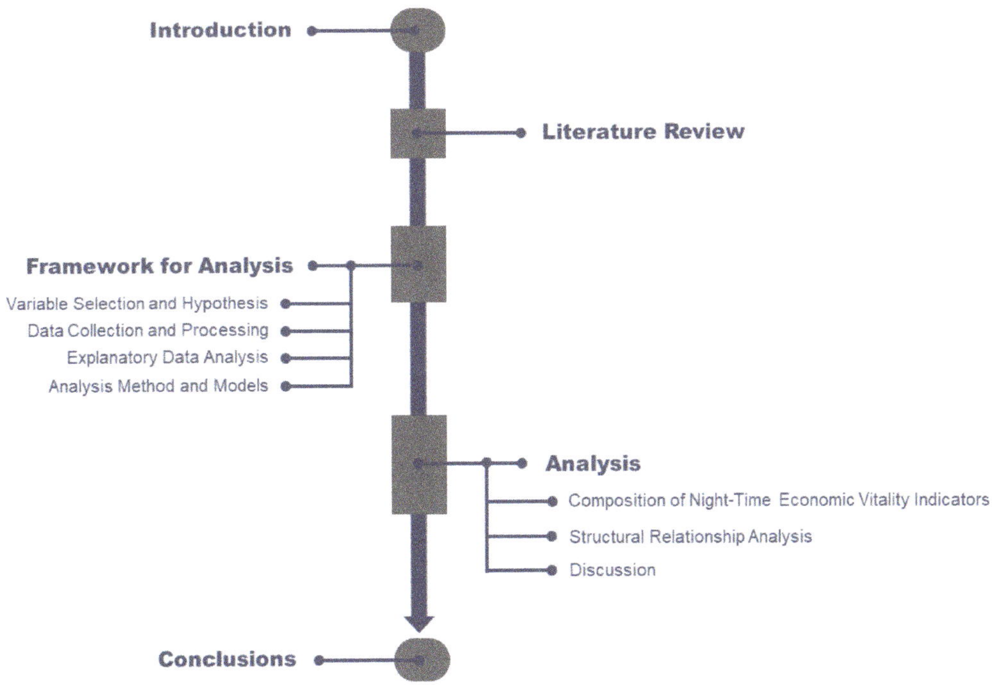

Figure 1. Flowchart of the study.

2. Literature Review

The term NTE emerged in the UK in 1995 when operating hours were extended to late night hours to revitalize the urban economy [9]. Since then, the concept has been used as a measure to understand a city's nighttime activities and has been treated as part of urban branding strategies, especially because young people flock to nighttime economic centers such as bars and clubs [10,11]. Successful nightlife places attract more foreign visitors to a city, and in addition to maintaining the vitality of the city center, promote the growth of the local economy [12].

According to Jane Jacobs [13], the ability to freely enjoy the nightlife of a city is an unequivocal social good. Similarly, when nightlife is aggregated, it creates a spatial basis for generating economies of agglomeration, which contributes to the city's overall social capital. The NTE has attracted extensive attention in major metropolitan cities such as New York, London, and Sydney because it secures urban competitiveness, increases sociocultural attractiveness, promotes urban development, and improves the urban vitality, in addition to boosting the city's economy, employment, and consumption [10,11]. In Asia, the NTE emerged as an issue in earnest when China hosted the 2019 Nighttime Economy Forum [14]. In Korea, the importance of nightlife has been recognized, and various tourism-focused projects (publication of night tourism guidebooks and the organization of the Seoul night goblin night market) for the public have been promoted; however, NTE terms were introduced only after the 2020 Night Tourism Forum [15].

With the growing importance of the NTE worldwide owing to COVID-19, many researchers have focused on this concept. Notably, the existing studies mainly covered the concept of NTE from the viewpoints of "entertainment and crime [16–18]", "behavioral patterns of people who have nightlife [19–21]", and "the night culture and social phenomenon [22–25]". In contrast, in Korea, primarily, survey-oriented studies to revitalize night markets or night tourism have been conducted recently from the perspective of tourism [26,27]. To analyze the NTE from the perspective of a city's social and economic revitalization, Lin et al. proposed the concept of NTEV by grafting the NTE into urban studies, developed an indicator using diverse urban data, and calculated an index of the NTEV in Zhejiang Province, China [5].

However, the NTE is not a standardized concept yet, because it addresses nighttime activities in various industries such as food and beverage, tourism, shopping, culture, and leisure [5]. One researcher defined the NTE as economic consumption in the fields of leisure, culture, entertainment, and food and beverage [28], whereas another researcher referred to it as day-to-day activities in urban public spaces, such as walking [29]. In addition, certain researchers emphasized the social aspect of the NTE [30], whereas others emphasized the economic aspect [5,11].

Definitions related to the timeslot of the NTE differ across countries and studies. One study defined the starting point of the night timeslot as the time at which people leave from work in the evening [31], whereas another study defined the nighttime slot as the interval between sunset and sunrise, that is, between 6 p.m. and 6 a.m. [10]. In addition, other researchers subdivided the NTE timeslot from 5 p.m. to 10 p.m. and nights after 10 p.m. [32,33]. At the national level, in the US, the interval between 6 p.m. and 6 a.m. is considered the nighttime [34]. In the UK, the nighttime is divided as follows: The interval between 6 p.m. and midnight is considered evening, and that between midnight and 6 a.m. is considered late night [35]. In Australia, the intervals between 6 p.m. and 9 p.m., 9 p.m. and 11 p.m., and 11 p.m. and 2 a.m. are considered early evening, evening, and late night, respectively [36].

Despite rich academic research on the NTE, most of the measurement scales have been devised based on qualitative indicators [19–25]. As quantitative indicators, the gross domestic product (GDP) and night-lighting data have been used with a focus on economic performance [37–39]: The GDP has been used as an official indicator of national growth, and night-lighting data, which represent the brightness of night lights, have been widely used by academicians in recent years as an alternative indicator because it represents the activities of people during nighttime [40]. However, GDP and night-lighting data are somewhat inadequate as indicators when they are uniformly applied to cities, which are characterized by the simultaneous occurrence of diverse economic, social, and cultural phenomena. Moreover, qualitative indicators do not fully reflect the characteristics of cities [5]. Studies related to the NTE of Korea, which focused on tourism, qualitatively measured people's behaviors and manners and the activities related to night tourism, night markets, and night festivals. The related indicators were designed based mainly on the results of surveys [26,27].

Considering these aspects, based on a literature review, we identified the following research gaps: (1) The NTE has been actively investigated, except in Korea, and the development of measurement indicators has been limited. Most of the developed indicators are qualitative, and only a few quantitative indicators exist, which can be applied to cities. (2) Korea's policies related to and academic interests in the NTE have mainly been centered around tourism, and urban studies remain to be performed. (3) The concept and definition of NTE vary across countries and focus industries. Moreover, a concept of the NTE in urban studies that reflects the characteristics of Korea and the associated indicators to measure it have not been developed yet.

To overcome these limitations, in this study, an analysis was performed considering the NTE as a factor that reflects the vitalization of a city. Instead of qualitative indicators, quantitative indicators that reflect the characteristics of Korea's NTE were constructed using urban statistical data. Furthermore, structural relationships of the NTE were established, reflecting the effects of COVID-19. The novelty of this study pertains to the empirical determination of the relationship between COVID-19, NTEV, and credit-card sales.

Before describing the analysis, we present an operational definition of the study objective. The objective of this study was to examine the NTE from the perspective of the city by using the concept of NTEV [5], which appeared with the application of the NTE concept in the field of urban studies. To measure the NTEV of the city, we defined the concept as "the degree of vitalization of the city's nighttime". Furthermore, we defined the NTEV timeslot as the interval between 7 p.m. and 8 a.m. The temporal definition of "night" in Korea is extremely diverse. Under the Labor Standards Act, working hours at night are from 10 p.m. to 6 a.m., and the dictionary definition of night refers to the time from sunset to sunrise. Moreover, the Seoul Metropolitan Government defines the floating population at night as the population between 7 p.m. and 8 a.m. [41]. Because the objective of this study was to measure the urban activity in the nighttime slot, that is, the NTEV, we defined nighttime as the interval between 7 p.m. and 8 a.m. based on the timeslot of the nightly floating population specified by Seoul Metropolitan Government and the definition that human nightlife begins from the time people leave work [31].

3. Analysis Framework

3.1. Variable Selection and Hypothesis

The measures and latent variables required for the analysis were constructed with reference to the literature (Table 1) and used to establish hypotheses. First, to confirm the effect of COVID-19, the COVID-19 construct was devised using the number of daily confirmed patients as a measurement variable.

We constructed the measurement variables of the NTEV by referring to studies such as those of Zikiriya et al., Xia et al., and Jeong and Jun [42–44]. Notably, Lin et al. used the nighttime electricity consumption, number of facilities, and online review data as NTEV measurement indicators [5]. Zikiriya et al. identified the urban vitality in the COVID-19 era considering the night-lighting data obtained using satellites [42]. Xia et al. and Jeong and Jun used the number of restaurants and night-lighting data as measures of floating population and credit-card sales, respectively [43,44].

The electricity consumption data for Korea in the night timeslot are not available because they are not segregated by the time zone. Consequently, we used night-lighting data instead of the electricity consumption variable, as an NTEV-related variable. In terms of operating-hour restrictions in response to COVID-19, the Seoul Metropolitan Government designated high-density entertainment facilities as Group 1 and has been managing them stringently. In other words, entertainment facilities, which are the most active at night in Seoul, have been the most adversely affected by COVID-19. In addition, because restaurants and businesses, which have been the focus of existing studies, mainly operate starting from daytime, we selected the number of entertainment facilities such as liquor and karaoke bars (entertainment facilities in Korea are stores that cook and sell food and alcoholic beverages, and they operate only at night) as a variable. Eventually, we used the night-lighting data, number of entertainment facilities, and nightly floating population as measurement indices constituting the NTEV.

To identify the structural relationship between COVID-19, NTEV, and credit-card sales, we considered credit-card sales as the dependent variable, with reference to the literature [5,45,46]. The reason is that credit cards represent the main payment option in many countries [47], and in Korea, the proportion (58.3%) of credit-card payments is higher than that of cash payments (21.6%). Moreover, in recent years, the number of cashless stores in Korea has increased [48]. Furthermore, in this study, the industry of credit-card sales was classified with reference to an existing study [45] that highlighted that the effect of COVID-19 on credit-card sales varied across industries. According to a classification provided by Shinhan Card Co., Ltd. (Seoul, Korea), these industries can be divided into 13 categories: restaurant and entertainment; distribution; food and beverage; clothing and merchandise; sports, culture, and leisure; travel and accommodations; beauty; life service; education and academy; medical care; furniture and home appliances; automobiles; and refueling industries. The furniture and home appliances and automobile industries, which are mainly sales-driven, are merged to obtain 12 categories. The differences across these 12 industrial groups are compared (Table 2).

Given this background, we aimed to evaluate the relationship between the number of confirmed COVID-19 patients and credit-card sales by industry. The influence of the number of confirmed COVID-19 patients on the decrease in self-employment sales has been widely discussed politically and academically [8,45,46], and thus, we established hypothesis Hypothesis 1. We established Hypothesis 2 to examine whether the number of confirmed COVID-19 patients negatively (−) affects the NTEV and Hypothesis 3 to evaluate whether the relationship between the NTEV and credit-card sales is affected by the number of confirmed COVID-19 patients as a moderating variable. Through these hypotheses, we attempted to identify the impact pathway of the number of confirmed COVID-19 patients, that is, direct, indirect, or moderating impact.

Hypothesis 1 (H1). *The number of confirmed COVID-19 patients has a negative (−) effect on credit-card sales.*

Hypothesis 2 (H2). *The number of confirmed COVID-19 patients has a negative (−) effect on the NTEV.*

Hypothesis 3 (H3). *In the relationship between NTEV and credit-card sales, the number of confirmed COVID-19 patients serves as a moderating variable.*

The Seoul Metropolitan Government has implemented a social-distancing policy as a measure to reduce the spread of COVID-19. This policy has been applied differentially to each facility. This objective is to prevent people from being active during night hours and encourage them to return home by limiting the operating hours of commercial facilities to 9 p.m. or 10 p.m. In addition, the Seoul Metropolitan Government has adjusted the number of spectators and events at cultural and sports facilities and recommended or mandated telecommuting for business facilities [49]. Notably, factory facilities related to the manufacturing industry, and residential facilities, have been excluded from these policies. Consequently, the effect relationships of COVID-19 and the NTEV differ depending on the region in which these facilities are concentrated. Because Korea's COVID-19 policy restricts the use of facilities, several studies have reported that the number of confirmed COVID-19 patients and sales decreased in areas with a high concentration of business and commercial facilities, but increased in areas with a high concentration of residential facilities [50,51]. In addition, because people's activities have revolved around residential areas after the COVID-19 outbreak, the movements and sizes of floating populations in residential areas have been more intense and larger, respectively, than those in other areas [50,51]. Therefore, to confirm the differences in terms of the density of facilities, we considered the density of each type of facility (residential, manufacturing, cultural, business, and commercial) as measurement variables and categorized them as (1) residential and manufacturing facilities and (2) cultural, business, and commercial facilities. This categorization was performed because Korea has restricted the operations of cultural, business, and commercial facilities under the regulatory policy in response to the pandemic, but the operations of residential and manufacturing facilities have not been restricted. Therefore, we classified the latent variables of the measurement variables as operationally restricted facilities and non-restricted facilities. Hypothesis 4 was established to examine the variation in the effect of the number of confirmed COVID-19 patients in the case of operationally restricted or non-restricted facilities (Hypothesis 4). Thereafter, we investigated whether credit-card sales (Hypothesis 4 + Hypothesis 1) and NTEV (Hypothesis 4 + Hypothesis 2) change with the number of confirmed COVID-19 patients in operationally restricted or non-restricted facilities, through mediation channels.

Hypothesis 4 (H4). *The impact of the number of confirmed COVID-19 patients varies depending on whether the operation of a facility is restricted.*

These hypotheses were focused on identifying the effects of the number of confirmed COVID-19 patients. To identify whether the spread of the pandemic influenced the considered structural relationship, the differences among the scenarios were compared by adding a structural relationship that excluded the number of confirmed COVID-19 patients. To this end, we attempted to identify the structural relationship related to COVID-19 from various viewpoints by checking for differences depending on the operating hours of operational restrictions on facilities, even in the absence of confirmed COVID-19 patients (Hypotheses 5 and 6).

Hypothesis 5 (H5). *The impact of the NTEV varies depending on whether the operation of a facility is restricted.*

Hypothesis 6 (H6). *The NTEV has a positive (+) impact on credit-card sales.*

To effectively examine the abovementioned structural relationship, we set the environmental factors as control variables (Hypothesis 7). Environmental factors that influence the population activity, urban vitality, and credit-card sales include measurement variables such as the minimum temperature, precipitation, and PM_{10} (Particle Matter 10 μm), as outlined by Yan et al., Keiser et al., and Kang et al. [52–54]. Finally, we established Hypothesis 8 to recognize that all of the previous influencing relationships differ by industry [45].

Hypothesis 7 (H7). *In the relationship between the NTEV, COVID-19, and credit-card sales, environmental factors serve as control variables.*

Hypothesis 8 (H8). *The structural relationship between the NTEV, COVID-19, and credit-card sales differs by industry.*

Table 1. Variables used in previous studies.

Variables			(1)	(2)	(3)	(4)	(5)	(6)	(7)	(8)	(9)	(10)	(11)	This Study
Dependent Variables	Credit-Card Sales	Credit-Card Sales by Industry					•	•	•	•			•	•
Independent Variables	Night Time Economic Vitality	Nighttime Electricity Consumption	•											
		Night-Lighting	•	•	•		•							•
		Nightly Floating Population					•				•	•	•	•
		Number of Restaurants			•									
		Number of Entertainment Facilities				•								•
		Number of Facilities	•									•		
	COVID-19	Number of Confirmed Patients		•					•			•		•
	Operating Restriction/ Non-Restricting Facilities	Residential Facilities										•	•	•
		Cultural Facilities												•
		Manufacturing Facilities												•
		Business Facilities										•	•	•
		Commercial Facilities										•	•	•
Control Variables	Environment	Minimum Temperature								•	•			•
		Precipitation								•	•			•
		PM_{10}								•	•			•
		PM_{25}									•			

(1) Lin et al., 2021 [5]; (2) Zikiriya et al., 2021 [42]; (3) Xia et al., 2020 [43]; (4) Hobbs et al., 2000 [19]; (5) Jeong and Jun, 2020 [44]; (6) Horvath et al., 2021 [46]; (7) Jo et al., 2020 [45]; (8) Kang et al., 2019 [54]; (9) Yan et al., 2019 [52]; (10) Kim., 2021 [50]; (11) Lim and Choi., 2022 [51].

Table 2. Industry classification of Shinhan Card Co., Ltd., and this study.

Industry Classification of Shinhan Card Co., Ltd.		Facilities Included in the Industry	Industry Classification of This Study	
1	Restaurant and Entertainment	e.g., Fast food chain; Cafe; Bakery shop	1	restaurant and entertainment
2	Distribution	e.g., Department store; Convenience store; Market	2	distribution
3	Food and Beverage	e.g., Butcher shop; Fisheries wholesale market; Flower market	3	food and beverage
4	Clothing and Merchandise	e.g., Optician; Jewelry shop; Offline fashion store	4	clothing and merchandise
5	Sports, Culture and Leisure	e.g., Movie theater; Indoor swimming pool; Bookstore	5	Sports, culture and leisure
6	Travel and Accommodations	e.g., Hotel; Duty free shop	6	travel and accommodations
7	Beauty	e.g., Hair shop; Cosmetics store	7	beauty
8	Life service	e.g., Laundry; Shoe repair shop	8	life service
9	Education and Academy	e.g., Reading room; Educational institute; English academy	9	education and academy
10	Medical care	e.g., Hospital; Pharmacy	10	medical care
11	Furniture and Home appliances	e.g., Home appliance store	11	Furniture, home appliances and automobiles
12	Automobiles	e.g., Automobile dealership; Tire sales department		
13	Refueling	e.g., Gas station	12	refueling

3.2. Data Collection and Processing

The spatial units for data collection were 424 administrative districts (dong) in Seoul. In July 2021, the Seoul Metropolitan Government changed the number of administrative districts to 425, but data for only 424 administrative districts are available. Therefore, we analyzed 424 districts. In terms of the spatial scale of the analysis units, the average area per administrative district was 1.42 km^2, given that the total area of Seoul is 605.2 km^2. The temporal target of this study was 2021, and to perform a cross-sectional analysis, we aggregated and analyzed one-year data.

We used the data of Shinhan Card Company (provided by the Seoul Metropolitan Government) as the credit-card sales data, i.e., the dependent variable. Among the independent variables, the entertainment facility variable representing the NTEV was computed by totaling the number of liquor and karaoke bars in operation as of December 2021. To reflect the floating population variable representing the population activity at nighttime, we used the data provided by the Seoul Metropolitan Government.

The illuminance values collected from the Smart-Seoul Data of Things (S-DoT) network were used as the night-lighting variable representing the nighttime brightness. The S-DoT data are real-time data provided by the Seoul Metropolitan Government for identifying and measuring various urban phenomena. As of December 2021, about 1100 monitoring sensors have been installed evenly throughout the 424 administrative districts of Seoul (Figure 2) [55]. The real-time data represent the actual nighttime brightness as the sensing data measured in minutes. We considered both the size of the nightly floating population and night-lighting values in our analysis by extracting only the data corresponding to the night timeslot (from 7 p.m. to 8 a.m.).

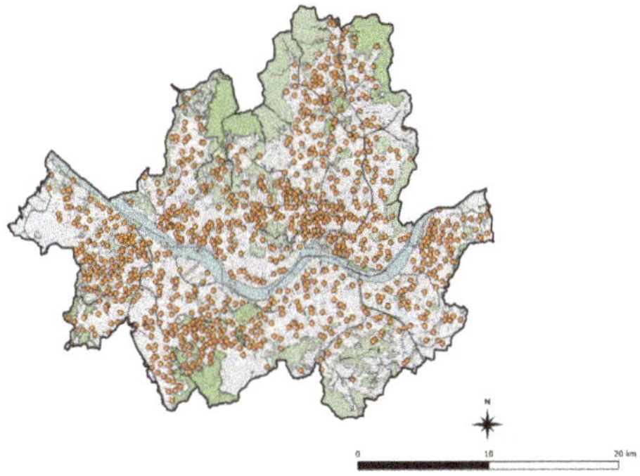

Figure 2. Distribution plot of Smart-Seoul Data of Things (S-DoT).

Moreover, we used data pertaining to the daily numbers of confirmed COVID-19 patients in 2021 provided by the Korea Centers for Disease Control and Prevention as the COVID-19 variable. Because these data are provided in units of 25 autonomous regions (gu), we requested each autonomous region to provide data in units of 424 administrative districts, which are the unit of analysis of this study (A gu is subdivided into several dong). Only 7 of 25 autonomous regions of Seoul provided the requested data. Therefore, to ensure data consistency, we estimated the data of the administrative district units by using the daily number of confirmed COVID-19 patients provided for the autonomous region units through population interpolation. To ensure the validity of population interpolation and reliability of the estimated data, we verified the accuracy of the population interpolation by comparing the relative errors between the estimated and actual data using the seven datasets of administrative districts units provided by autonomous agencies (Equation (1)). The accuracy of the estimated daily number of confirmed COVID-19 patients by administrative district was 98.96%; therefore, the information was considered useful.

$$\begin{aligned} \text{Accuracy}(\%) &= 100 - \text{elativeErrorRelative} \\ \text{Error}(\%) &= (|\varepsilon|)/\text{X} \times 100 \end{aligned} \tag{1}$$

The residential, manufacturing, cultural, business, and commercial facility variables, which were classified as operationally restricted and non-restricted facilities, were represented by Seoul's building data by use type, provided by the Ministry of Land. Notably, these data are point data, and all building data in Seoul are provided in the shp format. Therefore, we used the QGIS (Quantum Geographical Information System version 3.27) online open source program to extract the data provided for each building unit into administrative unit data.

The data of environmental variables can typically be acquired using three approaches: estimation from satellite images; determination using personal measurement means, or measurement using fixed weather-observation equipment [56]. In general, it is challenging to ensure the accuracy of satellite imagery data because of orbital cycles or cloud cover. Landsat data, which have intermediate resolution grades and are suitable for analysis, are often discontinuous because the orbital period is 16 d [57]. In addition, because these data are estimated using the surface radiation energy instead of being directly measured, they may differ marginally from the actual values [58]. Direct data acquisition using personal measurement means is difficult over a large area, which renders it challenging to grasp the trends across the entire city. Moreover, when using the data obtained from fixed weather-observation equipment such as automated weather station (AWS), spatial interpolation must be performed to extract data for a small spatial scale because typically only a few AWS exists in the region. Because the distance between the AWS equipment points is large, the estimated spacing values may differ from the actual values [58]. Considering these aspects, the actual S-DoT data of the minimum temperature and PM_{10} variables were used in this study. Because S-DoT does not provide precipitation data, the AWS data provided by the Korea Meteorological Administration for each autonomous district were collected, and the average daily rainfall in each administrative dong was estimated through spatial interpolation.

The credit-card sales, nightly floating population, night-lighting data, minimum temperature, and PM_{10} data, as variables used in this study, represented vast amounts of big data provided temporally. The credit-card sales data were provided on a daily basis for the 19,153-census output area, and the nightly floating population data were provided on an hourly basis for 424 administrative districts. The night-lighting data, minimum temperature, and PM_{10} data were collected in real time on an hourly basis using about 1100 sensors. Because each dataset was composed of micro units, data mining was performed by administrative district on a one-year basis, as shown in Figure 3.

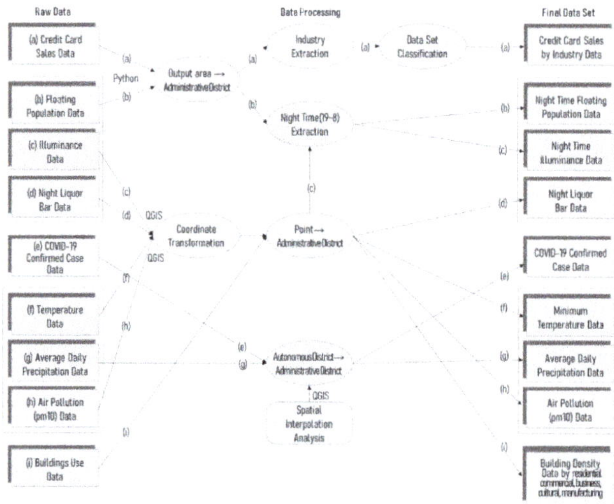

Figure 3. Data processing.

In particular, because the night-lighting, minimum temperature, and PM_{10} data obtained from the S-DoT network was expected to have missing values owing to the characteristics of sensing data, we attempted to eliminate any missing values identified in the data-review process.

3.3. Explanatory Data Analysis

3.3.1. Descriptive Statistics

Exploratory data analysis was performed to evaluate the accuracy and basic characteristics of the collected data. First, by conducting a descriptive statistics analysis using the SPSS program, the missing values, average values, minimum and maximum values, median values, and kurtosis and skewness of the data were confirmed (Table 3). In addition, data visualization was performed to visually examine the data of major variables such as COVID-19 confirmed cases, floating population, entertainment facilities, and five facility variables. Figure 4 shows the distribution and degree of data for 424 administrative districts in Seoul. The confirmed patients and floating population variables visualized the distribution degree of the population, and the five facility variables integrated all facilities to visualize the density of the entire facility. The number of samples of the entertainment facility variable was smaller than that of the other major variables: there were about 4000, and 101 of the 424 administrative districts of Seoul had zero data because there were no entertainment facilities. Therefore, the location of the entertainment facility variable was confirmed by visualizing the distribution of the facilities.

Table 3. Frequency analysis results.

Variables	N	Min	Max.	Avg.	S.D.	Skew.	Kurt.	Variables	N	Min.	Max.	Avg.	S.D.	Skew.	Kurt.
Credit-Card Sales 1: restaurant and entertainment	424	2.9949	88,370.35	2194.54	5996.40	8.80	107.31	Night-Lighting Data	424	0.00	16,019.84	287.60	917.23	14.097	222.741
Credit-Card Sales 2: distribution	423	0.3728	243,033.06	7429.11	26,843.92	6.89	50.85	Nightly Floating Population	424	4327.7196	73,743.06	24,003.87	10,354.77	0.925	1.502
Credit-Card Sales 3: food and beverage	424	0.5145	62,705.36	831.10	3816.55	12.35	178.55	Number of Entertainment Facilities	424	0.00	146.00	9.72	18.78	4.078	20.226
Credit-Card Sales 4: clothing and merchandise	424	0.2229	25,550.11	390.96	1837.39	9.29	103.32	Number of Confirmed Patients	424	2.6635	1285.00	452.21	187.37	0.874	1.741
Credit-Card Sales 5: sports, culture and leisure	424	2.4747	12,255.54	314.65	827.92	9.48	116.91	Residential Facility	424	0.0000	22.76	0.73	1.28	13.907	222.983
Credit-Card Sales 6: travel and accommodation	332	0.0035	79,756.90	1036.87	6566.57	9.77	103.06	Cultural Facility	424	0.0000	0.72	0.09	0.08	3.414	16.915
Credit-Card Sales 7: beauty	424	1.4245	14,536.46	138.53	741.49	17.65	338.72	Manufacturing Facility	424	0.0000	1.83	0.02	0.13	12.891	174.849
Credit-Card Sales 8: life service	424	0.4830	34,616.96	393.62	1820.31	16.11	297.53	Business Facility	424	0.0000	0.09	0.00	0.01	5.452	35.283
Credit-Card Sales 9: education and academy	424	0.9858	39,668.93	893.87	3019.33	7.44	74.16	Commercial Facility	424	0.0000	2.78	0.28	0.33	3.522	18.071
Credit-Card Sales 10: medical care	424	0.5095	108,389.96	2689.10	9548.28	8.21	77.03	Minimum Temperature	424	9.5003	16.44	12.75	0.93	−0.756	1.972
Credit-Card Sales 11: furniture, home appliances and automobiles	424	0.1044	1,149,857.31	3920.09	56,791.39	19.64	394.93	Precipitation	424	0.0308	1.40	0.18	0.18	3.727	18.402
Credit-Card Sales 12: refueling	280	0.6761	68,918.48	8887.12	9596.30	2.32	7.79	PM_{10}	424	0.3668	17.16	2.25	2.15	3.48	16.26

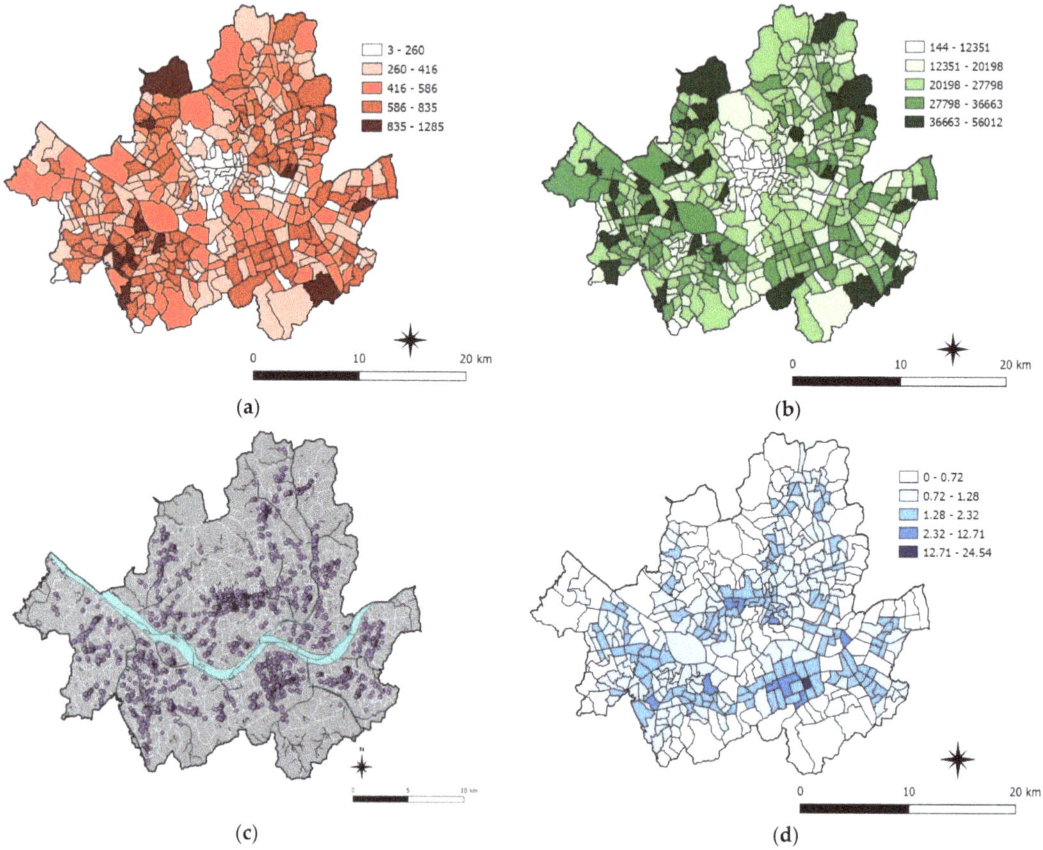

Figure 4. Data visualization of important variables. (**a**) distribution of COVID-19 confirmed patients; (**b**) distribution of floating population; (**c**) location of entertainment facilities; (**d**) density of five facilities.

According to the results, in terms of the credit-card sales by industry, which is a dependent variable, the sample sizes of the distribution, travel and accommodations, and refueling industries differed by 423, 332, and 280, respectively. Therefore, we deleted the three models corresponding to these industries based on the sample size of the industry, not the 424 administrative districts in Seoul. The resulting data were used for the analysis. In addition, we confirmed that the skewness (<3.0) and kurtosis (<7.0) exceeded the criteria, indicating non-normality of the data.

3.3.2. Normality and Preprocessing

Next, we performed quantile-quantile plot (Q-Q plot) and Shapiro–Wilk analysis by using R to confirm the normality of the data and distribution. The results of the Shapiro–Wilk analysis, which confirms the statistical normality, indicated the extremely small p-values of all the variables (Table 4) In the scatter plot of each variable in the Q-Q Plot indicated, the data points did not follow a straight line slope, which indicated that the data were not normally distributed (Figure A1).

Table 4. Shapiro-Wilk analysis results.

Variables	W	*p*-Value *	Variables	W	*p*-Value *
Credit-Card Sales 1: restaurant and entertainment	0.31158	2.2×10^{-16}	Night-Lighting Data	0.12087	2.2×10^{-16}
Credit-Card Sales 2: distribution	0.23756	2.2×10^{-16}	Nightly Floating Population	0.95555	5.303×10^{-10}
Credit-Card Sales 3: food and beverage	0.16137	2.2×10^{-16}	Number of Entertainment Facilities	0.52375	2.2×10^{-16}
Credit-Card Sales 4: clothing and merchandise	0.18961	2.2×10^{-16}	Number of Confirmed Patients	0.96143	4.165×10^{-9}
Credit-Card Sales 5: sports, culture and leisure	0.29631	2.2×10^{-16}	Residential Facility	0.22571	2.2×10^{-16}
Credit-Card Sales 6: travel and accommodation	0.14183	2.2×10^{-16}	Cultural Facility	0.69550	2.2×10^{-16}
Credit-Card Sales 7: beauty	0.10576	2.2×10^{-16}	Manufacturing Facility	0.09384	2.2×10^{-16}
Credit-Card Sales 8: life service	0.15037	2.2×10^{-16}	Business Facility	0.34267	2.2×10^{-16}
Credit-Card Sales 9: education and academy	0.28369	2.2×10^{-16}	Commercial Facility	0.66494	2.2×10^{-16}
Credit-Card Sales 10: medical care	0.25221	2.2×10^{-16}	Minimum Temperature	0.93564	1.446×10^{-12}
Credit-Card Sales 11: furniture, home appliances and automobiles	0.03860	2.2×10^{-16}	Precipitation	0.62332	2.2×10^{-16}
Credit-Card Sales 12: refueling	0.77614	2.2×10^{-16}	PM_{10}	0.95274	2.107×10^{-10}

* The e-value of the *p*-value means that the *p*-value is less than or equal to 10 to the power of −n, which indicates an extremely small numerical value that does not satisfy the significance level of >0.05.

To convert the units and ranges of different data into forms suitable for analysis and enhance the normality, we performed a normalization process by taking the log of the non-normal data. Thereafter, the abovementioned analysis process was repeated. The results indicated that the range of data was reduced through the use of log, although the normality of certain data did not increase (Figure A1). Thus, the exploratory data analysis indicated that the dataset used in this study did not follow the normal distribution.

3.4. Analysis Method and Models

We performed structural equation modeling (SEM) to clarify the relationship between COVID-19, NTEV, and credit-card sales, which has not been academically identified yet. SEM is a statistical technique designed to analyze structural relationships between correlation and theoretical causality among constituent concepts on the basis of metrics [59]. Because latent factors without measurement errors can be identified through confirmatory factor analysis, and the latent factor relationship can be simultaneously confirmed by a path analysis, the degree of explanation of a research model can be confirmed. This method is mainly used in exploratory studies to analyze multiple influences by simultaneously setting various independent and dependent variables or to identify the direct and indirect effects between the variables [59]. Notably, this method can enhance the analysis reliability by measuring the overall model fit, and handling data that are difficult to calculate (e.g., time-series data with autocorrelation errors, nonnormal distributions, and categorical variables).

According to the results of the exploratory data analysis, the dataset used in this study did not satisfy the conditions of the general structural equation from the standard viewpoint of distribution normality. The general structural equation pertains to covariance-based SEM (CB-SEM), as in the data used in CB-SEM, each variable must represent stationarity as a basic condition [60]. Considering this aspect, we performed PLS-SEM to address the nonnormal data encountered in SEM. The principal-component-based PLS-SEM method is less rigid in terms of the sample size and residual distribution requirements and is, thus, advantageous for analyzing data that do not follow a normal distribution [61]. Moreover, this method can be used to estimate the parameters more efficiently than typical CB-SEMs and offers higher statistical power [62]. In particular, in the application of formative indicators such as urban data to the model, model identification is facile, and the analysis is stable.

PLS-SEM was performed using the Smart-PLS 3.0 program. Figure 5 shows the structural relationship obtained in this study using the PLS-SEM method, and using the example of one of several industry-specific analysis models employed in this study.

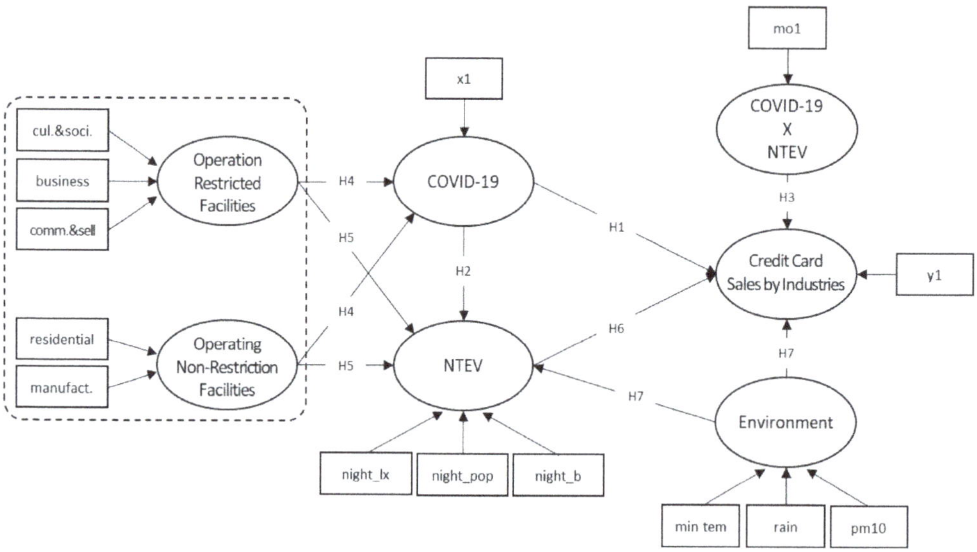

Figure 5. An analysis model used in this study.

The analysis models were composed of the potential variables representing the concept (internal variables) and measurement variables explaining the potential variables (external variables). The measurement of the relationship between these variables was set as the formative measurement model. A key consideration in PLS-SEM is the identification of the measurement indicators, including formative and reflective indicators. The formative indicators are causative indicators, i.e., they define the characteristics of the concept. In addition, a measurement variable induces a latent variable; homogeneity (correlation) between the measurement variables is low, and; these variables are mainly used in relationships in which an effect occurs when one measurement variable is removed. In contrast, reflective indicators are result indicators, i.e., the causal direction is directed from the concept to the indicator, and these indicators are signs of the construct. In other words, latent variables not only induce the measurement variables, but also stipulate that the measurement variables must be similar, such as survey questions [62].

The existing SEM studies mainly used reflective indicators owing to the lack of support for programs that analyze formative indicators or the difficulty associated with identifying models by using formative indicators. In addition, in the data or research to which formative indicators must be applied, reflective indicators have typically been applied. Notably, if the measurement indicators are set incorrectly in the SEM framework, model errors may occur, because the path coefficient and R^2 increase [59,61]. All the measurement variables used in this study were continuous variables based on urban data, and because the characteristics between the variables were independent, formative indicators were found to be more suitable than reflective indicators. Therefore, considering the data used in this study and objectives, we perform PLS-SEM using a formative measurement model and used all indicators as formative indicators.

In addition, to confirm the effects of the number of confirmed COVID-19 patients from various perspectives, we set the COVID-19-related construct as an exogenous latent variable, an endogenous latent variable, and a moderating variable. In PLS-SEM, because the moderating effect is confirmed as an interaction term, we added a moderating structure by performing mean-centering over the COVID-19 variable. This structural relationship is illustrated in Figure 4. Moreover, to identify the mediation effect of NTEV, we set the NTEV-related construct as an endogenous potential variable, which serves as both an independent variable and a dependent variable.

After setting up the basic study model, we classified and analyzed the analysis model for 12 industries: restaurant and entertainment; distribution; food and beverage; clothing and merchandise; sports, culture, and leisure; travel and accommodation; beauty; life service; education and academy; medical care; furniture, home appliances and automobiles, and; refueling.

When using a formative measurement model, the PLS-SEM analysis process is different from that of CB-SEM or reflective measurement modeling. Because the formative measurement model is free from measurement errors, the measurement variables must be independent and not correlated. Moreover, it is assumed that no error exists between the variables owing to the model characteristics [63,64]. In this context, the formative measurement model has criteria other than the assessment criteria, such as the validity, construct reliability and averaged variance extracted, used in general SEM (or reflective measurement models). As shown in Figure 6, the assessment procedure of the formative measurement model involves verification of the hypothesis of the structural model through path analysis after evaluating the measurement model in terms of the indicator validity, construct validity, outer weight, and outer loading. Therefore, using the Smart-PLS 3.0 program, we constructed the NTEV indicators and analyzed the structural relationships following the procedure of the formative measurement model (Figure 6).

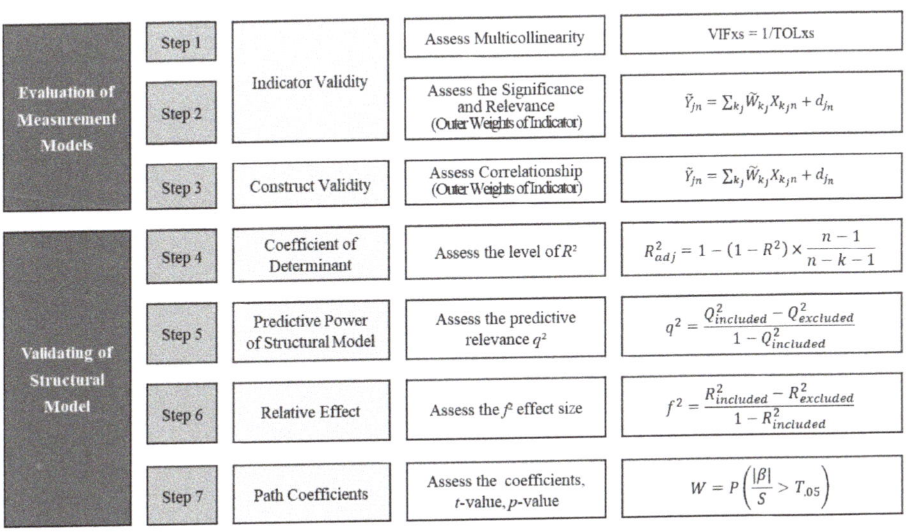

Figure 6. Assessment procedure of the formative measurement model (Step 7). Adapted from [59,62].

4. Analysis

4.1. Composition of NTEV Indicators

The Smart-PLS program was used to verify the NTEV indicators, as an objective of this study. All the variables used to identify the NTEV, i.e., the nightly floating population, night-lighting, and number of entertainment facilities, were set as indicators based on a review of the existing studies and established theories. The indicators were formative indicators with independent characteristics based on urban data. We performed a rigorous analysis to confirm the significance and suitability of these formative indicators and determine whether they appropriately reflect the construct.

Formative indicators can typically be assessed using the outer weights and outer loadings in bootstrapping analysis. If the t-value of the outer weights is greater than at least ± 1.65 at the 10% significance level in the two-tail test, or if the p-value is significant, indicator construction is considered to be possible. In contrast, if the value of the outer weights is not significant, the value of the outer loading must be 0.5 or higher. If the outer weight of an indicator is not significant, and the value of the outer loading is 0.5 or lower, the indicator is not suitable for forming a concept and must be discarded.

Therefore, we performed a bootstrapping analysis involving 5000 extractions to reduce errors and ensure consistency in estimation. In terms of the outer weights, both the t- and p-values were significant (Table 5), and the nightly floating population, night-lighting, and number of entertainment facilities were found to be suitable NTEV indicators, even without checking the outer loadings (Table 5).

Table 5. Verification of NTEV indicators (outer weights).

Construct	Indicators	Outer Weights	T-Value	p-Value
NTEV	Nightly Floating Population	0.588	24.002	0.000
	Nightly-Lighting	0.535	13.452	0.000
	Number of Entertainment Facilities	0.306	3.374	0.001

4.2. Structural Relationship Analysis

4.2.1. Evaluation of Measurement Models

To evaluate a formative measurement model using formative indicators, the validity of the measurement indicators and constituent factors of the model must be evaluated. In a formative measurement model, both the indicators and constituent factors must be independent and noncorrelated, because strong correlations are problematic from the viewpoints of methodology and interpretation [62,63].

The validity between measurement indicators is typically evaluated considering the multicollinearity, outer weights, and outer loadings. First, in terms of the multicollinearity, the variance inflation factor (VIF), defined as VIFxs = 1/TOLxs, must be 5.0 or less. According to a few researchers, the VIF must be equal to or less than 10, as in case of the reflective indicators, but it is not appropriate to apply the same acceptable reference values to reflective and formative indicators [65,66]. Because all the analysis models used in this study were formative measurement models that used formative indicators, we performed multicollinearity analysis with VIF = 5.0. For all the formative indicators (measurement indicators) constituting the 12 models, the VIF value ranged between 1.000 and 1.145, which indicated the lack of collinearity between the indicators. Thereafter, we analyzed the outer weights or outer loadings to evaluate the contributions and relevance of the formative indicators. This analysis was similar to the process of evaluating the construct validity of the NTEV indicators. The difference was that the previous measurement indicated the validity of the indicators constituting the NTEV concept, whereas this analysis was aimed at confirming the suitability of all indicators constituting the model. The suitability of the indicators reflected whether the corresponding construct of the multiple formative indicators (measurement indicators) was appropriate; thus, single formative indicators, such as the number of confirmed COVID-19 patients and credit-card sales, were not measured.

First, all the 12 models were checked using outer weights to verify the existence of the relative contributions of the formative indicators to the construct, that is, the relative importance levels of the constructs. For all the models, the PM_{10} variable of the environmental construct, manufacturing variable classified under the non-restricted facilities construct, commercial and business variables classified under the restricted facilities construct, and entertainment facilities variable of the NTEV construct were found to be not significant. If the values of the outer loadings were less than the reference value (0.5) and simultaneously nonsignificant, the indicator was required to be removed. We examined the absolute contribution of the indicators based on the outer loading values. The cultural variables classified under the restricted facility construct were not eliminated because the outer loading values were greater than 0.5 or significant. In particular, although these indicators were insignificant, they were important for the model validity [62]. We eliminated the PM_{10} variable under the environment construct, manufacturing variable under the non-restricted facilities construct, and business variable under the restricted facilities construct because they were nonsignificant and the value of the outer loadings was less than 0.5.

The outer weight values of the minimum temperature and precipitation variables under the environment construct and night-lighting data and entertainment facilities variables under the NTEV construct were insignificant in several models. According to the outer loadings, all variables except the minimum temperature variable of Model 6 were derived reasonably and were not removed. For the minimum temperature variable, the outer weights and outer loadings were insignificant, but this variable was not removed to ensure model consistency because it was an important indicator and was appropriately derived in several models simultaneously. The VIF values and outer weights values of the final indicators used in this study are summarized in Table 6.

Subsequently, we confirmed the validity between the constructs. For the formative measurement model, the correlation between all constructs must be less than 0.7 [67]. According to the analysis results, the relationship between the constructs was less than 0.7 for all models, which confirmed that the constructs composed of the formative indicators were independent of one another.

4.2.2. Structural Model Validation

Before the path analysis, we computed the R^2 and Q^2 values to measure the predictive accuracy and suitability, respectively, of the formative measurement model of PLS-SEM. Because the R^2 value indicates a higher level of prediction accuracy with a larger coefficient, and the standard for an acceptable R^2 value depends on the model complexity and the study premise, researchers must check the coefficient level of the overall research model, then decide the standard by referring to previous studies. In urban studies, values between 0.02 and 0.12 are considered weak, those between 0.13 and 0.25 are considered moderate, and those higher than 0.26 are considered strong [68]. According to the analysis results, most of the 12 industries exhibited moderate or strong model accuracy, and the COVID-19 construct of Model 6 and COVID-19 and credit-card sales constructs of Model 12 exhibited low accuracies (Table 7). Therefore, we excluded Models 6 and 12 from the path analysis because of their low predictive accuracy.

Table 6. Indicator validity results.

Constructs	Indicators	VIF	Model1	Model2	Model3	Model4	Model5	Model6	Model7	Model8	Model9	Model10	Model11	Model12
			Outer Weights	Outer Weights	Outer Weights	Outer Weights	Outer Weights	Outer Weights	Outer Weights	Outer Weights	Outer Weights	Outer Weights	Outer Weights	Outer Weights
Credit-Card Sales	Sales 1	1.000	1											
	Sales 2	1.000	-	1	-	-	-	-	-	-	-	-	-	-
	Sales 3	1.000	-	-	1	-	-	-	-	-	-	-	-	-
	Sales 4	1.000	-	-	-	1	-	-	-	-	-	-	-	-
	Sales 5	1.000	-	-	-	-	1	-	-	-	-	-	-	-
	Sales 6	1.000	-	-	-	-	-	1	-	-	-	-	-	-
	Sales 7	1.000	-	-	-	-	-	-	1	-	-	-	-	-
	Sales 8	1.000	-	-	-	-	-	-	-	1	-	-	-	-
	Sales 9	1.000	-	-	-	-	-	-	-	-	1	-	-	-
	Sales 10	1.000	-	-	-	-	-	-	-	-	-	1	-	-
	Sales 11	1.000	-	-	-	-	-	-	-	-	-	-	1	-
	Sales 12	1.000	-	-	-	-	-	-	-	-	-	-	-	1
NTEV	lux	1.145	0.250 (1.322)	0.000	0.207 (1.333)	0.351 (1.287)	0.569 (**)	0.740 (0.834)	0.055	0.508 (1.555)	0.180 (1.462)	0.340 (1.562)	0.374 (1.484)	0.284 (0.589)
	pop	1.117	0.000	0.009	0.000	0.000	0.000	0.000	0.000	0.000	0.000	0.000	0.000	0.000
	enter	1.027	0.000	0.028	0.139 (***)	0.000	0.000	0.000	0.000	0.000	0.152 (***)	0.000	0.000	0.434 (**)
COVID-19	covid	1.000	1	1	1	1	1	1	1	1	1	1	1	1
Restriction Facility	residential	1.013	1	1	1	1	1	1	1	1	1	1	1	1
Non-Restriction Facility	cultural	1.131	0.087 (**)	0.392 (***)	0.307 (***)	0.721 (**)	0.941 (**)	0.332 (*)	0.806 (**)	0.953 (**)	0.329 (***)	0.805 (**)	0.948 (**)	0.928 (1.080)
	commercial	1.131	0.000	0.04	0.020	0.000	0.000	0.000	0.000	0.000	0.021	0.000	0.000	0.079
Environment	min.tem	1.116	0.000	0.004	0.004	0.001	0.017	0.244 (-)	0.007	0.001	0.256 (0.635)	0.074	0.012	0.825 (0.644)
	precipi.	1.116	0.000	0.000	0.000	0.000	0.000	0.113(1.484)	0.000	0.000	0.009	0.014	0.000	0.286 (1.053)

( ) denotes the outer loading value of the nonsignificant indicator from outer weights. If the outer weights do not satisfy the condition, the outer loadings must satisfy either the coefficient value or the significance value. Coefficient values greater than or equal to 0.5 are indicated by numerical values, and the significant values are indicated by *, **, ***.

Table 7. Coefficients of determination of the models.

Models		R^2	Adj. R^2	Q^2
1	sales	0.548	0.544	0.503
	covid	0.150	0.146	0.093
	night	0.589	0.585	0.246
2	sales	0.367	0.361	0.264
	covid	0.147	0.143	0.087
	night	0.606	0.602	0.241
3	sales	0.301	0.296	0.264
	covid	0.148	0.144	0.089
	night	0.605	0.601	0.239
4	sales	0.387	0.383	0.361
	covid	0.150	0.146	0.094
	night	0.580	0.576	0.244
5	sales	0.498	0.495	0.480
	covid	0.149	0.145	0.093
	night	0.597	0.593	0.247
6	sales	0.354	0.346	0.319
	covid	0.120	0.114	0.100
	night	0.575	0.569	0.229
7	sales	0.508	0.505	0.487
	covid	0.149	0.145	0.092
	night	0.601	0.597	0.247
8	sales	0.369	0.365	0.312
	covid	0.150	0.146	0.093
	night	0.592	0.588	0.245
9	sales	0.284	0.279	0.246
	covid	0.148	0.144	0.089
	night	0.605	0.601	0.239
10	sales	0.403	0.399	0.363
	covid	0.149	0.145	0.092
	night	0.602	0.598	0.248
11	sales	0.274	0.268	0.233
	covid	0.149	0.144	0.093
	night	0.597	0.593	0.246
12	sales	0.037	0.023	−0.004
	covid	0.084	0.077	0.077
	night	0.649	0.644	0.238

The Q^2 value indicates predictive relevance. If the Q^2 value is 0 or higher, the standard is satisfied. According to the analysis, a negative (−) value was obtained for Model 12, which implied that the model had no predictive relevance (Table 7). For the other 11 models, the path model was noted to be a structurally acceptable measurement model [69].

Because this analysis was aimed at verifying the structural relationship of the models, if the predictive power of a measurement model was low, its reliability of the analysis result was low. Therefore, based on the results of previous analyses (evaluation of measurement models and structural model validation), we selected 10 models for the path analysis, after excluding Models 6 and 12 from the subsequent analysis.

Thereafter, we identified the structural relationships of the 10 industries through a path analysis. The results of hypothesis testing and path analysis conducted using the formative measurement model of PLS-SEM are presented in Table A1. Table A1 presents the results of not only the alternative hypothesis representing the research hypothesis, but also the null hypothesis and f^2 value indicating the degree of contribution of the exogenous latent variable to the endogenous latent variable.

The f^2 value indicates the effect size of the causative variable on the resulting variable. When the effect size is between 0.02 and 0.15, the effect of the exogenous latent variable is small. When the effect size is between 0.15 and 0.35, the exogenous latent variable has a moderate effect on the endogenous latent variable. When the effect size is 0.35 or higher, the exogenous latent variable has a strong effect on the endogenous latent variable. The effect size can be represented as "has" or "does not have" and large or small [69]. According to the analysis results, in the relationships in which the *p*-value of the path was insignificant, the f^2 value had no effect or small effect size (Table A1).

As shown in Table A1, we first verified only the hypothesized direct paths. The path analysis results for each hypothesis could be summarized as follows. According to Hypothesis 4, the areas with concentrated operationally non-restricted facilities had a positive (+) effect on the number of confirmed COVID-19 patients, whereas the areas with concentrated operationally restricted facilities did not affect the number of confirmed COVID-19 patients. These results were the same across all 10 models, and the result of Hypothesis 4 could be interpreted as the count of the number of confirmed COVID-19 patients in Korea. Because the number of confirmed COVID-19 patients in Korea was based on resident registration [70], the number of confirmed COVID-19 patients increased in the residential areas, whereas the cultural and commercial areas were not influenced. Therefore, Hypothesis 4, which stated that the effect on the number of confirmed COVID-19 patients differed with the concentration of operationally restricted or non-restricted facilities, was accepted.

Hypotheses 2 and 5 related to night economic vitality were tested. Hypothesis 2, which stated that the number of confirmed COVID-19 patients had a negative (−) effect on the NTEV, was rejected because a positive (+) result was observed for all models. In contrast, Hypothesis 5, which stated that the effect of the model on the NTEV differed depending on whether facilities are operationally restricted or non-restricted, was accepted for all models. Specifically, the results varied across the types of facilities: The operationally non-restricted and restricted facilities had a negative (−) and positive (+) effect on the NTEV, respectively.

The results of Hypotheses 2 and 5 could be interpreted as follows: First, as in the case Hypothesis 5 without a COVID-19 construct, if no pandemic occurred and the facilities were operating in the current state (if the operating hours, number of operations, and number of visitors to the facility were the same as those in the current limited state), the vitality of the night timeslot appeared to be active in areas with concentrated cultural and commercial facilities. Conversely, in residential areas, the vitality of the night timeslot tended to decrease. Moreover, according to Hypothesis 2, more confirmed COVID-19 patients in an area corresponded to a higher nighttime vitality in the area.

These results were more extensively interpreted by examining the mediated paths (restricted/non-restricted facilities → COVID-19 → night in Table A2). Table A2 shows the results of intermediate or indirect paths. The indirect path reflected the indirect effects between two or more variables through the statistical significance between the paths, although no hypotheses were established for this aspect [62]. Therefore, in addition to the hypotheses representing the direct path, we examined various paths through the indirect path.

In a path without the pandemic (Hypothesis 5), the NTEV was invigorated in areas with concentrated cultural and commercial facilities and suppressed in residential areas. In contrast, in the mediated path with the pandemic, the NTEV was invigorated in areas with concentrated residential facilities and not affected in areas with concentrated cultural and commercial facilities. These results highlighted that when the number of confirmed patients was considered, the scope of people's activities changed from cultural and commercial facilities to residential facilities. This finding is attributable to the fact that confirmed patients cannot leave the vicinity of their residences under Korea's COVID-19 regulation policy [70]; thus, people respond sensitively to the number of confirmed patients and reduce the scope of activities near their residences. Consequently, during the pandemic, in residential areas, the number of confirmed patients was high, and simultaneously, the NTEV increased. Moreover, in the areas with concentrated cultural and commercial facilities, no correlation was observed between the number of confirmed patients and NTEV. The result of Hypothesis 2 (COVID-19 had a positive effect on NTEV) could alternatively be interpreted as follows: In both the direct and indirect paths (mediated paths) from the operationally restricted or non-restricted facilities to the NTEV, the coefficient values were larger in the residential areas than those in the cultural and commercial areas, suggesting that the characteristics of the residential areas had a stronger effect on Hypothesis 2.

Hypothesis 1, which stated that the number of confirmed COVID-19 patients negatively (−) affected credit-card sales, was accepted because a negative (−) effect was observed in all nine industries, except the food and beverage industry. In other words, the number of confirmed COVID-19 patients adversely influenced the sales in most industries. In the case of the food and beverage industry, the sales were not affected by the number of confirmed COVID-19 patients because people continued to consume the products, regardless of the pandemic. Furthermore, according to the mediation path (COVID-19 → night → sales in Table A2), even if COVID-19 had an effect, the credit-card sales in all industries increased when using NTEV as the mediation path. These results highlighted that the NTEV factor is important for increasing sales across industries. Upon reconfirming this result based on the direct path between the NTEV and credit-card sales (Hypothesis 6), from which the number of confirmed patients of COVID-19 was removed, it was found that the NTEV had a positive (+) effect on credit-card sales. Thus, Hypothesis 6 was accepted for all models, and we confirmed that the NTEV had a strong positive effect on credit-card sales.

In addition, the paths formed according to the types of facilities were examined. When the COVID-19 factor was removed (restricted/non-restricted facilities → night → sales in Table A2), even when the NTEV was used as a mediated factor, credit-card sales decreased in residential areas but increased in areas with cultural and commercial facilities. When the COVID-19 factor was considered (restricted/non-restricted facilities → covid → night → sales in Table A2), unlike the previous results, credit-card sales increased in residential areas and were unaffected in areas with a concentration of cultural and commercial facilities. Similar to the results of Hypothesis 2 and 5, in the absence of the COVID-19 factor, people's consumption was centered in areas with a concentration of cultural and commercial facilities. In contrast, in the presence of the COVID-19 factor, people's consumption was centered in areas with a concentration of residential facilities. These results demonstrated that the scope of not only the activities, but also the consumption changed around residential areas due to COVID-19.

Hypothesis 3, representing the moderating effect, and Hypothesis 7, representing the control effect, were rejected for all models, except the distribution industry. In the formative measurement model of PLS-SEM, the moderating and control effects were interpreted as being present and absent if the path was significant and not significant, respectively. Therefore, Hypothesis 3, which stated that the number of confirmed COVID-19 patients had an effect as a moderating variable on the relationship between the NTEV and credit-card sales, was accepted only in the distribution industry (Model 2) owing to the significant effect in the negative (−) direction. For the remaining nine models, the hypothesis was rejected, confirming that the number of confirmed COVID-19 patients did not have any moderating effect. In addition, the control effect of the environmental factor (Hypothesis 7) appeared to be significantly positive (+) in the distribution industry, indicating that the control effect was present. In contrast, no effect was observed for the other nine models. The significant result obtained for the moderating effect of COVID-19 in the relationship between the NTEV and credit-card sales of the distribution industry indicated that sales decreased because of COVID-19 in typical distribution industries, such as large supermarkets and department stores. Moreover, the significant result obtained for the control effect in the distribution industry indicated that the environmental factors had a positive effect in terms of increasing sales in the distribution industry. This result is consistent with that of a previous study [71], which indicated that the distribution industry was negatively (−) affected by COVID-19 but positively (+) affected by environmental factors, such as temperature and precipitation, compared to other industries.

Finally, because the relationship between the paths was not the same across all the models, Hypothesis 8, which stated that the structural relationship of the models differed according to the industry, was accepted.

4.3. Discussion

According to the path analysis and hypothesis testing using 10 models with 10 indicators for each model, Hypothesis 4, Hypothesis 5, and Hypothesis 6 were accepted for all models, and Hypothesis 2 was rejected for all models. Hypothesis 1 was accepted for all models, except the food and beverage industry, and Hypothesis 3 and Hypothesis 7 were rejected for all models, except the distribution industry. Hypothesis 8 was accepted (the structural relationships differed by industry).

The structural relationship derived in this study can be interpreted as follows (Appendices B and C): First, the number of confirmed COVID-19 patients changes the scope of people's activities and consumption spaces. If the impact of COVID-19 is not considered, people's consumption and nighttime activities are enhanced in areas with a concentration of cultural and commercial facilities compared to those in areas with a concentration of residential facilities. In other words, if the operating hours of commercial facilities are shortened or the number of operations of cultural facilities is reduced (as in the current scenario) and the factor of the number of confirmed COVID-19 patients is absent, people would consume and engage in nighttime activities in areas with a concentration of cultural and commercial facilities. In contrast, if the COVID-19 impact spreads, and the number of confirmed patients increases, people's consumption and nighttime activity spaces may change from cultural and commercial facilities to residential facilities. These results are consistent with those of several previous studies [50,51] that indicated that people focused their activities in residential areas due to COVID-19.

Second, because of the effect of Korea's COVID-19 regulation policy, people's activities are concentrated around residential areas rather than cultural and commercial areas as the effect of COVID-19 intensifies. Korea has restricted the operating hours of cultural and commercial facilities as a part of its COVID-19 policy. Consequently, in the paths in which the number of confirmed COVID-19 patients was included, the activity patterns in the areas with a concentration of cultural and commercial facilities, where operations were restricted, and those in the areas with a concentration of residential facilities, where operations were not restricted, were reversed. These phenomena are attributable to the effect of the COVID-19 policy that limited the scope of people's activities to areas with a concentration of residential facilities.

Third, the NTEV is a major factor influencing the increase in the sales of various industries. In the direct path between the NTEV and credit-card sales, the NTEV had a positive effect on the credit-card sales. Moreover, in the mediated path between COVID-19, NTEV, and credit-card sales, the NTEV led to increased credit-card sales. In the direct path between COVID-19 and credit-card sales, the latter decreased owing to the number of confirmed patients, but in the indirect path between COVID-19, NTEV, and credit-card sales, the latter increased due to the NTEV input. Therefore, the analysis results of this study support the results of previous studies [5,12,72] that the local economy is vitalized when the local NTEV is activated.

5. Conclusions

The NTE invigorates night consumption markets and vitalizes cities. Therefore, major cities worldwide have taken increased interest in the NTE as a measure to boost urban economies, enhance citizens' leisure and tourism activities, and revitalize cities that have been affected by COVID-19 [73]. However, the understanding of and interest in the NTE and NTEV in Korea is inadequate. Moreover, NTE-related academic research in Korea has mainly been conducted in the field of tourism studies. In the field of urban studies, only limited research has been performed to measure the urban vitality through nighttime satellite imagery. None of the existing studies on the NTE have reflected the limited operating hours in response to the COVID-19 pandemic.

Therefore, this study has the following academic contributions to Korean research: We attempted to empirically analyze the concept of the NTE, which is being actively studied globally but has not been sufficiently reviewed in Korea. Moreover, we developed quantitative indicators of NTEV for Korea by applying the NTE concept to urban studies, which have otherwise focused mainly on the qualitative indicators used in tourism-related studies. This study is timely, in that, it exploratorily confirms the structural relationship between NTEV, COVID-19, and credit-card sales in Seoul, where the COVID-19 regulation pertaining to operating restrictions was applied the most strictly in Korea.

According to a comparison of the results of this study to those of previous studies, the relationship between NTEV and credit-card sales was identified in the same context as that in the studies of Lin et al. and Fu et al. [5,72]. In other words, we confirmed that the NTEV activates the consumption economy of the entire city [39,72,74]. Moreover, the analysis results of the relationship between COVID-19 and NTEV were similar to those reported in several previous studies. Jo et al. reported that the consumer behavior was strongly affected only in the early stages of COVID-19, and since then, daily life has been maintained to a certain extent as the pandemic has become commonplace [45]. Kim and Lim and Choi reported that people's activities increased in residential areas during the COVID-19 outbreak [50,51]. Thus, the analysis results of this study can be interpreted as being consistent with those of previous studies. In addition, the analysis results indicating that the influence relationships differ by industry are consistent with the results of previous studies [45,46]. Therefore, the academic implication of this study is to integrate the results obtained in the existing studies through a structural relationship.

The policy implications of this study, which would be valuable to managers and investors in the urban fields, are as follows: First, we confirmed that the COVID-19 pandemic hit the urban economy. Most industries, such as restaurant and entertainment; distribution; clothing and merchandise; sports, culture, and leisure; beauty; life services; education and academy, medical care, and; furniture and home appliances, experienced decreased sales due to COVID-19. We verified that Seoul's commercial district experienced a downturn owing to an increase in the number of confirmed COVID-19 patients and restrictions on operating hours, and assigned weight to the claim of economic damage to self-employment due to COVID-19 spreading. Second, we confirmed the importance of the NTEV. Our results indicated that the number of confirmed COVID-19 patients negatively affected credit-card sales, but if NTEV were to be used as a mediated factor, it was expected to have a positive effect. In other words, the NTEV is crucial for revitalizing the urban economy that has stagnated due to the pandemic, and policymakers must implement various projects to revitalize the night timeslot. Third, we confirmed the effectiveness of Korea's COVID-19 policy. An analysis of the facilities subjected and not subjected to operating restrictions under the social-distancing policy revealed that during the pandemic, people's activities and consumption were concentrated in residential areas, as opposed to cultural and commercial areas. Consequently, Korea's COVID-19 regulation policy, which restricted activities in cultural and commercial facilities, was effective in terms of enforcing quarantine. Fourth, the structural relationships differed across industries, which indicated that the government's response and policy measures must be tailored in the light of COVID-19.

This study represents a basic study on NTEV in Korea, focused on exploring and identifying the structural relationship between COVID-19, NTEV, and credit-card sales. We systematically analyzed the formative measurement model, which is relatively difficult to interpret and analyze among the PLS-SEM methods, using urban statistical data. Moreover, we applied the NTE theory, which has mainly been used in the tourism field, to urban studies. Therefore, this study can be rated as a high-quality study in terms of its research contribution and importance, pertaining to the expansion of structural equation data and techniques (use of a formative measurement model of structural equations in conjunction with nonnormal statistical data) and theories and topics (NTE and NTEV) to urban studies.

However, this study has a limitation, in that, it was not able to identify individual variables that affected credit-card sales by industry because the structural influence relationships between the constructs were identified owing to the exploratory nature of the study. In addition, the analysis results obtained in this study cannot be generalized because the effect of the COVID-19 policy was indirectly evaluated considering the restrictions and lack thereof on facility operation. Referring to the structural relationships presented in this study, future work can be used to perform time-series studies rather than cross-sectional studies and identify individual factors affecting credit-card sales or the NTEV by industry.

Author Contributions: Conceptualization: S.-a.K. and H.K.; methodology: S.-a.K.; validation: S.-a.K. and H.K.; formal analysis: S.-a.K.; investigation: S.-a.K.; resources: S.-a.K.; data curation: S.-a.K.; writing—original draft preparation: S.-a.K.; writing—review and editing: S.-a.K.; visualization: S.-a.K.; supervision: H.K.; project administration: H.K. All authors have read and agreed to the published version of the manuscript.

Funding: This research received no external funding.

Data Availability Statement: Not applicable.

Conflicts of Interest: The authors declare no conflict of interest.

Appendix A

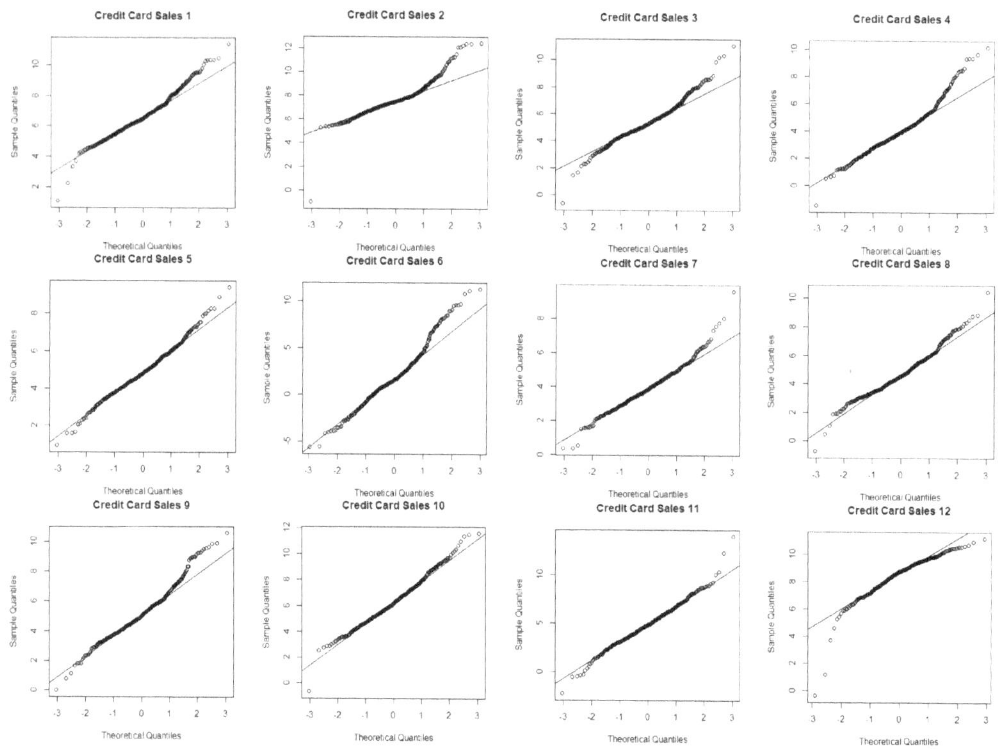

Figure A1. *Cont.*

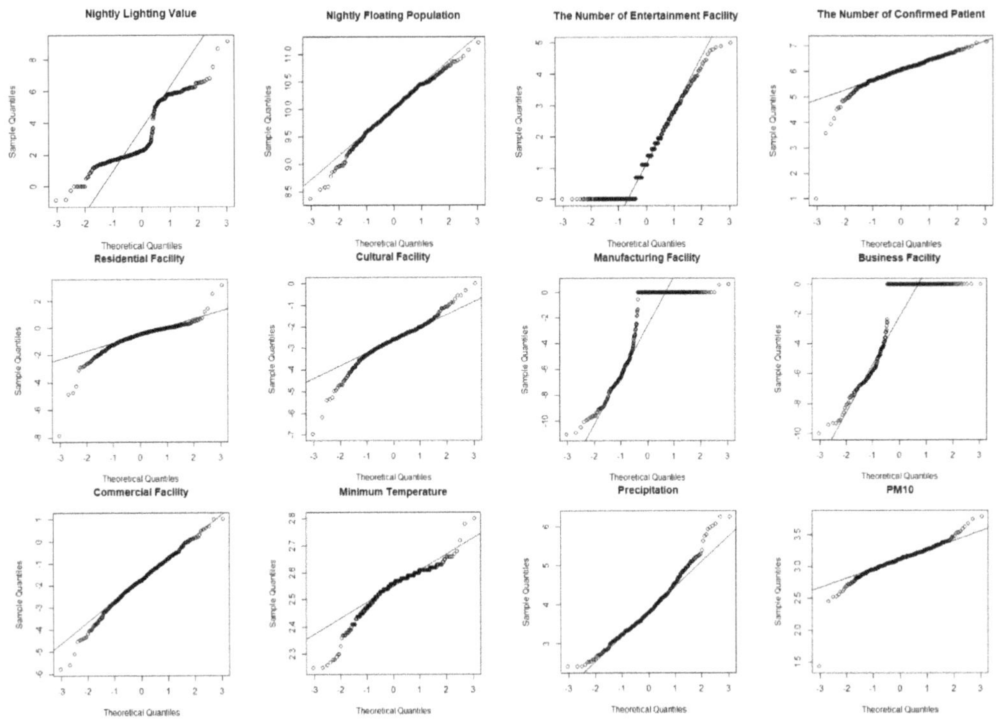

Figure A1. Q-Q Plot (Quantile-Quantile Plot) after log. Credit card sales 1 → restaurant and entertainment; credit card sales 2 → distribution; credit card sales 3 → food and beverage; credit card sales 4 → clothing and merchandise; sales 5 → credit card sales 5 → sports, culture and leisure; credit card sales 6 → travel and accommodation; credit card sales 7 → beauty; credit card sales 8 → life service; credit card sales 9 → education and academy; credit card sales 10 → medical care; credit card sales 11 → furniture, home appliances and automobiles; credit card sales 12 → refueling.

Appendix B

Table A1. Path and f^2 analysis results.

Model 1	Path Coefficients	t Statistics	f^2	Hypotheses	Hypotheses Test
COVID → sales	−0.415 ***	5.880	0.179	Hypothesis 1	H_0 Reject
					H_1 Accept
COVID → night	0.645 ***	11.441	0.693	Hypothesis 2	H_0 Accept
					H_1 Reject
COVID * → sales	−0.125	1.525	0.065	Hypothesis 3	H_0 Accept
					H_1 Reject
non-restric. → COVID	0.406 ***	3.389	0.167	Hypothesis 4	H_0 Reject
restric. → COVID	−0.062	0.902	0.004		H_1 Accept
non-restric. → night	−0.283 **	2.882	0.107	Hypothesis 5	H_0 Reject
restric. → night	0.494 ***	7.285	0.505		H_1 Accept

Table A1. *Cont.*

Model 1	Path Coefficients	t Statistics	f^2	Hypotheses	Hypotheses Test
night → sales	0.806 ***	14.085	0.864	Hypothesis 6	H_0 Reject H_1 Accept
evir → sales	0.217 ***	5.989	0.095	Hypothesis 7	H_0 Accept
evir → night	0.070	1.210	0.008		H_1 Reject
Model 2	**Path Coefficients**	**t Statistics**	f^2	**Hypotheses**	**Hypotheses Test**
COVID → sales	−0.174 **	1.985	0.016	Hypothesis 1	H_0 Reject H_1 Accept
COVID → night	0.730 ***	14.160	0.901	Hypothesis 2	H_0 Accept H_1 Reject
COVID * → sales	−0.127 *	1.770	0.053	Hypothesis 3	H_0 Reject H_1 Accept
non-restric. → COVID	0.402 ***	3.479	0.153	Hypothesis 4	H_0 Reject
restric. → COVID	−0.047	0.625	0.002		H_1 Accept
non-restric. → night	−0.232 **	2.568	0.069	Hypothesis 5	H_0 Reject
restric. → night	0.313 ***	3.293	0.199		H_1 Accept
night → sales	0.595 ***	7.233	0.252	Hypothesis 6	H_0 Reject H_1 Accept
evir → sales	0.110 **	2.498	0.017	Hypothesis 7	H_0 Reject
evir → night	0.100 *	1.768	0.017		H_1 Accept
Model 3	**Path Coefficients**	**t Statistics**	f^2	**Hypotheses**	**Hypotheses Test**
COVID → sales	0.043	0.548	0.001	Hypothesis 1	H_0 Accept H_1 Reject
COVID → night	0.723 ***	12.409	0.818	Hypothesis 2	H_0 Accept H_1 Reject
COVID * → sales	−0.027	0.576	0.002	Hypothesis 3	H_0 Accept H_1 Reject
non-restric. → COVID	0.402 ***	3.501	0.151	Hypothesis 4	H_0 Reject
restric. → COVID	−0.042	0.565	0.002		H_1 Accept
non-restric. → night	−0.205 **	2.050	0.048	Hypothesis 5	H_0 Reject
restric. → night	0.283 **	2.811	0.162		H_1 Accept
night → sales	0.503 ***	7.451	0.159	Hypothesis 6	H_0 Reject H_1 Accept
evir → sales	−0.005	0.107	0.000	Hypothesis 7	H_0 Accept
evir → night	0.129	1.319	0.024		H_1 Reject
Model 4	**Path Coefficients**	**t Statistics**	f^2	**Hypotheses**	**Hypotheses Test**
COVID → sales	−0.320 ***	4.483	0.086	Hypothesis 1	H_0 Reject H_1 Accept
COVID → night	0.626 ***	10.663	0.658	Hypothesis 2	H_0 Accept H_1 Reject
COVID * → sales	−0.068	1.162	0.014	Hypothesis 3	H_0 Accept H_1 Reject

Table A1. *Cont.*

Model 4	Path Coefficients	t Statistics	f^2	Hypotheses	Hypotheses Test
non-restric. → COVID	0.405 ***	3.362	0.168	Hypothesis 4	H_0 Reject
restric. → COVID	−0.063	0.946	0.004		H_1 Accept
non-restric. → night	−0.294 **	2.997	0.118	Hypothesis 5	H_0 Reject
restric. → night	0.521 ***	7.175	0.549		H_1 Accept
night → sales	0.713 ***	14.546	0.535	Hypothesis 6	H_0 Reject H_1 Accept
evir → sales	0.111 **	2.483	0.019	Hypothesis 7	H_0 Accept
evir → night	0.054	0.888	0.005		H_1 Reject
Model 5	**Path Coefficients**	**t Statistics**	f^2	**Hypotheses**	**Hypotheses Test**
COVID → sales	−0.348 ***	4.829	0.105	Hypothesis 1	H_0 Reject H_1 Accept
COVID → night	0.663 ***	11.909	0.706	Hypothesis 2	H_0 Accept H_1 Reject
COVID * → sales	−0.058	1.050	0.013	Hypothesis 3	H_0 Accept H_1 Reject
non-restric. → COVID	0.406 ***	3.442	0.165	Hypothesis 4	H_0 Reject
restric. → COVID	−0.060	0.845	0.004		H_1 Accept
non-restric. → night	−0.267 **	2.551	0.089	Hypothesis 5	H_0 Reject
restric. → night	0.459 ***	6.568	0.442		H_1 Accept
night → sales	0.835 ***	18.422	0.792	Hypothesis 6	H_0 Reject H_1 Accept
evir → sales	0.102 **	2.640	0.019	Hypothesis 7	H_0 Accept
evir → night	0.095	1.423	0.014		H_1 Reject
Model 7	**Path Coefficients**	**t Statistics**	f^2	**Hypotheses**	**Hypotheses Test**
COVID → sales	−0.211 **	3.070	0.037	Hypothesis 1	H_0 Reject H_1 Accept
COVID → night	0.695 ***	13.257	0.835	Hypothesis 2	H_0 Accept H_1 Reject
COVID * → sales	−0.048	0.856	0.009	Hypothesis 3	H_0 Accept H_1 Reject
non-restric. → COVID	0.406 ***	3.404	0.163	Hypothesis 4	H_0 Reject
restric. → COVID	−0.058	0.817	0.003		H_1 Accept
non-restric. → night	−0.279 **	2.885	0.107	Hypothesis 5	H_0 Reject
restric. → night	0.430 ***	6.020	0.384		H_1 Accept
night → sales	0.825 ***	16.955	0.744	Hypothesis 6	H_0 Reject H_1 Accept
evir → sales	−0.008	0.170	0.000	Hypothesis 7	H_0 Accept
evir → night	0.070	1.052	0.009		H_1 Reject

Table A1. *Cont.*

Model 8	Path Coefficients	t Statistics	f^2	Hypotheses	Hypotheses Test
COVID → sales	−0.351 ***	3.867	0.092	Hypothesis 1	H_0 Reject H_1 Accept
COVID → night	0.659 ***	10.808	0.720	Hypothesis 2	H_0 Accept H_1 Reject
COVID* → sales	−0.110	1.420	0.037	Hypothesis 3	H_0 Accept H_1 Reject
non-restric. → COVID	0.406 ***	3.421	0.166	Hypothesis 4	H_0 Reject
restric. → COVID	−0.061	0.866	0.004		H_1 Accept
non-restric. → night	−0.285 **	2.893	0.107	Hypothesis 5	H_0 Reject
restric. → night	0.479 ***	5.621	0.475		H_1 Accept
night → sales	0.680 ***	10.140	0.445	Hypothesis 6	H_0 Reject H_1 Accept
evir → sales	0.191 ***	4.784	0.055	Hypothesis 7	H_0 Accept
evir → night	0.070	1.200	0.008		H_1 Reject
Model 9	**Path Coefficients**	**t Statistics**	f^2	**Hypotheses**	**Hypotheses Test**
COVID → sales	−0.346 ***	4.268	0.055	Hypothesis 1	H_0 Reject H_1 Accept
COVID → night	0.721 ***	12.511	0.815	Hypothesis 2	H_0 Accept H_1 Reject
COVID * → sales	−0.077	1.433	0.017	Hypothesis 3	H_0 Accept H_1 Reject
non-restric. → COVID	0.402 ***	3.527	0.152	Hypothesis 4	H_0 Reject
restric. → COVID	−0.043	0.563	0.002		H_1 Accept
non-restric. → night	−0.207 **	2.079	0.049	Hypothesis 5	H_0 Reject
restric. → night	0.289 **	2.764	0.169		H_1 Accept
night → sales	0.712 ***	11.348	0.316	Hypothesis 6	H_0 Reject H_1 Accept
evir → sales	0.012	0.258	0.000	Hypothesis 7	H_0 Accept
evir → night	0.129	1.359	0.023		H_1 Reject
Model 10	**Path Coefficients**	**t Statistics**	f^2	**Hypotheses**	**Hypotheses Test**
COVID → sales	−0.179 **	2.302	0.022	Hypothesis 1	H_0 Reject H_1 Accept
COVID → night	0.682 ***	11.759	0.762	Hypothesis 2	H_0 Accept H_1 Reject
COVID* → sales	−0.079	1.396	0.021	Hypothesis 3	H_0 Accept H_1 Reject
non-restric. → COVID	0.406 ***	3.476	0.163	Hypothesis 4	H_0 Reject
restric. → COVID	−0.058	0.820	0.003		H_1 Accept
non-restric. → night	−0.263 **	2.567	0.087	Hypothesis 5	H_0 Reject
restric. → night	0.429 ***	5.390	0.387		H_1 Accept

Table A1. *Cont.*

Model 10	Path Coefficients	t Statistics	f^2	Hypotheses	Hypotheses Test
night → sales	0.727 ***	12.532	0.482	Hypothesis 6	H_1 Accept
evir → sales	−0.031	0.668	0.002	Hypothesis 7	H_0 Accept
evir → night	0.096	1.107	0.015		H_1 Reject
Model 11	**Path Coefficients**	**t Statistics**	f^2	**Hypotheses**	**Hypotheses Test**
COVID → sales	−0.237 **	2.937	0.034	Hypothesis 1	H_0 Reject
					H_1 Accept
COVID → night	0.670 ***	10.759	0.744	Hypothesis 2	H_0 Accept
					H_1 Reject
COVID* → sales	−0.056	1.360	0.008	Hypothesis 3	H_0 Accept
					H_1 Reject
non-restric. → COVID	0.406 ***	3.447	0.165	Hypothesis 4	H_0 Reject
restric. → COVID	−0.060	0.850	0.004		H_1 Accept
snon-restric. → night	−0.276 **	2.744	0.099	Hypothesis 5	H_0 Reject
restric. → night	0.458 ***	4.906	0.439		H_1 Accept
night → sales	0.596 ***	10.869	0.277	Hypothesis 6	H_0 Reject
					H_1 Accept
evir → sales	0.106 **	2.168	0.014	Hypothesis 7	H_0 Accept
evir → night	0.081	1.217	0.011		H_1 Reject

* $p < 0.05$, ** $p < 0.01$, *** $p < 0.001$

Appendix C

Table A2. Detailed path analysis results.

Path Coefficients	Model 1	Model 2	Model 3	Model 4	Model 5
non-restric. → night → sales	−0.228	−0.138	−0.103	−0.210	−0.223
restric. → night → sales	0.398	0.186	0.143	0.372	0.383
non-restric. → COVID → sales	−0.168	−0.070	0.017	−0.130	−0.141
restric. → COVID → sales	0.026	0.008	−0.002	0.020	0.021
non-restric. → COVID → night	0.262	0.293	0.290	0.254	0.269
restric. → COVID → night	−0.040	−0.035	−0.031	−0.039	−0.040
COVID → night → sales	0.520	0.434	0.364	0.447	0.553
non-restric. → COVID → night → sales	0.211	0.174	0.146	0.181	0.224
restric. → COVID → night → sales	−0.032	−0.021	−0.015	−0.028	−0.033
Path Coefficients	**Model 7**	**Model 8**	**Model 9**	**Model 10**	**Model 11**
non-restric. → night → sales	−0.230	−0.194	−0.147	−0.191	−0.164
restric. → night → sales	0.355	0.326	0.206	0.312	0.273
non-restric. → COVID → sales	−0.086	−0.142	−0.139	−0.073	−0.096
restric. → COVID → sales	0.012	0.021	0.015	0.010	0.014
non-restric. → COVID → night	0.282	0.267	0.290	0.277	0.272
restric. → COVID → night	−0.041	−0.040	−0.031	−0.040	−0.040
COVID → night → sales	0.573	0.448	0.513	0.496	0.400
non-restric. → COVID → night → sales	0.232	0.182	0.206	0.201	0.162
restric. → COVID → night → sales	−0.033	−0.027	−0.022	−0.029	−0.024

References

1. Bashir, M.F.; Ma, B.; Shahzad, L. A brief review of socio-economic and environmental impact of COVID-19. *Air Qual. Atmos. Health* **2020**, *13*, 1403–1409. [CrossRef] [PubMed]
2. Brookings. Available online: https://www.brookings.edu/blog/the-avenue/2020/03/17/the-places-a-covid-19-recession-will-likely-hit-hardest (accessed on 3 January 2022).
3. Khaliq, M. Impact of the coronavirus (COVID-19) pandemic on retail sales in 2020. *Off. Natl. Stat.* **2021**, *1*, 1–14.
4. Zuo, F.; Wang, J.; Gao, J.; Ozbay, K.; Ban, X.J.; Shen, Y.; Yang, H.; Iyer, S. An interactive data visualization and analytics tool to evaluate mobility and sociability trends during COVID-19. In *Human Computer Interaction*; Cornell University: New York, NY, USA, 2020.
5. Lin, V.S.; Qin, Y.; Ying, T.; Shen, S.; Lyu, G. Night-time economy vitality index: Framework and evidence. *Tour. Econ.* **2021**, *28*, 665–691. [CrossRef]
6. Zhang, Y.; Zhong, W.; Wang, D.; Lin, F.T. Understanding the spatiotemporal patterns of nighttime urban vibrancy in central Shanghai inferred from mobile phone data. *Reg. Sustain.* **2021**, *2*, 297. [CrossRef]
7. CNN. Available online: http://edition.cnn.com/2010/TRAVEL/10/26/seoul.guide/index (accessed on 3 January 2022).
8. Hankyoreh. Available online: https://english.hani.co.kr/arti/english_edition/e_business/961298 (accessed on 3 January 2022).
9. Chatterton, P.; Hollands, R. Theorising urban playscapes: Producing, regulating consuming youthful nightlife city spaces. *Urban Stud.* **2002**, *1*, 95–116. [CrossRef]
10. Beer, C. Centres that never sleep? Planning for the night-time economy within the commercial centres of Australian cities. *Aust. Plan.* **2011**, *48*, 141–147. [CrossRef]
11. Shaw, R. Beyond night-time economy: Affective atmospheres of the urban night. *Geoforum* **2014**, *51*, 87–95. [CrossRef]
12. Grazian, D. Urban Nightlife, Social Capital, and the Public Life of Cities. *Sociol. Forum* **2009**, *24*, 908–917. [CrossRef]
13. Jacobs, J. *The Death and Life of Great American Cities*; Random House: New York, NY, USA, 1961; Volume 41.
14. China Tourism Academy. Available online: http://www.ctaweb.org.cn (accessed on 3 January 2022).
15. Korea Tourism Organization. Available online: https://kto.visitkorea.or.kr/eng (accessed on 3 January 2022).
16. Hobbs, D.; Hadfield, P.; Lister, S.; Winlow, S. *Bouncers: Violence and Governance in the Night-Time Economy*; Oxford University Press: Oxford, UK, 2003; pp. 1–336.
17. Roberts, M. *Good Practice in Managing the Evening and Late Night Economy: A Literature Review from an Environmental Perspective*; Office of the Deputy Prime Minister: London, UK, 2004; pp. 1–54.
18. Philpot, R.; Liebst, L.S.; Møller, K.K.; Lindegaard, M.R.; Levine, M. Capturing violence in the night-time economy: A review of established and emerging methodologies. *Aggress. Violent Behav.* **2019**, *46*, 56–65. [CrossRef]
19. Hobbs, D.; Lister, S.; Hadfield, P.; Winlow, S.; Hall, S. Receiving shadows: Governance and liminality in the night-time economy. *Br. J. Sociol.* **2000**, *51*, 701–717. [CrossRef]
20. Hayward, K.; Hobbs, D. Beyond the binge in? booze Britain?: Market-led liminalization and the spectacle of binge drinking. *Br. J. Sociol.* **2007**, *58*, 437–456. [CrossRef]
21. Monaghan, L.F. Regulating 'unruly' bodies: Work tasks, conflict and violence in Britain's night-time economy. *Br. J. Sociol.* **2010**, *53*, 403–429. [CrossRef] [PubMed]
22. Hollands, R. Divisions in the dark: Youth cultures, transitions and segmented consumption spaces in the night-time economy. *J. Youth Stud.* **2002**, *5*, 153–171. [CrossRef]
23. Talbot, D. *Regulating the Night: Race, Culture and Exclusion in the Making of the Night-Time Economy*; Routledge: London, UK, 2007; pp. 1–164.
24. Eldridge, A. The urban renaissance and the night-time economy: Who belongs in the city at night? In *Social Sustainability in Urban Areas*; Routledge: London, UK, 2010; pp. 201–216.
25. Hadfield, P. The night-time city four modes of exclusion: Reflections on the urban studies special collection. *Urban Stud.* **2015**, *52*, 606–616. [CrossRef]
26. Song, H.; Kim, M.; Park, C. Temporal distribution as a solution for over-tourism in night tourism: The case of Suwon Hwaseong in South Korea. *Sustainability* **2020**, *12*, 2182. [CrossRef]
27. Kim, H.; Choi, S.; Park, H. An analysis in city tourist behavior at day and night time: Focused on Mokpo city in Jeonnam province. *Culin. Sci. Hosp. Res.* **2020**, *26*, 19–24.
28. McArthur, J.; Robin, E.; Smeds, E. Socio-spatial and temporal dimensions of transport equity for London's night time economy. *Transp. Res. Part A Policy Pract.* **2019**, *121*, 433–443. [CrossRef]
29. French of Ministry of Industry. Annexes. *Rapp. Énergies 2050* **2012**, 1–220.
30. Rowe, D.; Stevenson, D.; Tomsen, S.; Bavinton, N.; Brass, K. *The City after Dark: Cultural Planning and Governance of the Night-Time Economy in Parramatta*; University of Western Sydney: Penrith, Australia, 2008; pp. 1–44.
31. Bianchini, F. Night cultures, night economies. *Plan. Pract. Res.* **1995**, *10*, 121–126. [CrossRef]
32. Tiesdell, S.; Slater, A.M. Calling time: Managing activities in space and time in the evening/night-time economy. *Plan. Theory Pract.* **2006**, *7*, 137–157. [CrossRef]
33. Thomas, C.J.; Bromley, R.D.F. City-centre revitalisation: Problems of fragmentation and fear in the evening and night-time city. *Urban Stud.* **2000**, *37*, 1403–1429. [CrossRef]

34. NYC. Available online: https://www1.nyc.gov/assets/mome/pdf/NYC_Nightlife_Economic_Impact_Report_2019_digital.pdf (accessed on 25 January 2022).
35. Diplomacy, S.; Seijas, A. *A Guide to Managing Your Night Time Economy*; Sound Diplomacy: London, UK, 2018; pp. 1–37.
36. NSW. Available online: https://www.planning.nsw.gov.au/Policy-and-Legislation/Night-Time-Economy/Guide-for-establishing-and-managing-NTE-uses (accessed on 25 January 2022).
37. Rawski, T.G. What is happening to China's GDP statistics? *China Econ. Rev.* **2001**, *12*, 347–354. [CrossRef]
38. Doll, C.N.; Muller, J.P.; Morley, J.G. Mapping regional economic activity from night-time light satellite imagery. *Ecol. Econ.* **2006**, *57*, 75–92. [CrossRef]
39. Henderson, J.V.; Storeygard, A.; Weil, D.N. Measuring economic growth from outer space. *Am. Econ. Rev.* **2012**, *102*, 994–1028. [CrossRef] [PubMed]
40. Zhong, Y.; Lin, A.; Zhou, Z.; Chen, F. Spatial pattern evolution and optimization of urban system in the Yangtze River economic belt, China, based on DMSP-OLS night light data. *Sustainability* **2018**, *10*, 3782. [CrossRef]
41. Seoul. Available online: https://data.seoul.go.kr/dataVisual/seoul/ (accessed on 7 February 2022).
42. Zikriya, L.; Mahmood, K.; Zaidi, S.I.H.; Hussain, S.; Asim, M. Development of an indigenous scale on Resilience in Urdu. *Ilkogr. Online* **2021**, *20*, 7739–7746.
43. Xia, C.; Yeh, A.G.O.; Zhang, A. Analyzing spatial relationships between urban land use intensity and urban vitality at street block level: A case study of five Chinese megacities. *Landsc. Urban Plan.* **2020**, *193*, 103669. [CrossRef]
44. Jeong, S.Y.; Jun, B.W. Urban vitality assessment using spatial big data and nighttime light satellite image: A case study of Daegu. *J. Korean Assoc. Geogr. Inf. Stud.* **2020**, *23*, 217–233.
45. Jo, H.; Shin, E.; Kim, H. Changes in Consumer Behaviour in the Post-COVID-19 Era in Seoul, South Korea. *Sustainability* **2021**, *13*, 136. [CrossRef]
46. Horvath, A.; Kay, B.S.; Wix, C. The COVID-19 shock and consumer credit: Evidence from credit card data. *Soc. Sci. Res. Netw.* **2021**, *3*, 1–54.
47. Zhou, K.; Ye, J.; Liu, X.X. Is cash perceived as more valuable than digital money? The mediating effect of psychological ownership and psychological distance. *Mark. Lett.* **2022**, 1–14. [CrossRef]
48. Bank of Korea. Available online: http://www.bok.or.kr/ (accessed on 7 February 2022).
49. Seoul. Available online: https://mediahub.seoul.go.kr/archives/2002021 (accessed on 7 February 2022).
50. Kim, Y.L. A Big Data Analysis of Floating Population Network in the Seoul Metropolitan Area in the COVID Era. *Gyeonggi Res. Inst.* **2021**, *6*, 1–76.
51. Lim, H.J.; Choi, S.B. Analysis of the Effect of COVID-19 on Changes in Sales in Commercial Districts of Seoul, Korea. *Seoul Inst.* **2022**, *23*, 47–65.
52. Yan, L.; Duartea, F.; Wang, D.; Zheng, S.; Ratti, C. Exploring the effect of air pollution on social activity in China using geotagged social media check-in data. *Cities* **2019**, *91*, 116–125. [CrossRef]
53. Keiser, D.; Lade, G.; Rudik, I. Air pollution and visitation at US national parks. *Sci. Adv.* **2018**, *4*, 1613. [CrossRef] [PubMed]
54. Kang, H.J.; Suh, H.D.; Yu, J.M. Does Air Pollution Affect Consumption Behavior? Evidence from Korean Retail Sales. *Asian Econ. J.* **2019**, *33*, 235–251. [CrossRef]
55. Seoul. Available online: https://smart.seoul.go.kr/board/41/1243/board_view.do (accessed on 7 February 2022).
56. Sun, L.; Gao, F.; Anderson, M.C.; Kustas, W.P.; Alsina, M.M.; Sanchez, L.; Sams, B.; McKee, L.G.; Dulaney, W.P.; White, A.; et al. Daily mapping of 30 m LAI and NDVI for grape yield prediction in California vineyards. *Remote Sens.* **2017**, *9*, 317. [CrossRef]
57. U.S. Geological Survey. Available online: https://www.usgs.gov/ (accessed on 14 March 2022).
58. Kim, K.; An, Y. An Empirical study on the definition and classification methodology of urban heat island areas. *J. Korean Reg. Sci. Assoc.* **2017**, *33*, 47–59.
59. Zeng, N.; Liu, Y.; Gong, P.; Hertogh, M.; König, M. Do right PLS and do PLS right: A critical review of the application of PLS-SEM in construction management research. *Front. Eng. Manag.* **2021**, *8*, 356–369. [CrossRef]
60. Zhang, C.; Liu, Y.; Lu, W.; Xiao, G. Evaluating passenger satisfaction index based on PLS-SEM model: Evidence from Chinese public transport service. *Transp. Res. Part A Policy Pract.* **2019**, *120*, 149–164. [CrossRef]
61. Henseler, J.; Sarstedt, M. Goodness-of-fit indices for partial least squares path modeling. *Comput. Stat.* **2013**, *28*, 565–580. [CrossRef]
62. Hair, J.F., Jr.; Sarstedt, M.; Ringle, C.M.; Gudergan, S.P. *Advanced Issues in Partial Least Squares Structural Equation Modeling*; Sage Publications: New York, NY, USA, 2017; pp. 1–272.
63. Diamantopoulos, A. The Error Term in Formative Measurement Models: Interpretation and Modeling Implications. *J. Model. Manag.* **2006**, *1*, 7–17. [CrossRef]
64. Edwards, J.R.; Bagozzi, R.P. On the nature and direction of relationships between constructs and measures. *Psychol. Methods* **2000**, *5*, 155. [CrossRef] [PubMed]
65. Hair, J.F.; Ringle, C.M.; Sarstedt, M. PLS-SEM: Indeed a silver bullet. *J. Mark. Theory Pract.* **2011**, *19*, 139–152. [CrossRef]
66. Kock, N.; Lynn, G.S. Lateral collinearity and misleading results in variance-based SEM: An illustration and recommendations. *J. Assoc. Inf. Syst.* **2012**, *13*, 546–580. [CrossRef]
67. Bruhn, M.; Georgi, D.; Hadwich, K. Customer equity management as formative second-order construct. *J. Bus. Res.* **2008**, *61*, 1292–1301. [CrossRef]

68. Jingwen, M.; Shengchuan, Z.; Wu, L. Do Shrinking Cities Correlate with the Demographic Aging Process? Evidence from Shrinking Cities in China. *China City Plan. Rev.* **2022**, *31*, 33–42.
69. Hair, J.; Hult, T.; Ringle, C.; Sarstedt, M. *A Primer on Partial Least Squares Structural Equation Modeling (PLS-SEM)*; Sage Publications: New York, NY, USA, 2017; p. 207.
70. Korea Centers for Disease Control and Prevention. Available online: https://kdca.go.kr/ (accessed on 16 September 2022).
71. Han, S.L.; Moon, J. Impact of environmental changes on offline distribution channel sales. *J. Channel Retail.* **2020**, *25*, 31–51. [CrossRef]
72. Fu, H.; Shao, Z.; Fu, P.; Cheng, Q. The dynamic analysis between urban nighttime economy and urbanization using the DMSP/OLS nighttime light data in China from 1992 to 2012. *Remote Sens.* **2017**, *9*, 416. [CrossRef]
73. Seijas, A.; Gelders, M. Governing the Night-time City: The Rise of Night Mayors as a New Form of Urban Governance After Dark. *Urban Stud.* **2019**, *58*, 316–334. [CrossRef]
74. Chen, T.; Hui, E.C.; Wu, J.; Lang, W.; Li, X. Identifying urban spatial structure and urban vibrancy in highly dense cities using georeferenced social media data. *Habitat Int.* **2019**, *89*, 102005. [CrossRef]

buildings

MDPI

Article

Measuring Street Network Efficiency and Block Sizes in Superblocks—Addressing the Gap between Policy and Practice

Rim Anabtawi and Martin Scoppa *

Department of Architectural Engineering, Collage of Engineering, United Arab University, Abu Dhabi P.O. Box 15551, United Arab Emirates
* Correspondence: martin.scoppa@uaeu.ac.ae

Abstract: This paper uses quantitative methods to evaluate the application of street connectivity policies stated by Abu Dhabi's Urban Planning Council (UPC) on newly developed projects. The evaluation of the study was performed by measuring efficiency, i.e., how short and direct are paths between residential and nonresidential destinations to understand the ability of street networks to support sustainable transportation modes in the Capital District project. Efficiency is measured in twelve neighborhoods of the Capital District using Pedestrian Route Directness (PRD), a metric that meets Estidama—Abu Dhabi Green Rating System—walkability standards. Observation and analysis of the current stage of development show that more than 58% of the neighborhoods failed the route efficiency test to connect residential plots to one another. In addition, more than 40% of the neighborhood's residential plots could not efficiently connect to nonresidential plots. The study includes recommendations for policymakers and project developers to enhance the street infrastructure to correlate with Estidama ratings by taking advantage of sikkak, the alleyways system that is found in other neighborhoods in the city. Significantly, recommendations are based on rigorous quantitative analyses that can be used for implementation in real-world projects, thus strengthening the connection between policy and practice.

Keywords: superblocks urbanism; gulf urbanization; street connectivity and efficiency; walkability; sustainable urban development policy and practice

Citation: Anabtawi, R.; Scoppa, M. Measuring Street Network Efficiency and Block Sizes in Superblocks—Addressing the Gap between Policy and Practice. *Buildings* **2022**, *12*, 1686. https://doi.org/10.3390/buildings12101686

Academic Editors: Liyin Shen, Jorge Ochoa, Haijun Bao and Nikos A. Salingaros

Received: 30 June 2022
Accepted: 13 September 2022
Published: 13 October 2022

1. Introduction

Today, achieving the UN's sustainable development goals (SDGs) lies upfront in cities' development strategies. The advocacy for a more sustainable urban form is at the center of city planning agendas. A growing body of research provides evidence of a link between the sustainable urban form of cities and street connectivity [1–3]. Street systems can potentially increase urban transportation mobility and support walkability by efficiently linking spatially separated spaces when well-connected street networks are present [4]. The quality of street connections has been found to reduce car dependency, lower fossil fuel consumption, improve air quality, and enhance the overall quality of urban life [5].

After years of designing residential street networks with low levels of connectivity, multiple city planning agendas, visions, and green rating standards started to consider the contributions of improved connectivity [4]. As a result, street connectivity measures are now an established tool to achieve more sustainable transportation strategies for residential street networks. However, the application of connectivity measures highlighted in promising planning agendas and sustainability rating standards for new developments worldwide, especially in the Gulf region, is still understudied. This paper investigates the street connectivity of residential street networks in a newly developed sustainable urbanization project, the Capital District, Figure 1, in Abu Dhabi, United Arab Emirates (UAE). In addition, it focuses on retrofitting opportunities in the early stages of project development to bridge potential gaps between policy and practice.

The UAE has been experiencing rapid urbanization since 1970, and much urban growth and development tend to be made virtually instantly. This fast growth of the built-up area in UAE was possible using "superblocks" as an urban planning strategy. Superblocks are commonly used in the UAE. and Gulf Cooperation Council (GCC) countries such as Saudi Arabia, Bahrain, Kuwait, and others, as a planning system that helped the Arabian Gulf expand post-oil discovery [6]. Superblocks are designed as large areas of land enclosed with arterial avenues and are approximately 600×900 m in size. They are commonly used in residential neighborhoods in Abu Dhabi and are especially prominent in the Capital District project, the context of this study.

Interestingly, the new integrated public transport network proposed for the Capital District project incorporates advanced sustainable urban mobility strategies applied for the first time in Abu Dhabi, including high-speed rail, metro rail, and tram networks [7]. Once completed, the district is planned within a five-minute walk (300 m) from transit to all key destinations [8]. However, the project's current stage of development does not include any advanced transit systems yet, likely due to the current phase being focused on the development of twelve low-density residential superblocks which rely on their street networks to support walkability and cycling, as mentioned in the project proposal (USDM, 2015 P.63) [7].

Considering this, this research investigates the street connectivity of these twelve residential neighborhoods, looking at their role and impact on the overall mobility vision for the Capital District, particularly regarding its focus on creating an integrated multi-modal public transport network. Three different questions are addressed. First, how do the neighborhoods' street networks contribute to the overall mobility vision of the Capital District? This question is asked to assess the potential of those neighborhoods' street connectivity to be a part of the bigger urban mobility vision of the Capital District through a fully integrated transportation system. Second, what is the street network efficiency—i.e., to what extent can the network provide short and direct routes between plots in the low-density residential superblocks—of the Capital District? This question concerns the street network efficiency of developments constructed after the introduction of Estidama (Abu Dhabi's Green Building Rating System). It evaluates whether the superblocks' street connectivity performance meets the objectives and standards set not only by Estidama but and Abu Dhabi's Urban Planning Council (UPC). Third, what early retrofitting solutions are available for the street networks that do not meet UPC and Estidama standards? The third question concerns the impact of adding streets that cater to pedestrians, such as alleys and shared streets—respectively, sikkak and mushtarak in Arabic language, to the neighborhoods' street networks. In this case, the focus is on assessing their impact on the overall efficiency of the street system, and how they can be added after construction begins so that practice and policy are in better agreement.

By answering these three questions, this paper provides quantitative data to adjust and improve Urban Development Projects' street connectivity and efficiency of urban development projects before the urban form is finally established. In addition, the paper outlines recommendations to strengthen the connection between policy and practice through the continuous auditing and retrofitting of a residential project development.

2. Literature Review

2.1. Abu Dhabi's Superblock Development

Abu Dhabi's superblock neighborhoods were proposed first by British planner John Elliot in the 1960s, to the founding father of the U.A.E., Sheikh Zayed [9]. The early proposed superblocks were inspired by American planning ideas of the late 1920s, especially by Clarence Perry's Neighborhood Planning Unit (NPU) [10]. The neighborhood planning units in Abu Dubai were developed as components of a modular system that would work both as aggregations to form the larger, global city fabric and as independent "self-sustained" units where key land uses, such as mosques, schools, parks, and corner shops would support the local population.

As currently conceived and implemented, Abu Dhabi's superblock neighborhoods foster car dependency, and the transportation system is highly dependent on fossil fuels [6]. Therefore, Abu Dhabi is considered to have a high rate of car ownership. This high rate of car dependency makes it extremely important for Abu Dhabi to think of a future vision for its street system, such that automobile use is reduced and more sustainable mobility modes are supported and encouraged.

Fortunately, Abu Dhabi's government has been aware of the sustainability challenges brought by the predominance of motorized transportation. Multiple initiatives were outlined in Abu Dhabi's 2030 Vision, the city's forward-looking plan, as well as Estidama, Abu Dhabi's Green Building Standard, in a set of regulations to enhance different modes of transportation [10,11]. As a part of the Abu Dhabi 2030 regulation, The Urban Street Design Manual (USDM) was published to the public in 2010 and later updated in 2015 [12]. The manual included eight goals; one of the main goals is street efficiency, noting specifically short blocks and greater route choice as a means by which to achieve this (USDM, 2015, p. 27 [12]). Further, four different types of streets were introduced in the manual. These are: one-way streets (cars only), mushtarak (shared streets that serving both pedestrians and cars), Sikkak (pedestrian alleys), and shared access lane (cars and sidewalks) (USDM, 2015, pp. 77–79 [12]).

Mushtarak and sikkak are designed to enhance pedestrian movement within the neighborhood. Mushtarak (مُشْتَرَك) is the Arabic word for spaces shared by multiple modes of transport. A street concept similar to the popular Dutch's woonerf street introduced in the late 1960s, Mushtrak is designed to accommodate both cars and pedestrian movements [13,14]. Additionally, sikkak (سِكَّك) are characteristically present in superblocks in the UAE. and numerous other GCC countries' cities. Sikkak plays an essential role in enlarging the basic street network available to pedestrians and shortening superblocks' internal blocks. Their role has not been consistently studied; only recently have scholars tried to bring this issue to the foreground [15–17]. Scoppa et al. (2018) tested the street efficiency of ten different superblock designs, including orthogonal grids, Inward-looping street layouts, patterns with cul-de-sacs, and several other design variations [17]. The study found that sikkak make quite substantial contributions to street connectivity in all the tested network designs [17]. Additionally, the study noted that superblocks in Abu Dhabi have more sikkak than are necessary to ensure efficient connectivity and proposed a methodology for optimizing their provision, which is applied in this study.

Notably, the importance of sikkak has been underlined by Abu Dhabi's Urban Planning Council (UPC), the agency in charge of planning and managing the UAE.'s capital city's future growth. The UPC highlights the significance of sikkak in superblocks as critical pedestrian networks that improve access to services in neighborhoods (UPC, 2007, pp. 122, 154; UPC 2015, pp. 73, 91) [10]. Similarly, Estidama, Abu Dhabi's green building rating framework, encourages Sikkak to plan more sustainable neighborhoods by giving extra points for neighborhoods that improve walkability. Furthermore, Estidama defines sikkak as "key pedestrian routes" (Estidama, 2010 pp. 73–74, p. 166) [18]. Both street typologies enhance walkability and have been a critical component in efforts to support sustainable transportation modes in all new developments in Abu Dhabi. Especially, the design of residential networks is planned to enhance walkability and cycling as stated in the UPC and USDM [8,12] (UPC p. 51, 2009, USDM. p.71).

The UPC report also includes three significant challenges addressed in the design of pedestrian networks. First, designing smaller blocks to establish accessible and attractive pedestrian networks. Second, creating shaded zones to control the climate through the street and building orientation, and finally, land use distributions that enhance neighborhood diversity (UPC p. 51, 2009). Unfortunately, although those requirements and recommendations have been crystallized in multiple regulations and sustainable urban planning agendas for more than ten years, their application is still not evident in new and ongoing neighborhood projects and other large scale developments.

One of the most promising projects, designed and developed by Abu Dhabi's UPC, sets out to achieve high levels of street connectivity by following the Abu Dhabi 2030 Vision recommendation and Estidama Green Building. This project is the "Capital District" [7], and is regarded by the UPC as a demonstration project where numerous measures that Abu Dhabi developed for future sustainable development will be applied [16].

2.2. *The Capital District, Abu Dhabi*

The Capital District is a mega-development project currently under construction in Abu Dhabi, planned on a land area of forty-five square kilometers and designed for a population of three hundred and seventy thousand residents. The district is regarded as the physical development of the sustainable visions of the Abu Dhabi 2030 Plan [10]. The UPC planned the Capital District to enhance connectivity and promote walkability [8,10] (UPC, p. 51, 2009). The design of the capital district includes six major precincts: City Centre Precinct, Federal Precinct, Emirati Neighbourhood, Sports Hub Precinct, South Spine Precinct, and Palace Precinct, all of which can be seen in Figure 1.

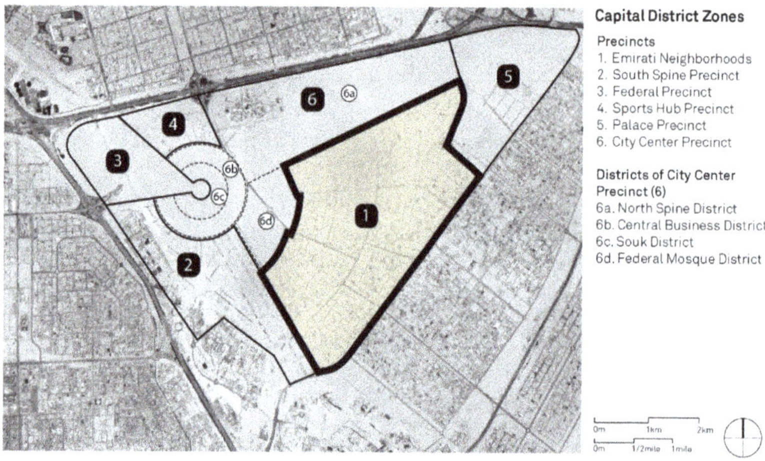

Figure 1. The Capital District Zones Diagram adapted by the authors from Abu Dhabi Urban Planning Council Report 2009 [8].

The Capital District's center is designed as a radial pattern of streets connecting the six major precincts. Five of which are designed as high-density developments with the plan of providing an extensive public transit system to connect them to the rest of the city and the larger region. The system will include high-speed rail, metro rail, and tram networks (UPC, 2015, pp. 48–49). The high-speed rail will connect the capital district to major locations in Abu Dhabi and other cities. Also, the proposed ten metro stations along the major spines of the district are designed to support the higher ridership associated to the higher built densities of these spines. Finally, the tram and bus networks will extend to the low-density development areas and connect with the higher-level transit system. Figure 2 illustrates the transit plan proposed by the UPC. Considering the different modes of transportation within the district, a more complex interconnected street system for Abu Dhabi was designed to enhance urban mobility with different street hierarchies and its cure Figure 3A. The low-density residential development called "Emirates neighborhoods Precinct" is planned to have amenities such as mosques, parks, and schools within walking distance. However, Figure 3 shows no pedestrian-only street or sikkak planned or laid out for the neighborhoods. Once completed, the twelve neighborhoods for Emirate national will be composed of villas for almost 3000 families. The precinct is made of plots planned to accommodate residential villas. Each neighborhood is designed to be self-sufficient, including all the necessary land uses, reflecting its inspiration to the neighborhood planning unit. The size and characteristics of each neighborhood differ largely. The main infrastructure and street network are currently established and completed as the first phase of the Capital District.

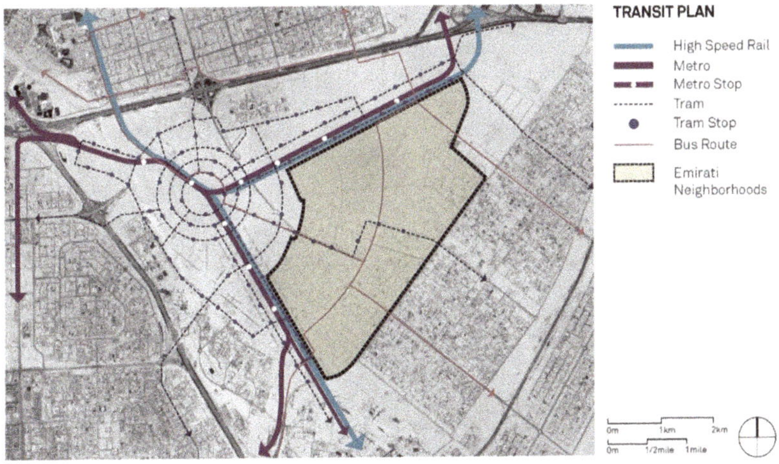

Figure 2. The transit plan of the Capital District. Diagram adapted by the authors from Abu Dhabi Urban Planning Council Report 2009 [8].

2.3. Street Connectivity Measures

As earlier noted, street network connectivity gained increased importance over the past years. In fact, considerable research has associated street connectivity with sustainable urban form development in cities, leading to increased research on the topic as well as increased used of connectivity metrics in practice [19–21]. As the body of knowledge grew, many metrics emerged as quantitatively testing tools for street connectivity [22]. Yet, studies show that no standard approach to testing connectivity exists [23]. For example, multiple studies focused primarily on density-based metrics, such as street, blocks, and intersections densities [24,25]. Urban planners usually prefer density measurements in regulations since they require simple calculations [4,25,26]. Thus, they are found in multiple sustainable rating codes for neighborhood design.

On the other hand, block size-based measures are regularly used in street connectivity research as well as regulatory frameworks. Block size metrics include block perimeter, area, and face length [26]. Just as density metrics, they are relatively easy to calculate and implement in development codes and regulations, and numerous studies have focused on block area and perimeter as a means to address connectivity [27,28]. In fact, multiple city regulations suggest limiting block perimeter to 400–900 m. or block area to 10 acres (~4 Has.). However, some geometrical flaws are evident when only using block perimeters or areas, which may reduce the efficiency of these metrics for land use regulations while also producing disproportionately long narrow blocks [29]. Considering this, several neighborhoods have adopted average block face length for new neighborhood development since it is more robust, not being distorted when different block configurations are tested. The standard block face is usually set at 100–200 m and applied to every neighborhood block. Understanding block sizes and their effect on permeability in street networks is essential. Nevertheless, a shortcoming of block size measures is that it is hard to understand how patterns or different block sizes fit together [26]. Consequently, studies have considered such measures unreliable street connectivity indicators because they are usually affected by the shape of the study area [25].

In addition, as shown by Peponis et al. (2008), substantially different street patterns could have the same density values, thus weakening the usefulness of these metrics, and are limited in terms of their ability to address the connectivity of the network [30]. This inability to detect street patterns makes block size and density measures alone unsuitable for this study. Indeed, these limitations are the reason for adopting a metric able to address connections between origins and destinations in this study, in what can be termed targeted connectivity analyses. Many studies have tested walkability as targeted connectivity of access to different locations using residential plots as origins. For instance, Altman-Hall measured the walking distance between residential plots and nonresidential plots, with the latter including schools, transit stops, and open spaces within neighborhoods [31]. Similarly, Song and Knapp tested access to bus and other transit stops, parks, and commercial spaces [32]. At the same time, Dill evaluated accessibility to transit stations only [24].

Other studies have tested street network connectivity using Pedestrian Route Directness (PRD) [33,34]. PRD was first proposed by Hess (1997); since then, it has been used more frequently in quantitative street connectivity studies [33]. PRD is defined as the ratio of the shortest network distance between given origin and destination pairs, to the straight-line or Euclidean distance between them. In doing this, this metric extends the concept of simple metric distance by introducing the notion of efficiency. Networks able to provide more direct routes—i.e., straighter, and less meandering routes—between origins and destinations, are more efficient networks in terms of supporting non-motorized mobility. This is the method used by the UPC to measure the quality of street connections in Abu Dhabi and will be further elaborated on in the next section, given that it is also the method adopted for this study. In fact, recent UAE-based studies have selected PRD to test the street connectivity efficiency in different superblock's street networks. Scoppa et al., 2018, tested PRD on ten different superblock street layouts, and found that orthogonal grids are highly efficient patterns, while patterns with cul-de-sacs may cause interrupted routes with low street efficiency [17]. This study also highlights the importance of alleys—sikkak—on improving the overall efficiency of the superblocks' street networks. Soon after, the same group of researchers further tested these neighborhoods' walkability potential by focusing on route directness to corners of the superblock, the points where superblocks connect and the points from where pedestrians can access surrounding areas. The study found that nearly all the tested neighborhoods have an efficient connection to the corners, providing further insight into the walkability of superblock street systems and their integration [35].

3. Methods

The study adopted a quantitative methodology based on the notion of route efficiency. In particular, the evaluation of walking routes in the superblocks that form the Emirati neighborhood precincts of the Capital District was based on the measurement of route directness. The study evaluated all the twelve superblocks within the emirate neighborhood precincts. Each Superblock has different characteristics and design configurations of street networks and characteristics. Figure 3A shows the position of the 12 neighborhoods and their current stage of development. At the same time, Figure 3B shows the street network of each neighborhood and dots representing the plots. More details about the characteristics of these twelve superblocks are introduced in Table 1.

The measure of network efficiency and directness used in this study is Pedestrian Route Directness or PRD. Proposed in the mid to late 1990's [33], this metric has seen increased use in research of UAE neighborhoods and superblocks [35]. Importantly, it forms part of Estidama—Abu Dhabi's Green Building Standards—regulations addressing walkability and sustainable urban development [18]. PRD is the ratio of the network distance to the Euclidean distance connecting an origin–destination pair of points. The lower this ratio, the more efficient the route. Calculations were performed based on the equation below.

$$PRD[i] = \frac{1}{n} \sum_{j \neq i}^{n} d_{i,j} / d_{i,j}^{Eucl} \quad (1)$$

where $PRD\ [i]$ is the pedestrian route directness of origin plot i, $d_{i,j}$ is the network distance separating origin plot i from destination plots j, $d_{i,j}^{Eucl}$ is the Euclidean or airline distance between the origin and destination, and n is the total number of plots in the Superblock. A graphic representation for a simple origin–destination pair is introduced in Figure 3A.

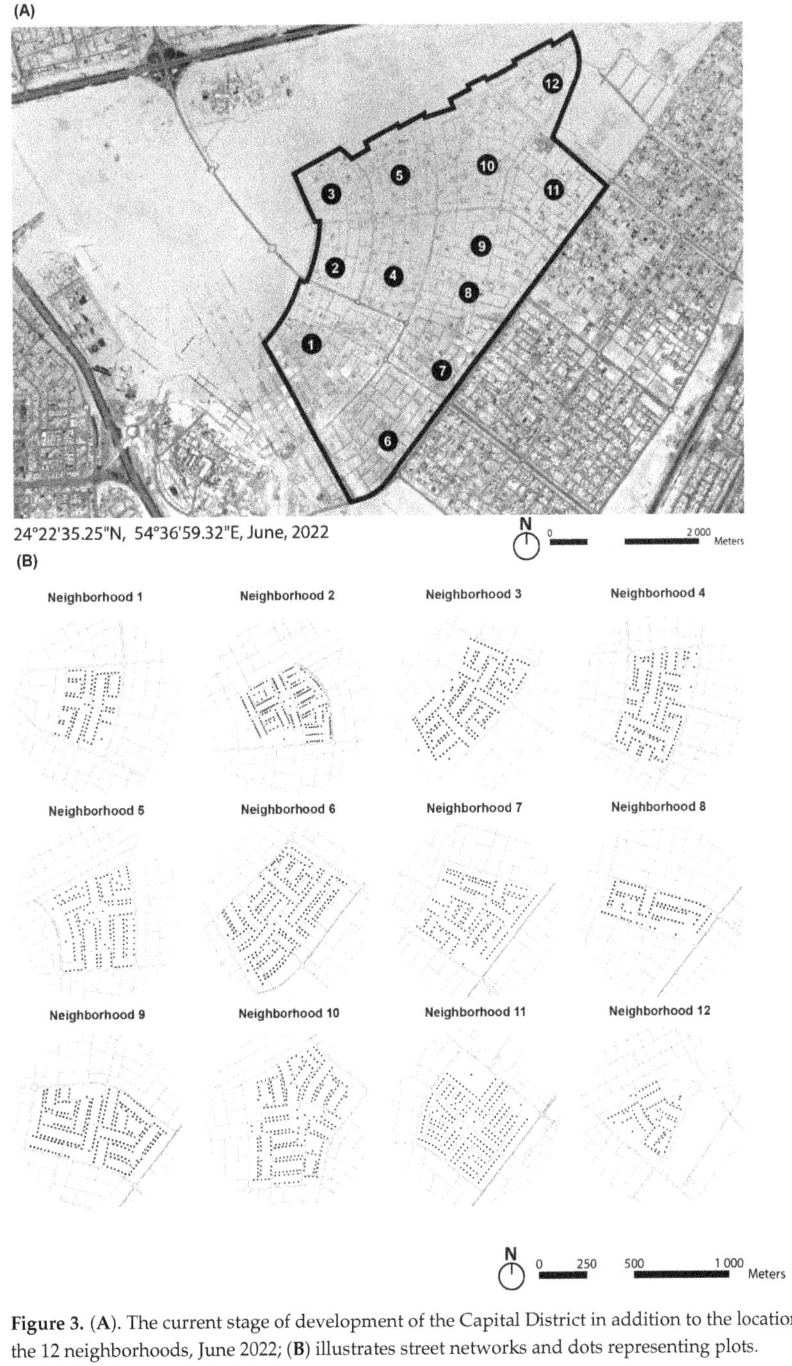

Figure 3. (**A**). The current stage of development of the Capital District in addition to the location of the 12 neighborhoods, June 2022; (**B**) illustrates street networks and dots representing plots.

Table 1. Descriptive statistics of the all-residential-plots-to-all-residential-plots route directness analysis.

Superblocks ID	Area (Ha.)	Width (Mts.)	Length (Mts.)	Number of Internal Blocks	Avg. Block Face Length (Mts.)	Avg. Block Perimeter (Mts.)	Avg. Internal Block Area (m^2)	Total Plot Number
Neighborhood 1	121.3	854.8	1835	27	187.9	941.2	45,699.3	241
Neighborhood 2	62.5	669.5	1088.6	14	187.2	894.4	44,628.8	133
Neighborhood 3	59.18	817.6	1006	24	153.9	793.0	32,966.6	254
Neighborhood 4	101.2	1238.3	713.5	48	167.2	789.3	36,015.2	198
Neighborhood 5	103.69	1157.5	1243.7	22	193.7	923.9	45,684.9	202
Neighborhood 6	165.39	1000.3	1321.2	31	195.5	1047.3	55,762.1	309
Neighborhood 7	120.6	1021.2	1248.8	25	188.2	924.9	46,967.4	211
Neighborhood 8	65.6	1237.6	879.6	13	197.3	927.8	47,490.5	114
Neighborhood 9	130.5	1395.7	933.4	24	203.2	1025.4	54,580.1	284
Neighborhood 10	99.1	1497.8	1608	34	109.4	935.8	21,454.7	305
Neighborhood 11	191.5	1204.4	1.131	24	205.0	993.7	55,975.2	235
Neighborhood 12	57.89	1000.2	800	13	186.7	912.1	45,955.0	105

The evaluation of this research was based on the ability of the twelve neighborhoods to support efficient connections between origins and destinations (O–D pairs) that the superblock residents would need or want to reach. Efficiency is understood in this study as the ability to provide short and direct connections between O–D pairs. The study included two sets of analyses between O–D pairs using two different networks illustrated in Figure 4b,c, Network 1 is the current network without any added sikkak while in Figure 4b, the added sikkak are shown.

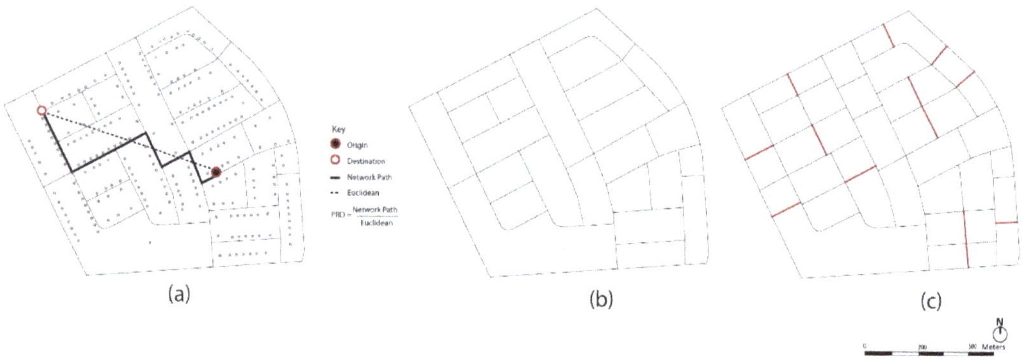

Figure 4. (**a**) An illustration of the route directness metric (PRD); (**b**) an illustration of the current network of the study (Network 1); (**c**) illustrates the current network with potential sikkak added (Network 2).

First, the study tested each plot's ability to connect to other residential plots, following an all-lots-to-all-plots rationale. The reason for considering all plots as origins as well as destinations for trips is based on the need to evaluate all possible routes within a given superblock, leading to a better understanding of the overall efficiency of the whole network, not just between single origin–destination pairs [15,36]. The second set of analyses observed the network's performance in providing direct access between all residential plots (the origins) and all nonresidential plots (the destinations). In this second evaluation, which we called all-residential-plots-to-all-non-residential-plots, the focus was placed on the evaluation of the efficiency of the land use distribution pattern as mandated by zoning regulations. Hence, the analyses focused on each neighborhood's ability to have connected pedestrian routes as per Estidama standards of a walkable community while also meeting universal walkable neighborhoods designs guidelines with accessible destinations within a 5 to 10 min walk, as per the original neighborhood planning unit (NPU) concept [11,37]. In addition, numerous previous studies suggest that, more direct routes connecting origins and destinations provide an incentive to walk as routes are shorter and, thus, more efficient [13,15,27,38–41].

In order to proceed with the calculation of PRD for the all-plots-to-all-plots and the all-residential-plots-to-all-non-residential-plots, it was necessary to build the street network maps, representing the street centerlines of each of the twelve neighborhoods studied. All superblock's maps were digitized using CAD and GIS software. Using these street centerline maps, and the points representing plot centroids, the data was ready for analysis. The analyses were performed using the ArcMap 10.8 GIS and used its Network Analyst module. As expected, the street centerlines represented the network, and the origin–destination matrix was built using the plot centroids.

As calculations proceeded, it was possible to estimate the two key values that make PRD. These are the network distance between each origin plot to each destination, as well as the straight—Euclidean—the distance between them. After all calculations were completed, the ratio of these two values was computed, and further evaluated following a pedestrian route directness test [38]. This test calculates the percentage of plots in a superblock whose PRD value is less than a 1.5 threshold. This threshold, utilized in Estidama regulations, indicates that plots have acceptable directness if they are, on average, no further than 1.5 times the shortest distance that connects them to other plots.

As earlier noted, two networks were used in this project. So, in addition to evaluating PRD and conducting PRD Tests on the base network (i.e., Network 1), we further evaluated the role of pedestrian network, sikkak, in providing efficient connectivity between origins and destinations. Previous local studies showed that sikkak break up long blocks in neighborhoods into smaller blocks, facilitating directness as demonstrated in several recent studies [17,35]. Considering these previous findings, the second network has added segments representing sikkak, as can be seen, in Figure 4c; sikkak were placed following a clear criterion. If the block's faces were over 200 m long, a sikka should be added in the middle to break long blocks into smaller ones. As mentioned before, previous studies and policies of block size regulations limit measures to 200 m block face from through street to through street [4,29]. In addition, a "continuity principle", adopted from previous studies, splits the blocks to create more continuous street centerlines [39,42].

A similar process was done on the twelve neighborhoods and then tested to study whether there were any improvements in network connectivity efficiency. The evaluation of the impact of the sikkak system in the Neighborhoods of the Capital District constitutes a key objective of this study. Currently, as shown in Figure 3A,B, the 12 neighborhood studies have no clear, planned sikkak, potentially missing the opportunity to create a better connected and more efficient system of pedestrian neighborhoods, as they are not yet built and could be added paths.

4. Results

As the analyses of all-residential-plots-to-all-residential-plots and all-residential-plots-to-all-non-residential-plots were completed for Networks 1 and 2, it was possible to evaluate the performance of each neighborhood in terms of providing efficient and direct paths between origins and destinations. It'ss important to note that the results are not comparable across the different superblocks studied, given that they have different characteristics in terms of size and shape. However, essential observations can be made to answer the study's questions. Table 2 shows that in Network 1—the network that does not include sikkak—the number of plots that passed the PRD test, i.e., had an average PRD value of 1.5 or less, varied between a maximum of 82.4% for superblock 12, and the lowest value of 16.4% for superblock 3.

These results demonstrate that the superblock street layout's design can significantly affect their connectivity efficiency. Likewise, to the noted maxima and minima, we can highlight that 7 out of 12 neighborhoods have more than 50% of their plots failing the directness test. In contrast, only one has passing plots percentages above 80%. As well as the distance between plots in each of these superblock neighborhoods differs significantly.

In fact, as outlined in the table, five neighborhoods have average trip lengths longer than 800 m and thus exceeding the standard 10 min walk.

Following the results obtained using Network 1, the evaluation of the role of sikkak as added to Network 2, is presented in the last three columns of Table 3. It is clear from the results that sikkak makes a remarkable contribution to the efficiency of the neighborhood networks. Without exception, the neighborhoods' percentage of passing plots exceeds 90% in ten of the studied neighborhoods, and only two cases show values below this percentage threshold and above 80%. Figure 4 illustrates the passing and failing plots in Superblock 3 using the two different networks.

Particularly noteworthy is superblock 3, shown in Figure 5, as well as neighborhoods 4, 5, and 6, which show many-fold increases in terms of passing plots and average PRD values. Consequently, the average trip distance also decreased in all neighborhoods, with only two neighborhoods offering average trip lengths above 800 m.

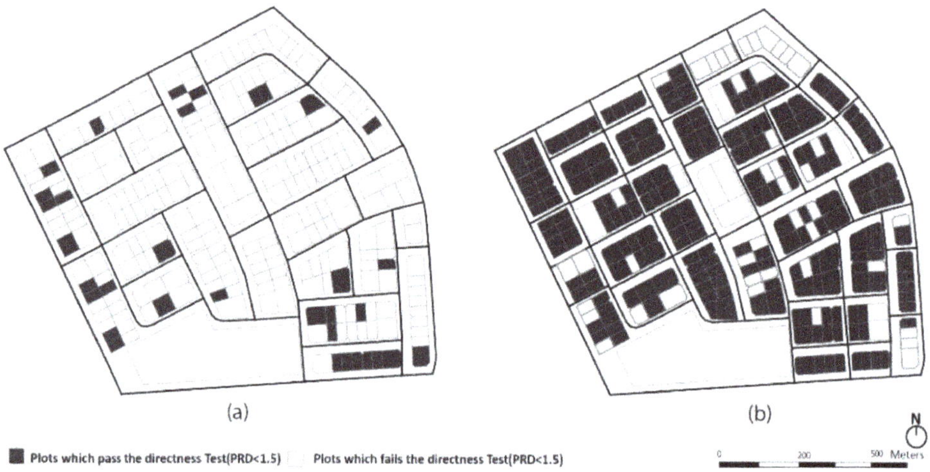

Figure 5. (**a**) Route directness results in terms of passing plots (shown in a darker color) using Network 1; (**b**) route directness results in terms of passing plots (shown in darker color) using Network 2, the network that included potential sikkak.

Similar to what occurred in the previous case, Table 3 shows that the efficiency of access to nonresidential destinations in the studied superblocks varies, but at least 5 neighborhoods show values below 50% of passing plots. However, and once again, it is worth noting the impact that sikkak has on improving the circulation efficiency provided by the road network when these alleyways are added.

A remarkable number of neighborhoods increase the number of plots passing the PRD test. In fact, eight neighborhoods achieve values above 90%, four with values above 80%. It'ss worth noting that the average distance length was reduced in all the cases resulting in only 2 neighborhoods above 800 m or a 10 min walk. Lastly, and as expected, besides a significant increase in the percentage of passing plots, the results obtained with Network 2 show substantial decreases in terms of the average PRD value for all the neighborhoods studied.

After outlining the results of both analyses, it is now possible to highlight the link between these street connectivity analyses and each network's general characteristics, focusing on the block size measure of each Superblock. A summary of the PRD results and block subdivisions is presented in Table 4. It is essential to note again that the superblocks are not directly comparable given variations in terms of their size and shape. However, important observations can be made regarding the contribution of Sikkak to the block size measures of the network.

Table 2. Descriptive statistics of the all-residential-plots-to-all-residential-plots route directness analysis of network 1 in columns (3–6). Results of using Network 2—the network that includes sikkak—are presented in columns (7–9).

Superblock ID	Residential Plots	Network 1				Network 2 (sikkak)			
		Passing Plots	% of Passing Plots	Avg. PRD	Avg. Trip Length (mts.)	Passing Plots	% of Passing Plots	Avg. PRD	Avg. Trip Length (mts.)
Superblock 1	232	106	45.7%	1.55	860.5	229	98.71%	1.32	766.4
Superblock 2	123	53	43.1%	1.50	589.7	117	95.12%	1.36	544.5
Superblock 3	238	39	16.4%	1.63	691.2	195	81.93%	1.41	571.5
Superblock 4	186	43	23.1%	1.68	848.7	173	93.01%	1.30	766.8
Superblock 5	192	56	29.2%	1.61	786.1	155	80.73%	1.43	695.5
Superblock 6	297	90	30.3%	1.84	977.8	277	93.27%	1.46	839.2
Superblock 7	198	126	63.6%	1.53	743.5	195	98.48%	1.30	688.8
Superblock 8	109	81	74.3%	1.39	633.6	109	100.00%	1.27	569.1
Superblock 9	274	126	45.9%	1.49	870.9	269	98.18%	1.32	786.1
Superblock 10	291	225	77.3%	1.43	887.8	291	100.00%	1.30	832.3
Superblock 11	226	159	70.3%	1.44	724.6	226	100.00%	1.30	724.6
Superblock 12	97	80	82.4%	1.40	516.1	95	97.94%	1.34	495.2

Table 3. Descriptive statistics of the all-residential-plots-to-all-non-residential-plots route directness analysis of Network 1 in column (3–6). Results of Network 2—the network that includes Sikkak—are presented in columns (7–9).

Superblock ID	Res. Plots	Non Res. Plots	Network 1				Network 2 (Sikkak)			
			Passing Plots	% of Passing Plots	Avg. PRD	Avg. Trip Length (mts.)	Passing Plots	% of Passing Plots	Avg. PRD	Avg. Trip Length (mts.)
Superblock1	232	9	90	38.79%	1.65	942.8	213	91.8%	1.32	807.8
Superblock 2	123	10	110	89.43%	1.39	464.6	117	95.1%	1.36	447.55
Superblock 3	238	12	98	41.18%	1.55	614.3	195	81.9%	1.41	549.02
Superblock 4	186	10	62	33.33%	1.65	900.7	177	95.2%	1.30	831.63
Superblock 5	192	12	121	63.02%	1.56	716.3	155	80.7%	1.43	664.19
Superblock 6	297	13	67	22.56%	1.75	977.5	280	94.3%	1.46	796.5
Superblock 7	198	5	112	56.57%	1.44	770.2	194	97.9%	1.30	526.66
Superblock 8	109	10	69	63.30%	1.48	694.1	88	80.7%	1.27	667.02
Superblock 9	274	14	179	65.33%	1.49	837.8	261	95.3%	1.32	742.1
Superblock 10	291	9	235	80.76%	1.46	896.2	285	97.9%	1.30	822.37
Superblock 11	226	8	72	31.86%	1.58	842.4	182	80.5%	1.30	695.6
Superblock 12	97	9	75	77.32%	1.40	545.5	91	97.9%	1.34	521.06

Table 4. Summary of the block size characteristics and the result of PRD for the two tested networks.

Superblock ID	Network 1						Network 2 (Sikkak)					
	Avg. Block Area (msq)	Avg. Block Face Length (mts)	Total Blocks	Avg. Block Perimeter (mts)	Avg. Street Length (mts)	ATA [1] Avg. PRD	Avg. Block Area (msq)	Avg. Block Face Length (mts)	Total Block	Avg. Block Perimeter (mts)	Avg. Street Length (mts	ATA [1] Avg. PRD
Superblock 1	45,699	187.9	27	941.2	15,135	1.55	28,695	125.1	43	686.5	11,983	1.32
Superblock 2	44,628	187.2	14	894.4	7862	1.50	28,583	142.4	22	684.1	9257	1.36
Superblock 3	32,966	153.9	23	793.0	10,927	1.63	19,964	118.6	38	567.1	12,456	1.41
Superblock 4	36,015	165.1	29	789.3	13,545	1.68	21,006	114.1	48	583.8	16,090	1.30
Superblock 5	45,684	190.9	22	923.9	12,219	1.61	28,716	137.9	35	686.2	14,065	1.43
Superblock 6	55,762	195.5	31	1047.3	17,996	1.84	27,992	149.8	58	683.8	22,619	1.46
Superblock 7	46,967	188.2	25	924.9	14,309	1.53	27,951	135.8	42	672.4	16,440	1.30
Superblock 8	47,490	197.3	13	927.8	8092	1.39	29,040	145.2	21	686.0	9222	1.27
Superblock 9	54,580	203.2	24	1025.4	14,637	1.49	25,764	125.0	51	651.1	19,253	1.32
Superblock 10	21,454	162.0	34	935.8	18,468	1.43	26,314	131.8	61	651.1	22,414	1.30
Superblock 11	55,975	205.0	24	993.7	14,148	1.44	31,050	155.9	43	686.1	17,003	1.30
Superblock 12	45,955	186.7	27	912.1	7598	1.40	23,897	128.1	25	614.4	9350	1.34

[1] A.T.A. stands for all-residential-plots-to-all-residential-plots.

On average, 15% additional street length was added to all the superblocks, reducing the average block face length by 28%, average block perimeter by 29% and average block area by 40%. Considering these results, as expected, Sikkak traversing long blocks increases the block density and enhances the street system's overall connectivity. It is also essential to look at the block length difference between superblocks. For instance, Superblocks 9 and 11 both had average block face lengths of more than 200 m, while all other superblocks had block faces of more than 150 m. on the contrary, when Sikkak was added, all the superblocks except superblock 11 were lower than 155 m.

5. Discussion

The study tested the street network efficiency of the twelve residential superblocks that make the Emirate Neighborhoods precinct of the Capital District project of Abu Dhabi. Two sets of analyses were conducted, uncovering the efficiency of the network in terms of connecting all plots in these neighborhoods, and between residential and non-residential plots by means of short and direct routes. The results provide valuable information by which to support several observations regarding the route efficiency that the neighborhoods provide.

First, the results highlight that only a few neighborhoods in Capital District currently provide short and direct routes between all possible pairs of origins and destinations. In fact, the results indicate that 7 out of the 12 neighborhoods studied failed the PRD test. More precisely, the test indicates that direct and efficient routes connecting the plots of the superblocks are characteristically absent in the majority of the neighborhoods. Similarly, 5 out of 12 neighborhoods failed the PRD test of providing efficient paths connecting residential and nonresidential plots. Indeed, in about half of the superblocks studied, reaching non-residential destinations involves route deviations that are larger than 1.5 times the shortest possible route. Taken together, these results show that there exist quite large variations in the street efficiency of the tested neighborhoods, and highlight the importance of addressing this matter if the Emirate Neighborhoods are to support the sustainable mobility vision of the Capital District project. In other words, the analyses bring forward that there exists an opportunity or optimizing the contribution of the Emirati Neighborhoods precincts to the ambitious sustainable urban mobility plans highlighted by the UPC for the Capital District. These results answer the first two questions outlined in the introduction, noting that the Emirates Neighborhood street networks are not all efficient, and that they will likely affect the overall mobility plans that the UPC set out to achieve.

Second, the neighborhoods' currently "as-built" status doesn't yet include alleys—i.e., sikkak—even though these have been noted to be key pedestrian infrastructure by the UPCs Urban Street Design Manual, Estidama rating system principles, and multiple recent studies of Abu Dhabi [7,11,14,15]. Following this observation, the study tested the addition of sikkak to answer the last question of the study. To do this, a tried and tested methodology previously applied in the study of Abu Dhabi superblocks was used, and actually enlarged by addressing the need to limit block face lengths to 200 m following international standards and research findings. As expected, given the previous results from tested neighborhoods with similar network designs [17], sikkak improved route directness where more than 80% of the plots pass the PRD test in the case of connections between residential plots to other residential plots as well as nonresidential destinations. However, unlike previous studies which focused on consolidated neighborhoods with already established plots, sikkak, and buildings, the Emirate Neighborhoods of the Capital District project can still be retrofitted as their construction is currently underway.

While these results provide actionable information to planning authorities, it is important to note that other properties of Abu Dhabi's Superblocks' physical form are not always covered in the city's sustainable development standards and manuals. Indeed, while the superblock framework, as a means to build cities and neighborhoods, has been adopted by multiple cities around the world and the Gulf, key urban theorists such as Alexander and Jacobs have long criticized it for creating fragmented and segregated neighborhoods that do not integrate well with their surroundings [40,43]. More specifically, according to Jane Jacobs, the large sizes that characterize superblocks were a major reason in isolating neighborhoods, especially when long blocks were present [41]. Recent studies considered scaling down the superblock to 400 m, resulting in more permeability between neighborhoods [44]. A recent example form practice regarding limiting sizes to about 400 × 400 Superblock can be found in the Barcelona superblock model, in which the sustainable mobility goals are constructed on the basis of shared streets, i.e., with cars and pedestrians sharing the right of way. Particularly, on this last point, it is worth noting that shared streets, or mushtarak in Arabic language, do feature in Abu Dhabi's planning strategies and standards when noting that pedestrians and pedestrianism are a priority for the city [45]. While this reduced superblock size seems optimal for supporting walkable distances with destinations reachable within five minutes walk, those superblocks are not yet being implemented in Abu Dhabi. In fact, the overall size of the neighborhoods is not currently directly addressed in any of the planning manuals and standards. Considering this, this study only tested the role of shorter blocks, as these are discussed multiple times in the UPC (UPC, pp. 51, 29, 41, 2009) and U.D.S.M (U.S.D.M., 2015, pp. 27, 77–79), noting that more clarity is needed regarding how short blocks should be as actual lengths are not currently discussed. This study shed light on the impact that block size regulations, specifically reducing block face length by adding alleys or sikkak, can have on the overall route efficiency that the street network provides.

After adding sikkak to block faces above 200 m, a quick assessment of the block subdivisions suggests some consistency between other block measures. For instance, the difference between the maximum and minimum average block perimeter of Network 1 is 258 m, while in network 2 the difference is narrowed to 119 m. Multiple city regulations suggest limiting block perimeter to 400–900 m or block area to 10 acres (~4 Has.) and keeping the average block face flexible. Further research may assist in testing different block size measures, limits, and standards for Abu Dhabi.

Lastly, The Capital District is a massive transit-oriented development project that, as it is still under construction, cannot yet be fully assessed. Still, this study's observations could inform and assist planning auditors and the UPC on the current situation of street efficiency of the project, so that the connection between policy and practice can be strengthened. Several phases of development are yet to be built in order for the Capital District project to be completed. As the project continues, additional studies would be needed in order to more comprehensively assess the extent to which policy and practice have actually merged in this ambitious project, especially with regard to its role in supporting sustainable mobility and transportation in particular, and sustainable urban development in general.

6. Conclusions

Over the last fifty years the NPU concept, materialized through superblocks, has played an essential role in Abu Dhabi's planning. The Abu Dhabi Planning Council recognizes the importance of planning more sustainable neighborhoods with more sustainable transportation modes in mind, as is reflected in the Capital District's plans. However, the challenge that remains is that of ensuring that the vision of sustainable mobility that underpins the Capital District project is fully and completely achieved.

This preliminary research into the street connectivity of the Emirate Neighborhoods area of the project was conducted to better understand the relationship between research, regulation, plans, and practice. Undoubtfully, narrowing the gap between policy and practice is considered a critical issue in all disciplines. In this paper, this gap is bridged by noting how slight additions to the total street network length by adding sikkak and shortening blocks could enhance the neighborhoods' street connectivity to support better walkability, encouraging individuals to use more sustainable and healthy transportation modes. In this study, the efficiency of the street networks of all the neighborhoods was quantified in terms of their ability to provide short and direct routes between origins and destinations. Precisely, their efficiency was measured using the Pedestrian Route Directness

(PRD) index and its associated PRD Test. The results of the study show that most of the tested neighborhoods failed this connectivity efficiency test. This might affect the overall urban transit-oriented development that the Abu Dhabi aims to achieve. Further, besides providing a clear picture regarding the efficiency of each neighborhoods' street network, this study evaluated the possibility of improving their efficiency by adding sikkak to the existing street system. The results reveal that all the studied neighborhoods can significantly increase their potential for walkability, and destinations could be more easily reached, if and when sikkak are added to them. Therefore, enhancing the street efficiency of each neighborhood will further support the urban mobility of the Capital District. Given these results, and in the interest of strengthening the link between policy and practice, this study recommends:

1. That the Neighborhoods in the Capital District are retrofitted with pedestrian walkways such as sikkak (pedestrian only alleys) or mushtarak (shared streets). also, the role of sikkak and mushtarak as key pedestrian infrastructure is further strengthened in planning new neighborhoods and retrofitting existing ones.
2. That block face length is evaluated as an additional standard for green building regulations that focus on neighborhood design in the UAE. In this case, more research, such as that presented in this paper, would be necessary to establish block face length limits and thresholds.
3. That the connection and integration of the different precinct of the project is ensured by actively and comprehensively testing route directness, as well as block sizes and lengths, thus perfecting the necessary merger of planning standards and planning practice.

To conclude, the UPC is developing sustainable community measures, standards, and codes, which are in line with those outlined by cities and regions worldwide. Such codes allow for urban development to achieve the urban form and density that is needed to support walking and transit, thus reducing automobile dependence. Notably, the work presented in this paper transcends the specific context of the United Arab Emirates and its cities. This is the case because they not only provide a means by which to address the larger call of Goal 11 of the United Nations Sustainable Development Goals with respect to Sustainable Cities and Communities, but also because they constitute a useful reference to other GCC countries' cities that share urbanization patterns and characteristics with the UAE.

Author Contributions: Conceptualization, M.S. and R.A.; methodology, M.S.; software, R.A., M.S.; validation, M.S., R.A.; formal analysis; investigation, R.A., M.S.; resources, M.S.; data curation, M.S., R.A.; writing—original draft preparation, M.S., R.A.; writing—review and editing, M.S.; visualization, M.S., R.A.; supervision, M.S.; project administration, M.S.; funding acquisition, M.S. All authors have read and agreed to the published version of the manuscript.

Funding: This research was supported by the United Arab Emirates University Start-Up Grant G00003328 and Sustainable Development Goals Research Program Grant 1984.

Acknowledgments: The authors would like to acknowledge the exceptional contribution of Architectural Engineering undergraduate students in this research, especially Hind Almheiri, Amna Aleghfeli, Shamma Alrashdi and Mira Aleghfeli.

Conflicts of Interest: The authors declare no conflict of interest.

References

1. Ewing, R.; Handy, S.; Brownson, R.C.; Clemente, O.; Winston, E. Identifying and measuring urban design qualities related to walkability. *J. Phys. Act. Health* **2006**, *3*, S223–S240. [CrossRef] [PubMed]
2. Berrigan, D.; Pickle, L.W.; Dill, J. Associations between street connectivity and active transportation. *Int. J. Health Geogr.* **2010**, *9*, 20. [CrossRef] [PubMed]
3. Talen, E. Sprawl Retrofit: Sustainable Urban Form in Unsustainable Places. *Environ. Plan. B Plan. Des.* **2011**, *38*, 952–978. [CrossRef]

4. Handy, S.; Paterson, R.G.; Butler, K. *Planning for Street Connectivity. Getting from Here to There*; Planning Advisory Service Report, No. 515; American Planning Association, Planning Advisory Service: Chicago, IL, USA, 2003.
5. Frank, L.D.; Engelke, P.O. The built environment and human activity patterns: Exploring the impacts of urban form on public health. *J. Plan. Lit.* **2001**, *16*, 202–218. [CrossRef]
6. Hashim, A.R.B. *Planning Abu Dhabi: An Urban History*; Routledge: London, UK, 2019.
7. Abu Dhabi Urban Planning Council. *Capital District. Abu Dhabi 2030 Vision*; Abu Dhabi Urban Planning Council: Abu Dhabi, United Arab Emirates, 2009; p. 153.
8. Abu Dhabi Urban Planning Council. *Capital District. Abu Dhabi 2030 Vision*; Abu Dhabi Urban Planning Council: Abu Dhabi, United Arab Emirates, 2007.
9. Abdo, R.; Batzel, G.M. Planning the Modern Arab City: The Case of Abu Dhabi. In *Reconsidering Jane Jacobs*; Routledge: London, UK, 2011; pp. 105–118.
10. Abu Dhabi Urban Planning Council. *Plan Abu Dhabi 2030: Urban Structure Framework Plan*; Abu Dhabi Urban Planning Council: Abu Dhabi, United Arab Emirates, 2007.
11. Abu Dhabi Urban Planning Council. *The Pearl Community Rating System*; Abu Dhabi Urban Planning Council: Abu Dhabi, United Arab Emirates, 2010.
12. Abu Dhabi Urban Planning Council. *Abu Dhabi Urban Street Design Manual*; Abu Dhabi Urban Planning Council: Abu Dhabi, United Arab Emirates, 2014.
13. Jonquiere, P. *Woonerf: An Environment for Man and Transport Together: The Present Aspects*; Japan, Tokyo, 1978.
14. Kraay, J.H. Woonerven and other experiments in the Netherlands. *Built Environ.* **1986**, *12*, 20–29.
15. Scoppa, M.; Anabtawi, R. Connectivity in Superblock Street Networks: Measuring Distance, Directness, and the Diversity of Pedestrian Paths. *Sustainability* **2021**, *13*, 13862. [CrossRef]
16. Alawadi, K.; Alameri, H.; Scoppa, M. Reclaiming Alleyways to improve network connectivity: Lessons from Dubai's neighborhoods. *J. Plan. Educ. Res.* **2020**. [CrossRef]
17. Scoppa, M.; Bawazir, K.; Alawadi, K. Walking the superblocks: Street layout efficiency and the sikkak system in Abu Dhabi. *Sustain. Cities Soc.* **2018**, *38*, 359–369. [CrossRef]
18. Abu Dhabi Urban Planning Council. *The Pearl Rating System for Estidama: Community Rating System*; Abu Dhabi Urban Planning Council: Abu Dhabi, United Arab Emirates, 2010.
19. Talen, E. Neighborhoods as service providers: A methodology for evaluating pedestrian access. *Environ. Plan. B Plan. Des.* **2003**, *30*, 181–200. [CrossRef]
20. Condon, P.M. *Seven Rules for Sustainable Communities: Design Strategies for the Post Carbon World*; Island Press: London, UK, 2012.
21. Jabareen, Y. Sustainable Urban Forms. *J. Plan. Educ. Res.* **2006**, *26*, 38–52. [CrossRef]
22. Ellis, G.; Hunter, R.; Tully, M.A.; Donnelly, M.; Kelleher, L.; Kee, F. Connectivity and physical activity: Using footpath networks to measure the walkability of built environments. *Environ. Plan. B Plan. Des.* **2016**, *43*, 130–151. [CrossRef]
23. Marshall, W.E.; Garrick, N.W. Effect of street network design on walking and biking. *Transp. Res. Rec.* **2010**, *2198*, 103–115. [CrossRef]
24. Dill, J. Measuring network connectivity for bicycling and walking. In Proceedings of the 83rd Annual Meeting of the Transportation Research Board, Washington, DC, USA, 11–15 January 2004.
25. Knight, P.L.; Marshall, W.E. The metrics of street network connectivity: Their inconsistencies. *J. Urban. Int. Res. Placemaking Urban Sustain.* **2015**, *8*, 241–259. [CrossRef]
26. Stangl, P. Overcoming flaws in permeability measures: Modified route directness. *J. Urban. Int. Res. Placemaking Urban Sustain.* **2017**, *12*, 1–14. [CrossRef]
27. Hooper, P.; Giles-Corti, B.; Knuiman, M. Evaluating the implementation and active living impacts of a state government planning policy designed to create walkable neighborhoods in Perth, Western Australia. *Am. J. Health Promot.* **2014**, *28* (Suppl. S3), S5. [CrossRef] [PubMed]
28. McDonald, K.; Oakes, J.M.; Forsyth, A.J. Effect of street connectivity and density on adult BMI: Results from the Twin Cities Walking Study. *J. Epidemiol. Community Health* **2012**, *66*, 636. [CrossRef] [PubMed]
29. Stangl, P. Block size-based measures of street connectivity: A critical assessment and new approach. *Urban Des. Int.* **2015**, *20*, 44–55. [CrossRef]
30. Peponis, J.; Bafna, S.; Zhang, Z. The Connectivity of Streets: Reach and Directional Distance. *Environ. Plan. B Plan. Des.* **2008**, *35*, 881–901. [CrossRef]
31. Aultman-Hall, L.; Roorda, M.; Baetz, B.W. Using GIS for evaluation of neighborhood pedestrian accessibility. *J. Urban Plan. Dev.* **1997**, *123*, 10–17. [CrossRef]
32. Song, Y.; Merlin, L.; Rodriguez, D. Comparing measures of urban land use mix. *Comput. Environ. Urban Syst.* **2013**, *42*, 1–13. [CrossRef]
33. Hess, P.M. Measures of Connectivity [Streets: Old paradigm, new investment]. *Places* **1997**, *11*. [CrossRef]
34. Moudon, A.V.; Hess, P.M.; Snyder, M.C.; Stanilov, K. Effects of Site Design on Pedestrian Travel in Mixed-Use, Medium-Density Environments. *Transp. Res. Rec.* **1997**, *1578*, 48–55. [CrossRef]
35. Scoppa, M.; Bawazir, K.; Alawadi, K. Straddling boundaries in superblock cities. Assessing local and global network connectivity using cases from Abu Dhabi, UAE. *Transp. Res. Part A Policy Pract.* **2019**, *130*, 770–782. [CrossRef]

36. Porta, S.; Crucitti, P.; Latora, V. The Network Analysis of Urban Streets: A Primal Approach. *Environ. Plan. B Plan. Des.* **2006**, *33*, 705–725. [CrossRef]
37. Perry, C.A. City planning for neighborhood life. *Soc. F.* **1929**, *8*, 98. [CrossRef]
38. Stangl, P. The pedestrian route directness test: A new level-of-service model. *Urban Des. Int.* **2012**, *17*, 228–238. [CrossRef]
39. Figueiredo, L.; Amorim, L. Continuity lines in the axial system. In *The Fifth Space Syntax International Symposium*; Delft University of Technology: Delft, The Netherlands, 2005.
40. Alexander, C. A City Is Not a Tree. In *A Pattern Language: Towns, Buildings, Construction*; Oxford University Press: New York, NY, USA, 1977.
41. Jacobs, J. *The Death and Life of Great American Cities*; Random House: New York, NY, USA, 1961; 458p.
42. Jiang, B. A topological pattern of urban street networks: Universality and peculiarity. *Phys. A Stat. Mech. Its Appl.* **2007**, *384*, 647–655. [CrossRef]
43. Plunz, R.; Sheridan, M. Deadlock Plus 50: On Public Housing in New York. In *Urban Planning Today: A Harvard Design Magazine Reader*; University of Minnesota Press: Minneapolis, MN, USA, 2006; pp. 14–23.
44. Mehaffy, M.W.; Porta, S.; Romice, O. The "neighborhood unit" on trial: A case study in the impacts of urban morphology. *J. Urban. Int. Res. Placemaking Urban Sustain.* **2015**, *8*, 199–217. [CrossRef]
45. Mueller, N.; Rojas-Rueda, D.; Khreis, H.; Cirach, M.; Andrés, D.; Ballester, J.; Bartoll, X.; Daher, C.; Deluca, A.; Echave, C.; et al. Changing the urban design of cities for health: The superblock model. *Environ. Int.* **2020**, *134*, 105132. [CrossRef]

buildings

MDPI

Article

The Principles of Design for Vulnerable Communities: A Research by Design Approach Overrunning the Disciplinary Boundaries

Emanuele Giorgi [1,*], Tiziano Cattaneo [2,3] and Karol Paulina Serrato Guerrero [1]

1 Tecnologico de Monterrey, Escuela de Arquitectura, Arte y Diseño, Campus Chihuahua, Chihuahua 31300, Mexico
2 Department of Civil Engineering and Architecture, University of Pavia, 27100 Pavia, Italy
3 College of Design and Innovation, Tongji University, Shanghai 200070, China
* Correspondence: egiorgi@tec.mx

Abstract: Current changes are making communities, cities, and territories increasingly vulnerable. Urban architectural interventions have the power to intervene this situation, directly reducing vulnerabilities or backing social initiatives. Urban and architectural interventions, however, are also those that take a longer time to be implemented and to impact society. For this, these interventions must be sustained by broad and transversal visions, as well as referring to the temporal context of the coming decades. For these reasons, the research project "Design for Vulnerables" aims to define which methodologies should be adopted to reduce urban vulnerabilities in the coming decades. A design workshop, set in a vulnerable community in the northern Mexico, was organized, documented, and analyzed. Based on the research by design methodology, the research highlighted current issues, transversal to urban-architectural design, which influence urban vulnerabilities. This multidisciplinary approach made it possible to generating a set of principles of Design for Vulnerables, graphically represented by a re-interpretation of the Krebs cycle.

Keywords: urban vulnerabilities; vulnerable communities; multidisciplinary approach; disciplinary boundaries; design workshops; research by design; Design for Vulnerables; Krebs cycle design

Citation: Giorgi, E.; Cattaneo, T.; Serrato Guerrero, K.P. The Principles of Design for Vulnerable Communities: A Research by Design Approach Overrunning the Disciplinary Boundaries. *Buildings* **2022**, *12*, 1789. https://doi.org/10.3390/buildings12111789

Academic Editors: Liyin Shen, Jorge Ochoa and Haijun Bao

Received: 3 September 2022
Accepted: 13 October 2022
Published: 25 October 2022

1. Decades to Come: Challenges for Urban Vulnerable Communities

The current crises, which are impacting contemporary society and which, in the coming decades, will turn into important global challenges, make it urgent to deeply consider what characteristics cities and territories must adopt [1,2]. Undoubtedly, the city, the place of maximum expression of human phenomena [3], need be placed at the center of a discussion that concerns different scientific and humanistic disciplines [4–9]. Cities must again be the place that allows human flourishing and the enhancement of the communitarian environment [10]. This has important implications for policies makers, designers, architects, engineers, and, more in general, for all those people who have an impact on the built environment. It is inappropriate to think that society can address the current challenges with the current processes and policies, which partially are the generators of many of the problems themselves [11]. This implies having to define new working methodologies that must be even more innovative when it comes to intervening in vulnerable communities [12]. These contexts and the concept of vulnerability itself are studied and discussed by the international scientific community, which highlights (1) how it is more appropriate to indicate this situation with references to the plural vulnerabilities and (2) how all living beings are subject to some levels of vulnerabilities.

1.1. Urban Vulnerabilities

All the new contemporary challenges imply developing new considerations on "being vulnerable", which has become an ever more varied and complex concept. Each academic field developed a specific concept of vulnerability (related to its own way to study the social and natural environment) and a theoretical definition—more specific than the vague "measure of possible future harm". In the scientific literature, the concept of vulnerability is a very complex one, because it can be used in different fields to analyze specific aspects of different disciplines, with definitions serving specific methods and indicators [13]. Thus, innumerable facets of vulnerability can be met, and therefore it can be safely referred to as "vulnerabilities", to correctly indicate these different aspects that can be assessed. In general, we can refer to the concept of vulnerabilities as those conditions by which an event can be detrimental to the physical, emotional, or economic well-being of a person or community [14]. The observation by Wolf et al. helps in understand a common pattern in the assessing methodologies of different disciplines, which can be grouped into three types: "evaluate harm for projected future evolutions, evaluate the current capacity to reduce harm, or combine the two" [15].

Moreover, in academic literature, the concept of vulnerability is often associated with environmental risk [16]. This allows us to highlight how these events are the ones that endanger the psychophysical well-being of a person or a community more than any other. However, it is wrong to consider that the concept of vulnerability should be limited to these environmental risks. In contrast, reflecting on the state of vulnerability means analyzing social, economic, or cultural aspects that are at the base of the well-being of people and individuals.

Due to the complexity of this concept [15,17], the importance of its contextualization [18], the relativity of the concept itself [19] and the goal of this research, the authors tried to keep the approaches to vulnerability as wide as possible. Differently from other studies, which aim to define design principles for specific situation of vulnerability (environmental risks, flooding, earthquake, climate change, etc.), this research aims to keep in sight several concerns (political, economic, social, and health, among others). All these social problems are further aggravated in extreme conditions, where the lack of social ties is added to serious basic problems, such as overcrowded housing, ethnic discrimination, poverty, or unemployment. Furthermore, as also shown by the COVID-19 outbreak and the need for social distancing, the lack of social ties led to several serious situations, such as domestic violence or isolation [20,21].

For all these reasons, the scientific disciplines refer to "vulnerable communities" (urban or rural) as those communities that are more limited in being able to respond to changes that will impact the society [22,23] and they represent that sector which will increasingly suffer from changes in the short and long term. Therefore, designing for these contexts requires a new way to approach the concepts of "design" and "vulnerabilities". The authors consider that considering—during this specific research—very specific conceptualizations, definitions, or assessments of vulnerabilities, could limit the spectrum of applications. Even if several definitions, as those of W. Neil Adger, require that to define vulnerability in communities, indicators must be considered along the time [17], for the purposes of this research, the authors considered specific indicators in a defined moment.

1.2. *Definition of Urban Vulnerability used by the Research*

According to the previous analysis, a universal definition of "vulnerability" can be considered as a "potential state, whose equilibrium can be compromised by a disturbing event". Based on this general definition, everyone must be considered vulnerable. Nevertheless, persons with less political, economic, or technological power must be considered more vulnerable than those who have the power to reduce the imbalance introduced by the disturbing event.

Moreover, to be not too restricting or too vague, to define a "vulnerable community", for the purposes of this research, a community should be based on these characteristics:

- Limited economic resources;
- Limited political weights and excluded from the principals political decisions;
- Scarcity of basic services (light, water, sewer system, etc.) and public services (transportation, garbage management, etc.);

- Environmental emergencies (pollution);
- Social isolation and segregation for the formal city.

1.3. Looking for a Definition of "Design for Vulnerables": Current Gap, Research Objective, and Contribution

Currently, in vulnerable communities (as previously defined), it is not easy to outline guidelines for the design. In particular, it can be common to start with a wrong approach and set up an inappropriate community interaction strategy. Recent approaches comprehend community participation as the main way to an appropriate sustainable development design in vulnerable communities [24–26]. However, the current reality makes this approach no longer sufficient: new complexities (1) of the urban and social phenomena (which imply a new design vision) and (2) of the possible futures (which make forecasts unpredictable) make it urgent to update the methodology of how design should approach these vulnerable contexts. It is necessary to update methodologies that can lead a designer during the initial stages of the project, to properly define needs, hopes, strategies, and solutions. Based on this interpretation of the current design problems in vulnerable areas, the research project "Design for Vulnerables" was started, with the aim to understand which dimensions must be considered when planning urban-architectural interventions in these contexts. A multidisciplinary approach is an urgent need to define the first approach to planning and design in vulnerable communities. This research aims indeed to understand how design solutions and methodologies should evolve to propose suitable solutions for all these kinds of communities, where new environmental stimuluses can create uncertain futures and potential harms.

This hypothesis, supported by the results, is represented at the end of the paper, through a four steps map—challenges, understanding, focusing, and strategies. The process of "Design for Vulnerables" must contemplate different scales (global and local) and act with different focuses (goals and tools). The goal of this representative hypothesis is to establish an interrelation between these steps, scales and focuses, where Anthropocene, technology, person, and environment are the four main connectors in multiple dominions.

2. Knowledge Gap and Emergencies That the Research Aims to Fill

According to the previous considerations, the relevance of this research is mainly related to the current existing gap in the academic literature and to the need to fill it. Thus, the development of a new methodology for design can be facilitate. This section explains why the Design for Vulnerables research project aims to define which design methodologies should be adopted to reduce urban vulnerabilities in the coming decades, generating a set of principles of Design for Vulnerables, graphically represented by a re-interpretation of the Krebs cycle.

2.1. Existing Knowledge Gap

Currently, the academic literature does not collect texts and research that (1) investigate the role of design in "vulnerable contexts", as defined in this research, or (2) are based on an inter-disciplinary vision of the concept of "vulnerability".

The authors performed a deep review of the academic literature, looking for the existing knowledge in the field of design for vulnerable communities. Scientific publications and outreaches were analyzed to understand the relevance of the research project. The lack of holistic and multidisciplinary approach is particularly relevant in the most cited articles on this topic, in the areas of social sciences, environmental sciences and arts and humanities. Among all the studied material, for clarity and readability, the authors decided to present here just the 10 most cited articles, which represent the most significant resources for the academic knowledge. In fact, if we consider the most cited Scopus indexed articles, based on these limits (TITLE-ABS-KEY (architecture AND vulnerable AND community); from 2015 to present; Subject Area: Social Sciences, Environmental Sciences; Arts and

Humanities; Document Type: Article, Conference Paper, Book Chapter), we can observe how the concepts relating "vulnerability" and "design" are limited to very specific aspects:

1. "2011 AERA Presidential Address: Designing Resilient Ecologies: Social Design Experiments and a New Social Imagination"—2016, 58 citations, vulnerable ecologies and nondominant communities [27];
2. "Queering women, peace and security"—2016, 50 citations, sexual and gender-based violence [28];
3. "Survey, HBIM and conservation plan of a monumental building damaged by earthquake"—2017, 18 citations, conservations and earthquakes [29];
4. "Citizen science-informed community master planning"—2020; 15 citations, flooding [30];
5. "Importance of soft canopy structure for labrid fish communities in estuarine mesohabitats"—2017, 13 citations, habitat and fishing [31];
6. "Utilization of the Maryland environmental justice screening tool: A Bladensburg, Maryland case study"—2019, 12 citations, environmental justice and GIS [32];
7. "Policy innovations for pro-poor climate support"—2020, 9 citations, climate adaptation and infrastructures [33];
8. "Slum upgrading and climate change adaptation and mitigation: Lessons from Latin America"—2020, 8 citations, Climate change and Informal settlements [34];
9. "The governance of adaptation financing: Pursuing legitimacy at multiple levels"—2017, 7 citations, climate adaptation and governance [35];
10. "Sunshine, temperature and wind: Community risk assessment of climate change, indigenous knowledge and climate change adaptation planning in Ghana"—2020, 6 citations, climate adaptation and indigenous knowledge [36].

As can be observed, these major scientific products have a very specific slant and do not address the issue of design challenges in vulnerable communities for the coming decades, based on a holistic and multidisciplinary approach. A scientific product recently published by the same authors is "Design for Vulnerable Communities" [12], which makes an effort to collect the interdisciplinary visions generated by the Round Tables, which are part of this research. However, the book does not present the results of this research and does not reach the conclusions presented in this paper, since the purpose of the two publications are radically different.

Based on this important gap in the academic literature, it seemed timely to develop this research. This necessity comes, in particular, by the fact that the initial hypothesis is that Design for Vulnerable Communities represents an urgent call to our discipline, for which analysis and proposals can no longer be derived from activities confined within disciplinary boundaries.

2.2. *Emergencies for Vulnerable Contexts*

Although the contemporary global condition is absolutely the best in the history of mankind (long life expectancy, smallest percentage of people living in extreme poverty, etc.), the contemporary world is literally altered by epochal changes that have a huge qualitative and quantitative impact on the planet and the humanity [37]. Climate change and uncontrolled technological development offer important elements for reflection to understand contemporary conditions of vulnerability and think of effective intervention solutions. Climate change already counts with a structured academic literature relating design solutions and vulnerable communities. Technological development is still barely discussed in the academic literature of design for vulnerable communities.

2.2.1. Impact of Climate Change on Vulnerable Communities

Anthropogenic changes in the natural environment have been known since the earliest human activities (agriculture and early rural settlements) [38]. The enormous quantitative change of recent decades, however, has maintained this catastrophic impact, shifting its effects from a limited and almost insignificant scale to a global and extremely significant dimension and with important repercussions in many fields, from the environment to society. This is such a strong impact that the economic and social systems that led to this situation are strongly questioned [11,39]. The change in climatic phenomena can be observed, among other things, in the increase in temperatures, in a new distribution of extreme atmospheric phenomena (hurricanes, storms, etc.) or in changes in sea currents [40]. All these phenomena, beyond causing deleterious changes in the natural environment, are contributing to social changes that, although little studied at this time, have very deleterious effects on the structure of society and on the well-being of vulnerable communities [41]. Due to climate change, the world of production is changing and will change more and more, both agricultural production [42] (for example) and the production of services. There are many implications for poverty [43], for well-being and health (clean air, clean water, enough food and safe shelter) [44,45], as well as on migratory processes [46] and on community security [47]. It is very clear how necessary and indispensable it is to consider these changes when an urban-architectural intervention is going to be proposed.

2.2.2. Impact of Uncontrolled Technological Development on Vulnerable Communities

If the exponential growth of human activities is producing unprecedented changes in the ecosystem, the impetuous technological development is shaping many scenarios that were unthinkable until a few years ago. Thus, nowadays, this is a highly debated topic because, day by day, it has increasingly important repercussions on everyone's life and because it questions many of the certainties upon which contemporary society has been formed (production, social relations, services, spatial dimensions, temporality of life, etc.).

An interpretation of technological development has connotations of positivity and considers that the relationship with technology will be directed to a support for a healthy human flourishing; in contrast, a second interpretation sees in the unbridled development of the technological system even a threat to the entire humanity. Regardless of these two interpretations, although they have a more long-term perspective and are extremely relevant in other contexts, what must be highlighted here is how, for the most vulnerable communities, technological development is the key to getting out of conditions of vulnerability, where physical and environmental dimensions are a barrier [48,49]. If vulnerable communities lose this opportunity to take advantage of technological development to get out of their vulnerable condition, their vulnerability will become even stronger and the social, economic, and cultural differences could be insurmountable. Technological ignorance is presented as one of the serious dangers that hang over the future of vulnerable communities, showing itself, perhaps even more dangerous than illiteracy. In both cases, the urban-architectural design has very important responsibilities in proposing environments that are useful to face these changes. This leads to the need to discuss the current concept of urban vulnerabilities and what the role of the designer should be. In the last decades, starting from the works of Giancarlo De Carlo in Italy, participative design is considered as one of the most appropriate and sustainable ways to approach design in communities. However, the complexity of the contemporary challenges implies going over these methodologies and defining new ways to interact with vulnerable communities.

2.3. *Contemporary Design and Multidisciplinary Dimensions*

Moreover, although the world of construction is one of the human activities that is most slowly aligned with social transformations, architectural design has always represented one of those human activities that is most sensitive to changes in culture and social phenomena. For this reason, given the upheavals that are taking place, it is very essential that urban-architectural design be able to question itself, become an active recipient of new needs, and thus prove to be capable of rethinking its being, its strategies, and its methodologies of work. Economic aspects, related to design, have a core role in this vision [37,50]. Of course, also anthropological studies [51,52], geographical issues [53,54], environmental sciences [40], or urban studies [55–59] have generated much knowledge that can apport to the discussion. For this reason, understanding the phenomena that characterize our territories is a priority: as these realities are becoming increasingly complex, the question that the research project Design for Vulnerables aims to understand is "how can design contribute to empowering vulnerable communities in the years to come?" As Papanek wrote in his seminal book in 1973 (originally, in Sweden, in 1970) [60], *"in an era of mass production in which everything must be planned and thought through, design has become the most powerful tool with which man shapes things. his tools and environments (and, by extension, society and himself). This demands great social and moral responsibility from the designer. It also calls for a greater understanding of people on the part of design practitioners and a greater understanding of the design process on the part of the public. [...] Design must become an innovative, highly creative and interdisciplinary tool that responds to people's true needs. It needs to be more research-oriented, and we need to stop desecrating the earth itself with poorly designed objects and structures"*.

As Papanek shows, in addition to being innovative and creative, design must become an interdisciplinary tool in order to find solutions that respect people and the planet. Today, in a society in which the fields of knowledge, responsibilities, and relationships are more complex than in 1970s, having an interdisciplinary design becomes an even more current requirement. This means leaving purely disciplinary works/knowledge: all those that deal specific questions and problems with the same method and approach [61]. The approaches that are not limited to a single area of knowledge, the "non-disciplinary knowledge" [62] and that have acquired special importance in the medical and nursing fields [63], they can assume various characteristics depending on the relationships that are structured between the different disciplines. In this context, characterized by new challenges for the planet, by unprecedented concepts of vulnerabilities, and by new responsibilities for design practice, a "non-disciplinary" approach can help to understand the state of vulnerabilities and to propose suitable solutions in vulnerable communities. This research aims to understand how much the design practice results receptive of an initial "non-disciplinary" approach.

3. Materials and Methods: Research by Design

The research presented in this paper is the result of the first year of work in the vulnerable community Paso del Norte (Chihuahua, Mexico). The deep interaction with residents and the wide participation of designers and interdisciplinary experts have been the main characteristics of a design workshop that allowed to generate a final definition of Design for Vulnerables. To understand what dimensions must be considered in order to propose urban architectural interventions in vulnerable contexts, a design workshop was held based on three fundamental actions (Figure 1): (1) Design groups, composed by international designers and residents in the vulnerable community, (2) Experts Round Tables, carried out by international experts, to introduce interdisciplinary perspectives about vulnerabilities, and (3) Real Life Web Lab, which allowed permanent communication between designers and members of the community during the pandemic. Results have been validated and compared to synthesis the principles of Design for Vulnerables.

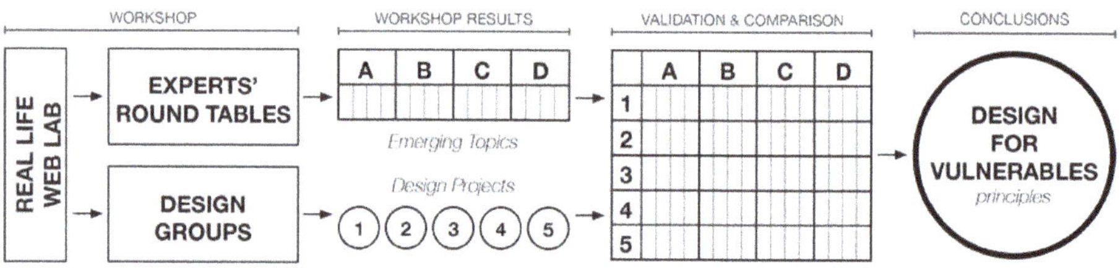

Figure 1. Scheme of the research flow.

3.1. Research by Design

This research, which uses the design workshop process and results as a research laboratory, is based on the research by design methodology. This methodological approach aims to use design as a process to foster dialogue between stakeholders (designers, citizen legislators, and researchers) and to sensitize both local government authorities and citizens about possible design solutions that are determined based on environmental, social, and economic patterns, and not merely on land use [64]. The research by design approach developed from Dutch practice at the Faculty of Architecture in Delft [65]. The research by design approach was defined by Hauberg [66] and Roggema [67] as follows: "*Research by design is a type of academic research through which design is explored as a method of inquiry, through the development of a project and also exploring the different means with which a project is carried out: sketches, mapping, among others*". Furthermore, research by design is a strategy, as Hauberg (2011) stated: "*It is used to describe the various ways in which design and research are interconnected when new knowledge about the world is produced through the act of designing. The methodology aims to generate desirable, perhaps unexpected, urban prospects rather than likely, but less desirable, urban developments*" [35]. Nassauer and Opdam [68] asserted that design is a common ground for researchers and practitioners to bring scientific knowledge to decision-making on landscape change, demonstrating that the pattern-process paradigm should be extended to include a third part, called "design". In this research project, the research by design method was applied for the regeneration of the Paso del Norte community.

According to Schoonderbeek, the term "research by design" can move to indicate three different situations or categories of relationship between research and architecture: (1) considering design as an act of research; (2) considering the design as the object of the research that is developed according to a controlled methodological process or (3) considering the design as a possible beneficiary of a research process that can provide useful information to the design process [69]. In the case of Design for Vulnerables, what the authors wanted to achieve was that, through design, they could activate research activities on the urban quality of the Paso del Norte neighborhood. Thus, the methodological process of research by design, in this case, must be understood under the first category of design as an act of research: a design based on defined methodological processes and specific instruments that can, thanks to the observations that are generated in the process and to the comparable data that are obtained, provide answers to a specific research question.

3.2. *Design for Vulnerables Research Project*

Design for Vulnerables is a research project supported by the Observatorio de Ciudades of Tecnológico de Monterrey (Guadalajara, Mexico), started in 2021. A first context of study was the vulnerable community of Paso del Norte, in the city of Chihuahua (Guadalajara, Mexico), which will be followed by studies in other locations in the same state of Chihuahua (Ciudad Juárez, Mexico) and in the southern state of Chiapas (Guadalajara, Mexico).

Several universities and laboratories participate in the research project as promoters, as well as two different faculties of the Tecnológico de Monterrey (which is the host institution): the School of Architecture, Art and Design and the School of Humanities. The Design for Vulnerables activities can be observed on the project web page: "https://www.designforvulnerables.com/" (accessed on 15 August 2022) [70].

3.2.1. Paso del Norte, Chihuahua, Mexico: A Vulnerable Community

The first study context of the project has been the vulnerable community Paso del Norte (PDN) in the city of Chihuahua. Chihuahua is the capital of the homonymous state, which is the largest one of the Mexican Federal Republic, located in the central border with the United States of America. For this reason, the state and the capital play an important role in the management of migratory phenomena that cross the American continent from south to north (and from north to south). Specifically, the city of Chihuahua, which is about 300 km from the border, is the scene of a transit migration. That is, most of the migrants who arrive in the city stop for a few days to rest, waiting to reach Ciudad Juárez at the border. This implies, unlike the border city, that the vulnerable communities of the capital Chihuahua are not urban areas that host important groups of migrants who move to the US, or who, in contrast, seek to return to their country of origin. In these communities, the most relevant migratory phenomenon, on the other hand, refers to permanent or seasonal internal migration, with people moving from rural areas to cities, mainly to look for work.

Specifically, PDN is a peri-urban colony, where about 2000 people live. It has been formed over the last 70 years, alternating formal and non-formal processes, mainly thanks to the mentioned migration.

For Mexico, the main indicators, and criteria to define a vulnerable community come from the National Institute of Statistic and Geography (INEGI) (Instituto Nacional de Estadística y Geografía). Thus, today, PDN can be considered a vulnerable community according to the previously defined focus:

- Few economic resources: the majority of the population works in the industrial sector (with an average income of 250 USD/month [71] or in domestic cleaning (average income 200 USD/month) [71];
- Limited political weights and excluded from the principal political decisions: in the opportunities of "participatory budget" promoted by the municipality, Paso del Norte has been excluded from financing and the majority of public interventions have been financed and promoted by the community itself;
- Scarcity of basic services (light, water, sewer system, etc.) and public services (transportation, garbage management, etc.): less than the 30% of the streets are paved; there are no public transportation stops in the neighborhood; garbage collections comes irregularly once a week; around the 70% of houses has connection to drainage and 80% has connection to electricity [72];
- Environmental emergencies (pollution): the community is located between two canyons, which are used as illegal landfill (Figure 2), and is divided from the formal city by Sacramento River, which is showing higher and higher levels of pollution;
- Social isolation: the highway and the river divide the community form the formal city, creating a perception of division and isolation from the city of Chihuahua.

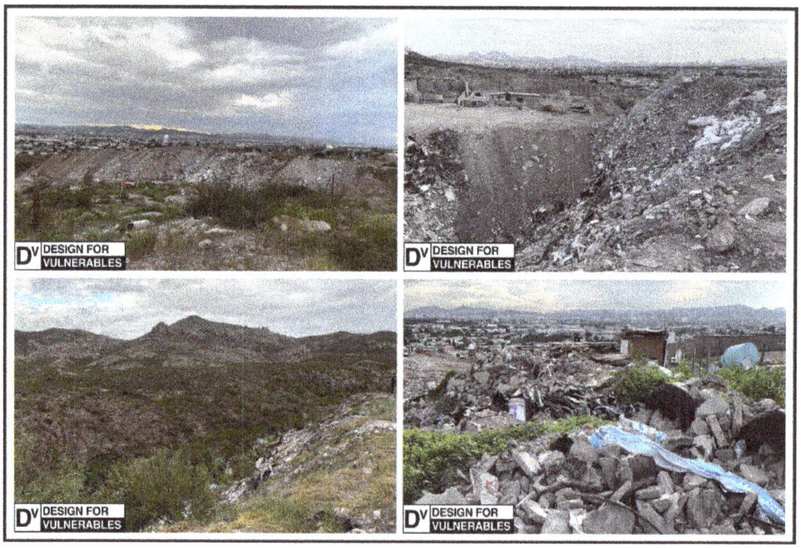

Figure 2. Canyons around Paso del Norte used as landfill.

For all the references and other details, please, visit the project web page www.designforvulnerables.com (accessed on 15 August 2022).

A characteristic of this community and one of the main reasons for its vulnerability is its semi-isolation from the formal city. PDN was set on the slopes of the mountains that defines the eastern border of the urban area of Chihuahua, located on the side of the

Rio Sacramento (one of the two main waterways of the city). Moreover, in recent years, alongside the watercourse, a high-traffic road was developed, contributing to relegating the community outside the formal urban area. This division means so much to the perception of belonging to a reality different from the formal city.

For some years, Tecnologico de Monterrey has been working in this community with social activities coordinated by the Professor Virginia Aceves and her association Accionética. These activities allowed to generate confidence in the educational institution, allowing to carry out research activities directly with the residents of PDN. In fact, as previously introduced, a key moment of this first study of the Design for Vulnerables project was the multidisciplinary workshop which was based on the possibility of constant dialogue between the participants (designers, interdisciplinary experts, and residents of Paso del Norte).

3.2.2. Real Life Web Lab

To allow this dialogue to take place in the best possible way, even during the isolation imposed by the COVID-19 pandemic, the research group structured a Real Life Web Lab. The purpose of this laboratory was to allow participants to be able to have an immersion, albeit virtual, in the life of the community, thus recreating that experience of approaching the reality of study, typical of the in-person workshops. The activities of the Real Life Web Lab began with a first Zoom broadcast from the community (December 2020), in which members of the research group showed the community to the participants, observing the most relevant urban areas and interviewing residents of the community. The activities of the Real Life Web Lab continued, mainly through WhatsApp groups, with constant discussions between participants outside the community and residents.

The Real Life Web Lab tool was created primarily to cope with the conditions imposed by the pandemic. Despite this, it has proven to be an excellent tool for allowing dialogue in a structured way and between people, who cannot coincide in the same place. In addition, the Real Life Web Lab allowed to record the interactions between participants and to document them in a more structured way. Indeed, the Real Life Web Lab compiled a series of videos, documents, and proposals that emerged from the working groups.

Throughout the six weeks of the workshop, the teams worked on five activities defined within the framework of the "Real Life Web Lab" (Appendix A). These weekly activities were necessary to guide the working groups in the development of a final proposal, standardizing the points of discussion, the methodology of analysis, and development of the proposal. This with the aim of being able to easily observe differences and similarities among the final proposals.

According to the research by design methodology, being able to use very clear and defined design instruments is key to having an objective and reliable research process [73]. For this reason, the authors decided to be very clear with the structuring of the design methodology. The required weekly activities were directed towards deep knowledge of the community and the development of ideas for the improvement of the future.

3.2.3. Interdisciplinary Round Tables

If the Real Life Web Lab aimed at providing participants with knowledge about the context, while not being physically present, the Interdisciplinary Round Tables aimed at providing participants with multidisciplinary knowledge, while not being experts in different topics. For this reason, four round tables, where at least one member of each design group should be present, were organized to present and discuss interdisciplinary issues. These four round tables were organized during the first two weeks of the workshop, in order to provide the design groups with the theoretical multidisciplinary foundations at the beginning of their activities. The goal was that designers could start their process with a theoretical basis expanded by discussion with interdisciplinary experts.

The structure of these round tables consisted of four moments (Appendix B): (1) presentation by the moderator of the round table, with introduction of the discussed topic, paying particular attention to its relationship with planning in vulnerable communities and to the relevance that is expected in the next decades; (2) thematic presentations by experts, aimed at presenting both examples of studies or interventions in vulnerable areas, as well as providing a vision and a methodology to be able to interpret vulnerability; (3) discussion among the invited experts coordinated by the moderator of the round table to facilitate the emergence of points of contact between the different disciplines, and (4) moments of individual discussion between the experts and the working groups (by means of Zoom's breakout rooms), with the aim of discussing particular aspects of urban-architectural analysis in Paso del Norte.

All the round tables have been recorded and uploaded for free use in the project web page. These records represent the main activities' products, while the results of the interactions between experts and designers represent the activities' impact. The main output of the Round Tables is the list of "Emerging Topics" that has been synthesized by the authors. Since the goal was just to empower the designers with multidisciplinary views, no other documentation (surveys, reports, etc.) has been generated from these activities.

3.2.4. Design Groups

Deep knowledge of the area of study, given by the Real Life Web Lab, and deep knowledge of the global phenomenon that may interact with the reality of the vulnerable community, given by the Experts Round Tables, were the basis for the discussion of the proposal for urban-architectural intervention within the design groups. These working groups were defined before the beginning of the workshop. All the members of the design groups had different backgrounds, and it was sought to have in each team at least: (1) one resident of Paso del Norte, (2) an architecture student, (3) an architecture professor, (4) an active professional architect in Chihuahua, (5) a recent graduate of architecture degree, and (6) an active professional in a reality different from Chihuahua.

As members of the design groups, 28 people attended the workshop as members and 8 persons as mentors. They participated from:

- Professional practice (as professional designers or studios): 10 Mexican professionals (Chihuahua and León) and 1 Spanish professional (Barcelona).
- Universities: from Italy (University of Pavia) and Mexico (Tecnológico de Monterrey in Chihuahua, Tecnológico de Monterrey in León, ISAD, Universidad de La Salle)
- Laboratories and Schools: Sustainable Territorial Development (Tecnológico de Monterrey) and UPLAB (University of Pavia).

All the participants, who did not know the context of Paso del Norte, received introductions to the workshop topics thanks to the Real Life Web Lab (Appendix C). The reason for organizing the design groups with participants with different backgrounds cam from the need: (1) to standardize the groups and to more easily compare the proposals; and (2) to offer, in each of the design groups, different visions coming from the different levels of the professional career (current student, recent graduate student, local professional, and international professional).

At the end of the workshop, each team submitted a formal proposal for intervention in the community. One aspect that assumes a very strong relevance in the Design for Vulnerables design workshop is the participation of residents in the discussion and design activities. Although participation, as a design methodology, is researched and applied on many occasions of theoretical and practical exercises, this is still a methodology that requires constant development and attention, in order to be effective [74]. According to Aish, in participatory design, two aspects must be considered: (1) satisfaction of the people for the final result and (2) "customized" balance among technical, functional, economic, social, and cultural concerns [74].

4. Results and Discussion

4.1. Interdisciplinary Round Tables: Emerging Topics

The Experts' Round Tables underlined several interesting outputs for the designers. These outputs can be observed as emerging topics that interdisciplinary experts consider as the most urgent issues according to their disciplines. For this reason, the main output of the Expert' Round Tables can be considered this list of emerging topics. With the aim to define this list, after the Round Tables, for several weeks, the authors carried out an in-depth analysis of the issues that emerged during the round tables. Starting from the recordings and the supporting graphic material (mainly the presentations), the authors extrapolated the themes that emerged and proceeded to group them according to the similarity of the conveyed message. Twenty categories came out from this grouping process (human impact on the environment, climate change and its consequences, energy poverty, etc.). Later, these twenty groups were clustered into four broader categories. This process made it possible to synthesize the messages that the interdisciplinary experts shared with the designers. The four categories that collect the twenty emerging topics are presented below. What is interesting to discuss, based on this list, is that, speaking of vulnerability, many disciplines traditionally away from architecture can propose useful reflections for the practice of architectural design. To facilitate the reading of this paper, just the four categories and the names of the twenty emerging topics are presented here. The whole definition of each one of them can be founded in Appendix D or on the research project's web page.

Challenges: to Design for Vulnerables, it is important to have in mind the new changes (and uncertainties), originated in the new geological era of the Anthropocene, that hit people and vulnerable communities. Defining the challenges helps to lead the understanding of the global phenomena. (C1) Human impact on the environment; (C2) Climate change and consequences; (C3) Health environment; (C4) Technological development; (C5) Political responsibilities.

Understanding: to Design for Vulnerables, it is important to understand the phenomena and the variants that define vulnerable conditions. Understanding global phenomena helps to define the focus for vulnerabilities in local communities. (U1) Human Development Index (HDI); (U2) Economic poverty; (U3) Energy Poverty; (U4) Strategic Alliances.

Focusing: to Design for Vulnerables, it is important to define the focus on the local dimension, to observe this phenomenon on a smaller scale. Focusing helps to elaborate strategies at local level. (F1) Digitization and Remote Sensing; (F2) Business Awareness; (F3) Social inclusion; (F4) Urban food system; (F5) Segregation and socio-spatial justice.

Strategies: to Design for Vulnerables, it is important to elaborate strategies to solve the challenges present in local vulnerable communities. (S1) Temporary relief and lasting solutions; (S2) Technology as instruments of citizen participation; (S3) Holistic approach; (S4) Integration with the formal environment (S5) Heritage and residual spaces; (S6) Opportunities for entrepreneurship.

Based on this list of emerging topics, one of the main peculiarities of this research can be observed: challenges, understanding, focusing, and strategies highlight issues that are already addressed by the academic literature in the field of design. The peculiarity to be underlined here is that these issues have never been considered together and within a process of design with vulnerable communities.

4.2. Design Groups: Design Projects

As a result of the activities that the design groups developed along the workshop, five proposals for intervention in vulnerable communities resulted. These represent, then, a set of five strategies to empower vulnerable communities. These strategies were presented as a formal intervention proposal in front of the community and the moderators of the round tables. Regarding the design process, it is important to underline as these five approaches have been directly defined by the five design groups. No thematic input has been given by the authors to the designers: these approaches are the results of different analysis and research promoted within each single group.

These five approaches, which, as said, have been generated by each design group without any input by the authors, could be summarized as follows:

- Team 1 seeks to enhance visual and physical connections and rehabilitate existing public spaces, to increase community resilience, thus fostering a sense of belonging and community;
- Team 2 wants to promote the local sense of belonging to innovate social relations, promote circular economy activities, working with a new neighborhood council, the community involvement of young people, and regenerating infrastructure and public spaces in Paso del Norte;
- Team 3 designs effective management and social cohesion strategies, reorganizing the Neighborhood Council and proposing social self-motivation activities, and optimizing shared public spaces, and proposing a community pavilion that can serve as a place of cohesion and community management;
- Team 4 focuses on the reforestation of large areas of the community, as it seeks to enhance the natural heritage of Paso del Norte, understanding it as a "common good", a cohesive element of the community, and an opportunity for territorial integration. Thus, a territorial corridor is created as a source of new social activities, coordinated from a community "operation" center;
- Team 5 wants to take advantage of natural and landscape resources to offer new business opportunities. Resorting to ecotourism strategies, use of social media and incentives for a natural evolutionary change, it seeks to promote a natural community empowerment to improve the sense of belonging and, finally, provide instruments to reduce the vulnerability of the community.

4.3. Validation and Comparison between Design Projects and Experts Round Tables

Once the workshop was completed, and the design solutions presented, it was possible to proceed with a comparison between the Experts Round Tables' outputs (synthesized by the authors in 20 emerging topics and grouped in 4 categories) and the five design proposals.

This comparison is, therefore, a post-project exercise that has the three objectives: (1) deepening the relations between the four categories of the emerging topics (hereinafter referred to as "The relations among emerging topics"); (2) understanding which typologies of design solutions are considered relevant by designers when intervening in a vulnerable reality (hereinafter referred to as "Typologies of design solutions") and (3) understanding the receptivity to integrate emerging topics in the proposals (hereinafter referred to as "The receptivity of the emerging topics").

These three goals allow us to converge, therefore, towards a synthesis of the principles of Design for Vulnerable Communities, which is the ultimate goal of this research. The results contributed to generate the graphic synthesis of the Krebs cycle of Design for Vulnerables. Starting from these results, the experimentation of this synthesis will start through the application to some similar projects already scheduled in Mexico for the second half of 2022 (Ciudad Juárez, Chiapas, Chihuahua city center).

4.3.1. Validation

This comparison served as a process for validating the results too. In fact, the same designers made the association between the principles that emerged from the round tables and the design principles adopted by their design teams. Therefore, the designers validated the "emerging themes" summarized by the round tables and they directly validated the synthesis of the project proposals. If the authors of the research had been the ones who had carried out the synthesis of the project proposals, errors would have easily been created and could have missed some project nuances, thus limiting, or exaggerating the complexity of the proposals.

4.3.2. Comparison

The comparison was made by means of a matrix defined by the emerging topics, grouped in the 4 main categories (columns) of challenges, understanding, focusing and strategies and the 5 design projects. After the workshops, these projects have been analyzed, by the designers itself, through the categorizes of "goals" (G), "interventions" (I) and "elements" (E) (lines) to facilitate the association between design solutions and emerging topics. To avoid erroneous associations between design solutions and emerging topics, the authors asked to the design groups to analyze their own projects. Since the purpose of this research is to define the dimensions and the relations involved in the general process of "Design for Vulnerables", the authors intend this exercise of comparison as a way to extract principles, synthetizing characteristics and relations among the four main emerging topics. The results are summarized in the following table (Figure 3). Here, the matches between emerging topics and design solutions are represented by the filled cells (1.1, 1.2, 1.3, etc.), whose full meanings are unfolded in Appendix E, in order to facilitate the reading of the paper.

In addition, even just with the present/absent quality shown in Figure 4, some considerations for each project can be raised.

Project 1 "Networks and nodes"

The project proposes some clear objectives, reducing environmental contamination, moving the attention of the local government toward the community, and integrating the community (to the formal city and within itself). Sustainable and regenerative approaches guide the interventions to reach these goals, while the river and the landscape become the two most relevant elements to work with. For this first team, some considerations deserve to be highlighted. No references have been made to: (1) Climate change and its consequences; (2) Technological development; (3) Human Development Index; and (4) Resilience of the Urban Food System, while, differently from other groups, they pay attention to Digitalization and Remote Sensing as a way to focus on the design for vulnerable communities.

Project 2 "Sense of belonging"

This team focuses its attention on challenges of Human Impact on the Environment, Health Environment, and Political Responsibilities. According to their proposal, kids' participation in the communitarian life and public gardens have a principal role in the design for vulnerable communities. In addition, no attention is given to the issues of: (1) Climate change and its consequences; (2) Technological development; (3) Digitalization and Remote Sensing; (4) Resilience of the Urban Food System; and (5) Technology for Citizens' participation.

Project 3 "Community management"

This third group defines four priorities related to global challenges: (1) control of the garbage management; (2) renovation of hygienic infrastructures; (3) technology as means of training the community; and (4) strong partnership with local government. To reach these goals, particular relevance is given to temporary relief (at least, design, financing, and construction) and lasting solutions (hub for workshops and teaching). Furthermore, as most of the other groups, no attention is given to the issues of: (1) Climate change and its consequences; (2) Digitalization and Remote Sensing; (3) Resilience of the Urban Food System. Moreover, differently to the other projects, this group does not consider the issues of (4) Energy Poverty; (5) Social Inclusion and Health; and (6) Integration with the formal environment.

Project 4 "Ecological corridor"

The fourth group centers on the challenge related to the "Human Impact on the Environment", focusing on "Business Awareness" and "Social Inclusion and Health", while proposing strategies mainly related to "Heritage and Residual Spaces". In particular, the environmental issues are related to the design of an ecological corridor which can connect the community with the formal environment, enhancing the existing the cultural and natural landscape heritage. As the other groups, no attention is paid to (1) Climate change and its consequences; and (2) Resilience of the Urban Food System. Moreover, no attention is given to (3) Technological development; (4) Human Development Index; (5) Technology for Citizens' participation.

Project 5 "Tourist route"

This fifth project refers mainly to the development of a route for tourism connecting the community to the natural resources in the natural landscape surrounding the community. The main goals refer to creating awareness about caring for the ecosystem and to improve the social environment, as well as enhancing technological capacities and political responsibilities. As in almost all the other groups, references are missing to the (1) Climate change and its consequences; (2) Digitalization and Remote Sensing and (3) Resilience of the Urban Food System.

DFV		Challenges					Understanding				Focusing					Strategies					
		Human impact on the Environment	Climate change and consequences	Health Environment	Technological Development	Political Responsibilities	Human Development Index	Economic Poverty	Energy Poverty	Strategic Alliances	Digitization and Remote Sensing	Business Awareness	Social inclusion and health	Resilience of the urban food system	Segregation and socio-spatial justice	Temporary relief and lasting solutions	Technology for citizen participation	Multidisciplinary and holistic approach	Integration with the formal environment	Heritage and residual spaces	Opportunities for Entrepreneurship
Project 1	Goals			1.2		1.3													1.13		
	Interv.	1.1						1.4		1.6		1.4	1.8			1.10		1.12		1.14	
	Elem.								1.5		1.7				1.9		1.11				1.15
Project 2	Goals	2.1		2.3		2.5		2.9					2.14		2.17				2.21		
	Interv.	2.2				2.6		2.10	2.11			2.13	2.15			2.19		2.20			2.23
	Elem.			2.4		2.7	2.8			2.12			2.16		2.18					2.22	
Project 3	Goals	3.1						3.6				3.8			3.9	3.10					
	Interv.			3.2	3.3					3.7						3.11	3.12				3.15
	Elem.					3.4	3.5											3.13		3.14	
Project 4	Goals	4.1		4.4								4.9	4.11								4.19
	Interv.	4.2				4.5		4.6		4.8			4.12			4.14		4.15		4.17	
	Elem.	4.3							4.7			4.10			4.13				4.16	4.18	
Project 5	Goals	5.1		5.2				5.6				5.8	5.9								
	Interv.					5.4	5.5					5.8			5.10	5.11			5.14	5.15	5.16
	Elem.				5.3				5.7								5.12	5.13			
TOT		8	0	6	2	7	3	6	4	4	1	7	7	0	6	6	3	5	4	6	5

Figure 3. Table to summarize the comparison between round table outputs and proposals. Numbers are placed as references for detailed explanations (Appendix E).

5. Discussion Generated by the Comparison

As declared at the beginning of this paper, the research's aim is to update methodologies that can lead a designer during the initial stages of the project in vulnerable communities to properly define needs, hopes, strategies, and solutions. The comparison presented in Figure 4 allowed us to discuss about new needed methodologies. Moreover, before discussing the outputs of this comparison, it is appropriate to make a consideration regarding the current approach to design in and for vulnerable communities, which is often characterized by the following aspects [60,75,76]:

- Vulnerable situations are seen as places where design is excluded, rather than situations that must be intervened in (for ethical responsibility) and "opportunities" to renovate the discipline;

- Technology is considered inappropriate to vulnerable contexts and seen as an imposition, rather than a strategic opportunity to improve the life quality in vulnerable communities;
- Design solutions mainly come from disciplinary field, rather than looking for solutions with a wider interdisciplinary sight.

Within this context, the comparison resumed in the table highlights how the role of the architects and the research methodologies for interventions in vulnerable communities need to radically change. While some of the emerging issues can be considered proper of the discipline, others are totally new. The comparison can highlight three aspects that are discussed in the following sections: (1) the relations among "emerging topics", which allow to better understand their meanings and the theoretical principles of Design for Vulnerables; (2) the typologies of design solutions, which allow to understand which are the strategies that could be considered as guidelines for Design for Vulnerables; (3) the receptivity of the emerging topics, which allow to understand which interdisciplinary topics have been assimilated by the architectural practice and, instead, which still need more incentives for a proper Design for Vulnerables.

5.1. The Relations among Emerging Topics

New methodologies to drive the principles of design in vulnerable communities need to be based on emerging topics, coming from multidisciplinary fields of knowledge. The matrix validation process highlights how it is appropriate to condense the emerging topics into four categories. This structure also allows to highlight some aspects that are listed here:

a. The four main emerging topics can be considered as working areas. This means that challenges, understanding, focusing, and strategies must be considered as key moment of the process of Design for Vulnerables. While emerging topics underline the interdisciplinary vocation of these four topics, the design projects underlined as these four topics are partially considered in the design processes.
b. Interventions consider different scale of work. Design for Vulnerables does not mean focusing just on the local community because a global sight is required to clarify challenges and understanding vulnerabilities.
c. Design for Vulnerables means to keep under control aims and goals.
d. The importance given to formal environment, landscape resources, heritage, and public spaces represent an attitude of deep interest toward the potentialities of the context.
e. Multidisciplinary analysis and research capacities are the basis of conscious interventions in emergency contexts.

As shown in the literature review, there is no prior research discussing this holistic view of the problem and an overall design method. The results of this research project highlight how this vision is appropriate and allows the development of a coherent and global discussion on emerging issues for design in vulnerable communities.

5.2. Typologies of Design Solutions

Any new methodology to drive the principles of Design for Vulnerables must be defined from some typologies of interventions. For this reason, the matrix can be useful also to propose a list of guidelines and project-actions for vulnerable communities. Of course, this section of typologies of design solutions strongly depends by the context and by the characteristics of vulnerabilities of Paso del Norte. Moreover—without being ultimate universal solutions—they can give an idea of topics and issues that can be useful to contemplate while approaching vulnerable communities. Therefore, these actions could (and should) contribute to a paradigm shift with respect to previous design approaches.

a. Interests in enhancing the programs of users, be human beings, animals, plants, groups/communities, or any other human–nature combination.

b. Abandonment of anthropocentrism and redefinition of human activities in mutual equilibrium with the environment, allowing landscape and natural resources to assume a central role in the regenerative development of the community.
c. Inclusion and legitimation of different languages and aesthetic repertoires, accepting the ordinary. Designer should become "translators" and "educators" of the residents, who are the true participants and protagonists of the transformation.
d. Proposing solutions which could allow solving multiple problems, minimizing the creation of new needs and maximizing new opportunities.
e. Experimentation with the community to produce results or working hypotheses better than an exercise of mere theoretical application.
f. All architecture deserves the attention of designers, no matter how small, peripheral, or academically irrelevant it may seem at first sight: it is the representation of a local culture rich in values, which should be valued as a heritage of knowledge and a genuine expression of relationships social and environmental aspects of a community.
g. Promotion of the reuse and circular recycling of any waste or material already used to create new components for architecture, in combination with the sharing of skills and competences of local inhabitants. Likewise, attention to the architectural potential of public spaces and areas, whose rehabilitation within an urban-architectural process can help create new relationships with the formal city (services, connections, etc.).
h. Design of spaces and architectures that can be transformed over time, adapting to change, and offering flexibility to the entire community.
i. Rejection of a romantic/nostalgic attitude, so the use of any technology will be supported and encouraged, with the aim of real empowerment of communities and all inhabitants.

In contemporary scientific literature, there are several different approaches that introduces reflections such as those presented here in the previous points. Nevertheless, a methodology merging all these approaches is missing, since this research presents a new focus (vulnerable communities in the next decades) which has not been taken in consideration before. Moreover, in some cases, based on an old way to analyze design methodologies, these emerging approaches could seem even antithetic. For example, philosophies related to the abandonment of anthropocentrism arrive even to reject integration of technological devices in sustainable solutions, as highlighted by Cole [77] and Zhang [78]. In contrast, this research shows how integrating technology to "no-anthropocentric" solutions represents a valid method to design for vulnerables.

5.3. The Receptivity of the "Emerging Topics"

The new methodology that the research aims to define, must also be based on the receptivity that design groups show during the design process, so as to understand which emerging topics are willing to be considered and which ones need deeper discussion. Regarding the way the designers elaborated proposals containing references to the "emerging topics" that they approached during the round tables, it is appropriate to underline how some topics have been integrated to the proposals, while other have not. In the design phase:

a. less attention has been dedicated to the issues of "climate change" and "digitalization".
b. more attention has been given to the issues of "human impact on the environment", "political responsibilities", and "social inclusions and health".

The fact that no group has introduced any issue related to climate change can be considered quite strange since climate change was a recurring theme during the presentations and that, in contemporary design practice, great relevance is attributed to this topic. Perhaps the fact that in the studied context (Paso del Norte) the emergency is mainly connected to social aspects meant that attention was not focused on environmental emergencies and on the risks associated with climate change.

Even the lack of attention to the issue of digitization could seem something strange even if more understandable, since too little attention is given to the digital issue as a phenomenon with a high impact for society: the consciousness of how much is necessary to integrate digitization both in the design process and in the functional program of spaces in vulnerable communities is still too low [79]. The lack of attention to issues of climate change and digitalization must raise alarm about the inability of the design world to meet the revolutionary and unprecedented changes (positive and negative) that are impacting society. This implies that more efforts must be made to encourage the integration of these issues into architectural practice. These results and concerns are in line with the results presented internationally [80,80–82].

On the other hand, the higher attention to the social aspects of an architectural intervention can reflect the fact that during the analysis of the context, the main emergencies that have been found are related to social problems and the lack of attention by the local political system. In fact, it could be said that these issues have been leaders in the international design landscape of the last decade.

6. Krebs Cycle of Design for Vulnerables: Discussion about Approaches to Design in Vulnerable Communities

Inspired by the principles of the Krebs cycle of creativity (KCC), by Neri Oxman [83], the authors want to abstract the principles that emerged from this research activity, considering that this tool must be superimposed on the contextual realities, as very well explained by Samantha Winter during the Round Tables [10]. In fact, the elements used to generate this abstraction come from exercises applied to a very specific study context (Paso del Norte). This means that with this abstraction, the authors aimed to summarize only the basic concepts for the "Design for Vulnerables", their characteristics and relationships (Figure 4).

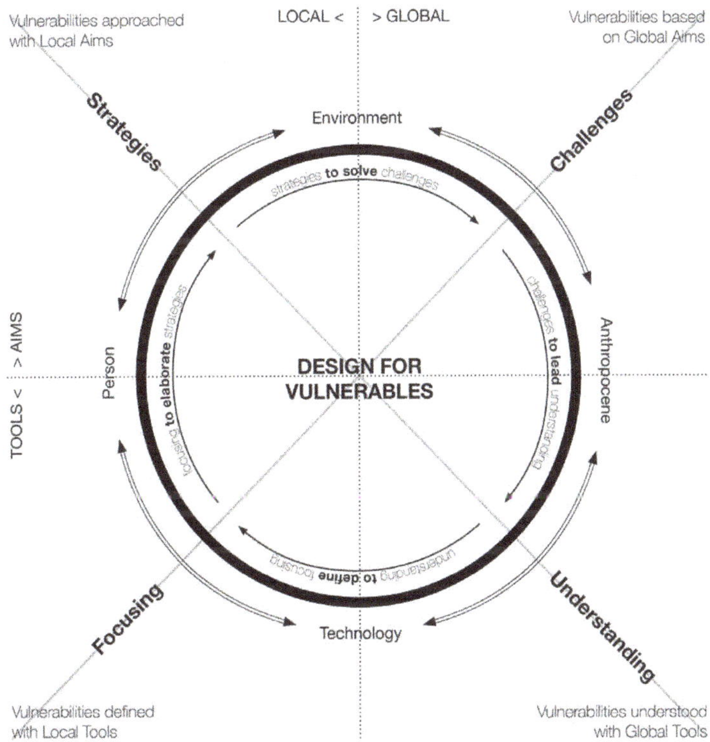

Figure 4. Krebs cycle of Design for Vulnerables.

As the matrix shows, the issues that emerged from the discussion with interdisciplinary experts, as well as the design process, revealed that there are four main work areas on which the "Design for Vulnerables" process should be based. The first area of work represents understanding the current challenges on a global level (challenges), followed by a second area of interpretation and measurement of phenomena (again with reference to global concepts) (understanding). A third area of work is related to focusing at the local level on the characteristics of the vulnerable community (focusing), so to be able to enter the fourth phase, when local solutions are provided to the initial challenges (strategies). The comparison exercise with the projects made it possible to highlight the characteristics and relationships of these areas. As in the case of KCC, these characteristics and relationships can be described with these aspects.

6.1. Each Area Is a Different Combination of Scales (Global and Local) and Focuses (Goals and Tools)

The quadrant is divided vertically between a local scale (left) and a global scale (right): "Challenges" and "understanding" belong to the global scale, since both areas deal with global issues; in contrast, the areas of "focusing" and "strategies" bring the work to the local level of the community. Similarly, the quadrant is divided horizontally between "aims" (top) and "tools" (below): "Challenges" and "strategies" are found in the quadrants of the "aims", as the work in both areas is specifically dictated by the pursuit of goals (contemporary challenges and people's well-being, respectively). "Understanding" and "focusing" are in the quadrants of the "tools", as they need technical tools to define vulnerabilities levels (Figure 5A).

6.2. Each Area Has a Different Purpose

The role of challenges is to clarify the main issues that are creating potential conditions of vulnerabilities in our contemporary society (climate change, technology, politics, etc.); it "converts" environmental conditions into Anthropocene questions. The role of "understanding" is to measure the vulnerabilities, based on global indexes and scales (energy, poverty, development, etc.); it "converts" Anthropocene questions into technical measurements. The role of "focusing" is to measure the vulnerabilities on a local level, where technical tools are applied to the life and the daily activities of people (entrepreneurship, social inclusion, food systems, etc.); it "converts" the technical measurements into person's necessities. The role of "strategies" is to define the best way to reduce vulnerabilities on a local level; it "converts" person's necessities into environmental conditions, representing the data that initiated the KCC in Challenges (Figure 5B). At this 'Cinderella moment'—when the hands of the KCC strike midnight—new environmental conditions inspire new challenges. The last sentences are a re-elaborated version from Age of Entanglement, by Neri Oxman [83].

6.3. Each Area Provides Additional Value to the Design Process

It is unthinkable to consider that an intervention can focus exclusively on one area of the process: all depend on the previous one and allow the next one to develop. It is impossible to "understand" the phenomena of vulnerability if the contemporary "challenges" have not been clarified. Similarly, it is impossible to "focus" on the vulnerability characteristics of the local community without "understanding" the phenomena of vulnerability. Therefore, intervention "strategies" cannot be defined without knowing the vulnerability characteristics of the local community. Finally, global "challenges" cannot be solved without knowing which strategies are necessary to intervene at a local level (Figure 5C).

6.4. The Relationship between Two Contiguous Areas Passes through a Conceptual Dimension

The connection between two contiguous workspaces is a specific conceptual dimension. "Challenges" and "understanding" are linked by the dimension of the Anthropocene, which represents the new reality to which humanity must get used to. "Understanding" and "focusing" are connected by the dimension of technique and technology, which "normatively" characterizes (today) the system of evaluation of reality. "Focusing" and "strategies" are connected by the "person", or rather the "community": as the focus becomes local, they have the person as a dimension of implementation. Finally, "strategies" and "challenges" relate to each other by the environment dimension, which represents the place of implementation of the "strategies" and the dimension in which the "challenges" take place (Figure 5D).

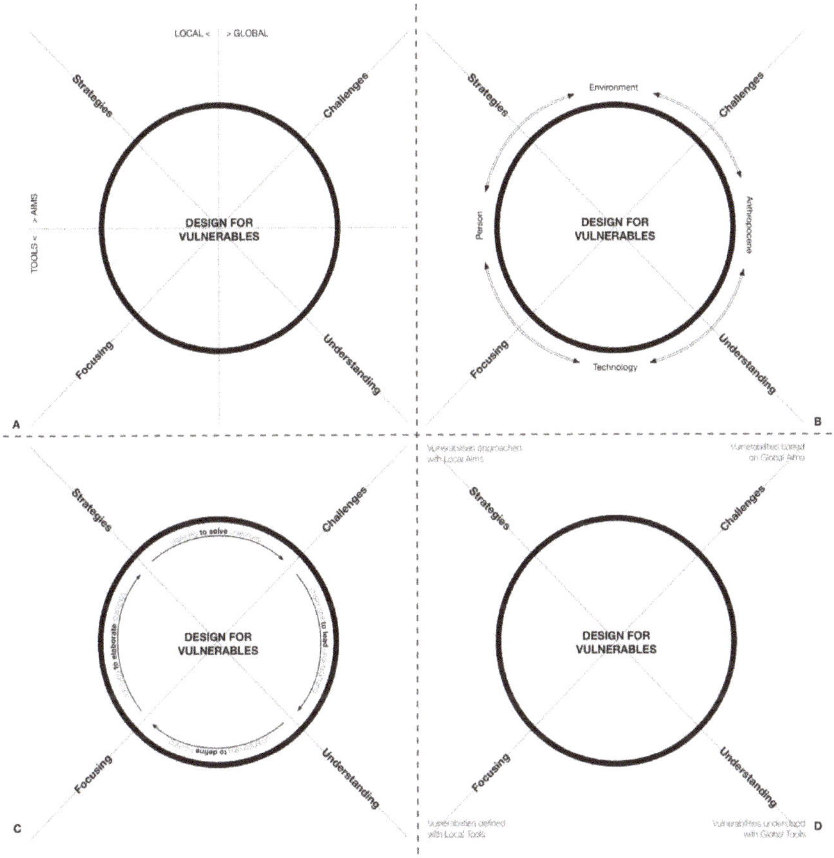

Figure 5. Four reading of Krebs cycle of Design for Vulnerables: (**A**) Each Area Is a Different Combination of Scales (Global and Local) and Focuses (Goals and Tools); (**B**) Each Area Has a Different Purpose; (**C**) Each Area Provides Additional Value to the Design Process; (**D**) The Relationship between Two Contiguous Areas Passes through a Conceptual Dimension.

7. Conclusions and Recommendation

7.1. Contribution and IMPACT

The contributions of this paper lie in proposing a new methodology to approach the first steps of Design in Vulnerable Communities. While the academic literature and the design practice have both important gaps when considering design approaches in vulnerable communities, with an interdisciplinary view and a long-term focus, this research project works in this gap and allowed to analyze the issue of design in vulnerable communities in the coming decades. As shown in the existing knowledge gap, the so-called "challenges", "understanding", "focusing", and "strategies", have been already addressed in different fields of knowledge. Moreover, no research is considering them together to define a methodology for design in vulnerable communities.

The project results, graphically expressed by the reinterpretation of the Krebs cycle", show how the process of "Design for Vulnerables" must contemplate, in particular in the first stages, different scales (global and local) and act with different focuses (goals and tools). Issues related with Anthropocene, technology, person, and environment are the four main connectors, in multiple dominions, between different steps, scales, and focuses. Operating with multidisciplinary view in each of the four "working areas" (challenges, understanding, focusing, and strategies), can enrich the process with potential energy, allowing to easier define the aims or better decide the appropriate tool to approach vulnerabilities. In this process, we can appreciate the analogy with the Krebs cycle, where each compound generates energy (and values) to the process.

7.2. Research Limitations

Of course, there is a basic aspect that is worth tracing again: the need to superimpose an abstract tool such as this one, on local realities. Thanks to this overlap, the Krebs cycle of Design for Vulnerables will highlight which challenges, issues, or opportunities will be the most relevant for each context. The importance of the context is absolutely not to be forgotten, since it is the basis of any approach to the issue of vulnerability. During one of the round tables, Samantha Winter (Columbia University, New York, NY, USA) masterfully described this necessity of contextualizing the studies when indagating for vulnerabilities [10].

Some limitations exist in the development of the research. Some of them may lie in the very methodology of "research by design" [73,84]: for the knowledge creation process to be considered research, the methodology must be explicit, openly communicated, and reviewed [85]. In some cases, this communication with the participants may have been limited, in particular with the residents of the vulnerable community—due to the limitations in the availability of technology in the neighborhood and to the pandemic. In different circumstances, when the workshop could have been carried out face-to-face, the participation could have been more effective, in terms of collaboration, exchange, and creation of knowledge.

In this research, suitable solutions are not tested against uncertain futures. This limitation will be overcome through future research, by applying approaches similar to those of Salas and Yepes [86] and Hall et al. [87]

7.3. Research Development

The results obtained so far, however, show how design for vulnerable communities must be considerably open to interdisciplinary knowledge and discussions. Future developments of this research will be directed towards a deeper understanding of (1) the role that multidisciplinary engagement plays in the changing reality of contemporary vulnerable communities and (2) the role that technology will play in facilitating these much-needed new design practices. For this reason, the very next step will be consolidating the Krebs cycle of Design for Vulnerables. To do this, the authors will apply in the following semester the same methodology and the circle to other cases, with different characteristics: Ciudad Juárez (city in the border with USA), Chiapas (southern state of Mexico), and Chihuahua city center (in an urban context). Then, the authors will adapt the circle according to the new concurrent data structures and, finally, they will ensure that the circle is mature enough to be usable for external users. Moreover, some interventions are planned in all these communities and the authors are committed to measure the results obtained with these interventions. Therefore, the ultimate step will be making the Krebs cycle of Design for Vulnerables digital.

Author Contributions: Conceptualization, E.G. and T.C.; methodology, E.G. and T.C.; validation, E.G. and T.C.; formal analysis, E.G. and T.C.; resources, K.P.S.G.; data curation, E.G.; writing—original draft preparation, E.G.; writing—review and editing, E.G., T.C., and K.P.S.G.; visualization, E.G. All authors have read and agreed to the published version of the manuscript.

Funding: The research presented in this book was performed thanks to the support of all the residents of Paso del Norte community and funded by the Fondo de Investigación 2020–2021 of Observatorio de Ciudades" of the School of Architecture, Art and Design of Tecnológico de Monterrey—2020/2, through the research project "Design for Vulnerables", with a duration from October 2020 to December 2021.

Data Availability Statement: The data presented in this study are openly available in the project webpage www.designforvulnerables.com.

Acknowledgments: The research project was performed within a long-term international collaboration among the School of Architecture, Art and Design of Tecnologico de Monterrey (Mexico), the China Lab. for Architecture and Urban Studies of the University of Pavia (Italy), and the Environmental Futures Lab. at the College of Design and Innovation, Tongji University in Shanghai (China), under the supervision of Tiziano Cattaneo and Emanuele Giorgi. Special thanks to the colleagues who participated in this project: Arq. Pablo Hernández Quiñones, Arq. Pablo Rentería-Rodríguez, Ing. Alfredo Mauricio Flores Herrera, and Virginia del Socorro Aceves Tarango.

Conflicts of Interest: The authors declare no conflict of interest.

Appendix A

Appendix A presents the activities performed by the design groups along the six weeks of workshop (Figure A1).

"Mapping Paso del Norte" (week 1): based on knowledge of the area and discussion with residents, each group analyzed and mapped some characteristics of the community (colors, sharing, history, landscape, and production) with the aim of understanding its implications in the life of the colony. Based on the team's topic (team 1—colors; team 2—landscape; team 3—shearing; team 4—history; team 5—production), the participants have to: (1) produce a thematic map of Paso del Norte; (2) relate it to "community" issues.

"Here is where we live" (week 2): the members of the community presented where they live and the public spaces where they spend their free time, what they do, what their work and skills are. So the activities consisted in mapping: (1) use of public and private space; (2) relationship with neighbors; (3) mobility and connections; (4) dreams and nightmares.

The results of these first two phases were shared among all the working groups. So, to start the proposal phase, which took the three following phases.

"Paso del Norte today" (week 3): had the purpose of providing various analyzes on the current state of the community, in order to highlight the aspects in which intervention is most needed. With reference to the contemporary situation, the participants have to prepare: (1) SWOT analysis; (2) mapping of urban phenomena; (3) mapping of the main actors; (4) analysis of community levels.

"Paso del Norte tomorrow" (week 4): consisted in considerations over the community in near, median, and far future, developed with the same analysis tool as the previous week. The aim is to highlight the most urgent aspects to intervene. With reference to an expected situation (2025, 2030, and 2050), the participants had to prepare: (1) SWOT analysis; (2) mapping of urban phenomena; (3) mapping of the main actors; (4) analysis of community levels.

"Let's do it" (weeks 5 and 6): formal development of an intervention proposal (urban, architectural, economic, etc.). The participants must develop an intervention proposal composed of: (1) description; (2) objectives; (3) reasons; (4) methodology and actors; (5) impacts; (6) phases; (7) costs; (8) promotion.

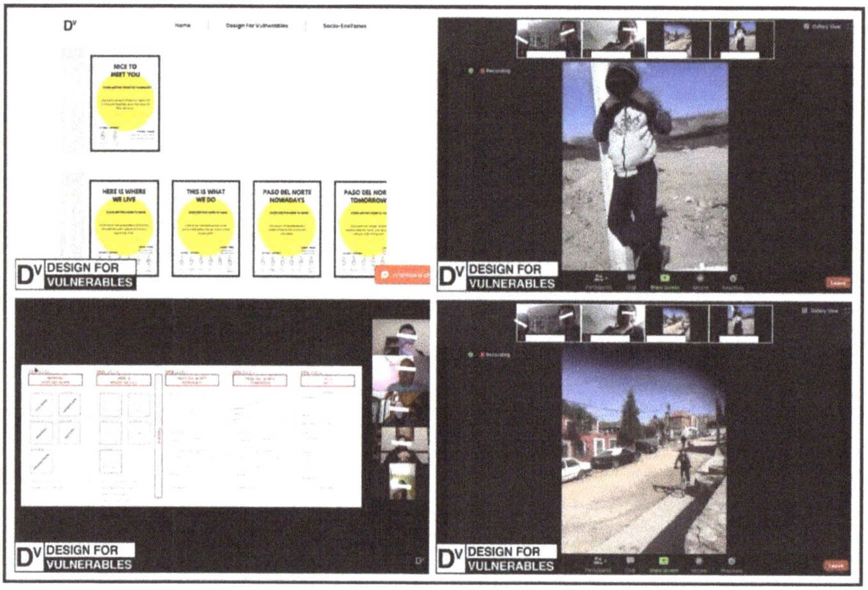

Figure A1. Real Life Web Lab activities.

Appendix B

The four round tables that were organized are presented in Appendix B and the phases of the round tables, as well as the interaction between experts—designers—community is represented in the picture (Figure A2).

The meaning of vulnerability (Thursday, 7 January 2021) served to present the main interpretations of the concept of vulnerability, under different disciplinary perspectives. At the table, mainly theoretical aspects were presented, with several demonstrations of real and application cases. Moderator: Miguel Ángel Montoya (Tecnológico de Monterrey, School of Architecture, México). Participants: Samantha Winter (Columbia University, USA); Ardeth Barnhart (Boston University, USA); Viviana Barquero (Tecnológico de Monterrey, EAAD, School of Architecture, México); Luis Fernández (Tecnológico de Monterrey, Sustainability, México); Gustavo Merino (Tecnológico de Monterrey, Escuela de Gobierno, México); Marco Morandotti (University of Pavia, Italy).

Strategies (Friday, 8 January 2021) was a moment to discuss what strategies design practice has been adopting in recent years to solve problems in vulnerable communities. Moderator: Aleksandra Krstikj (Tecnológico de Monterrey, School of Architecture, México). Participants: Ersel Kripa (Texas Tech El Paso, USA); Stephen Mueller (Texas Tech El Paso, USA); Carlos Gotlieb (ENSAP Bordeau, posgrado Rebulding the Wolrd, France); Nivaldo Andrade (Bahia Federal University, Brazil); Giulio Verdini (Westminster University, UK); Ioanni Delsante (Huddersfield University, UK); Carlo Berizzi (University of Pavia, Italy).

Global to Local (Thursday, 14 January 2021) allowed to analyze how global problems come to impact the life and well-being of communities and people. Moderator: María Elena de la Torre (Tecnológico de Monterrey, School of Architecture, México). Participants: Simone Lucatello (Instituto Mora, México); Mariajulia Martinez (Tecnológico de Monterrey, SDGs Initiative, EGADE, México); Jeremy Cheval (École Urbaine de Lyon, France); Christiane Molina (Tecnológico de Monterrey, EGADE, México); Roberto De Lotto (University of Pavia, Italy); Andrea Marinoni (Artic University, Norway); Paolo Ceccarelli, (ILAUD, Italy); Pilar Guerreri (ILAUD, Italy).

Social Entrepreneurs (Friday, 15 January 2021) It was an occasion to present social entrepreneurship solutions in vulnerable contexts, with examples from China and Mexico.

Moderator: Pablo Hernandéz (Tecnológico de Monterrey, School of Architecture, México). Participants Jingyi Lu (PINWU studio, Deputy Director of Rong Design Library, China); Ni Minqing (Directora DESIS LAB, Tongji University, China); Cindy de la Torre (Tecnológico de Monterrey, Emprendimiento, México); Alejandro Delgado (Busuleba A.C., México).

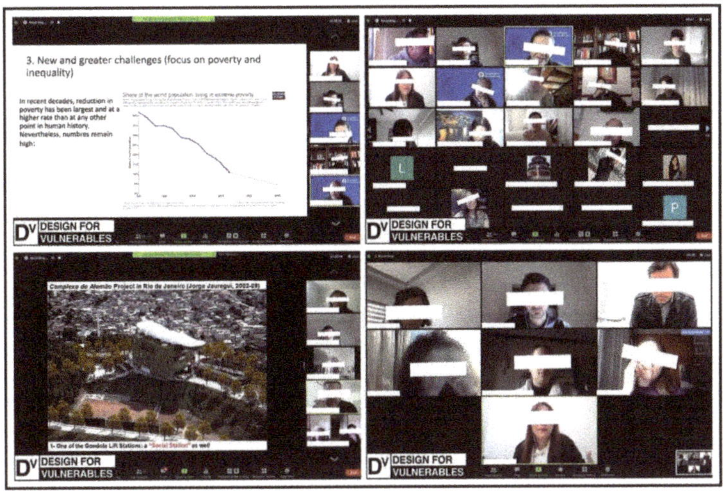

Figure A2. Interactions between experts and working groups during the experts' round tables.

Appendix C

Appendix C presents the summary of the projects elaborated by the design groups and presented to the community. In the figure, some pictures of the presentations are shown (Figure A3).

Project 1: "Networks and Nodes"

The community of Paso del Norte is undoubtedly characterized by very strong community ties stemming from a long history of residents with their community. However, environmental risks, insecurity, and pollution are causing these ties to weaken. The disintegration of these relationships also has repercussions on the community's public spaces, which are becoming less used or neglected. The main need in Paso del Norte is to recreate a sense of community that allows residents to face contemporary challenges together. To achieve this, however, it is necessary to revalue the physical spaces in which the community was formed. Therefore, the proposal focuses on the urban quality of public spaces (streets, plazas and urban fronts) trying to allow universal accessibility to the whole community, providing a strong identity.

Design Project 2: "Paso Del Norte, new generations and sense of belonging"

The proposal starts from a social observation about the importance of the youngest segment of the population: to recover a strong sense of belonging to the community that lasts for a long time, it is necessary to organize activities to involve the youngest groups of residents in the life of the community to (1) give them a sense of responsibility towards the social environment of their neighborhood, which will allow them to be more responsible towards the common good, (2) value them and make them feel that they are an important part of the community. The sense of belonging is the main aspect to work in this proposal and the strategy to achieve it is the involvement of people, starting with the youth. This involvement can be facilitated through physical interventions in the neighborhood, starting with the basic services that should be guaranteed to all neighbors, the cleaning of the filthy and polluted areas of the neighborhood and the regeneration of common spaces.

Design Project 3: "Restructuring of the neighbors' council and community pavilion Paso del Norte"

To address the existing problems in Paso del Norte community, this proposal takes into account: (1) a restructuration in the organization of the neighbors' council so that all residents can feel part of this structure, (2) having more responsibilities inside the life of the neighborhood to (3) increase the number of activities that take place within it. More activities and more community life in the neighborhood require more dignified and effective meeting spaces. Therefore, the organizational proposal goes hand in hand with (4) the proposal of a pavilion that can host the most important activities of the community. By strengthening the community within, the proposal also seeks (5) to implement opportunities for connection with external associations, thus ending marginalization.

Design Project 4: "Paso del Norte, Ecological Corridor"

The natural resources of the neighborhood are the opportunities to strengthen the community identity of Paso del Norte. The Sacramento River is no longer considered a barrier to the city and a segregation reason, it has become a natural element of opportunity to insert Paso del Norte into a territorial scale system. Likewise, the Nombre de Dios mountain range ceases to be the landscape background of the neighborhood and becomes part of an ecological corridor that detonates the economic development of the community, its visibility at a territorial level and the improvement of the environmental quality of the context. Re-establishing the floral and landscape "functionality" of this corridor brings the need to consolidate the physical elements of the neighborhood, particularly infrastructure and services. In addition, a community center is envisioned in the neighborhood to facilitate meetings and activities among neighbors, as well as a "center of operations" of the corridor.

Design Project 5: "Paso del Norte Route"

Considering the advantages of territorial and landscape connections of Paso del Norte towards the Sierra Nombre de Dios, this proposal indicates the development of a hiking area a possible strategy for the strengthening of the Paso del Norte community. The natural context becomes a tourist attraction that allows residents in the community to develop economic activities, starting on the main street of the neighborhood (José Fierro Street) and extending throughout the community. The eco-tourist activities, promoted by social networks and organized in the context close to the colony, are intended to become an economic spillover for the community.

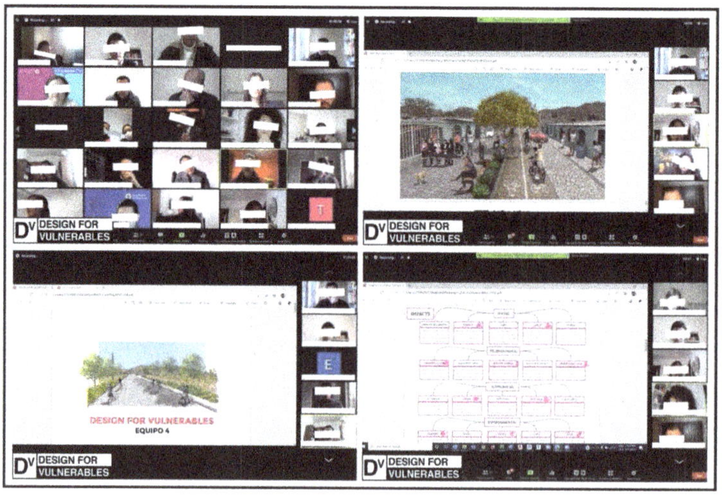

Figure A3. Design activities and presentation of the final proposals.

Appendix D

Challenges

C1—Human impact on the environment: since the potential impact of human actions increases more and more, the influence they can have on the social and environmental context is always greater. Knowing how to propose actions that limit potentially negative impacts on the environment appears, therefore, to be a challenge for interventions in vulnerable communities.

C2—Climate change and consequences: mitigation, adaptation, and resilience are the main three concepts for responding to the consequences of climate change (COP23) [88]. Knowing (1) how to choose which of these three options best suites to the intervention context and (2) which strategy is the most appropriate to the vulnerable reality, is a challenge that will become more and more relevant in the coming decades. In fact, the effect of climate change in vulnerable communities is undoubtedly a global emergency. Therefore, knowing how to consciously intervene in these situations is (and will increasingly be) a main challenge in these contexts.

C3—Health environment: The uncontrolled development during the recent decades has seriously endangered the quality of the environment in which most vulnerable communities live. Pollution, lack of basic services, and poor education are the main causes of environments with poor levels of health. Improving the environment and raising awareness on healthy quality of life represent new challenges for the society in the coming decades.

C4—Technological development: The technological capabilities, which are becoming more and more preponderating, open a panorama of unprecedented opportunities for vulnerable communities and a worrying scenario of an increased gap between the more and the less vulnerable sectors of the society. For this reason, offering interventions able to bring technology closer to vulnerable communities takes on a very important role in the community empowerment processes [89,90].

C5—Political responsibilities: Political attention to vulnerable communities is often reduced due to the low weight that these realities can assume at the electoral level. This situation, added to an increasingly scarce decision-making power represents a very significant challenge for interventions in vulnerable communities. In fact, these interventions must propose solutions capable of activating processes of political responsibility.

Understanding

U1—Human Development Index (HDI): to understand the state of vulnerability, it is proposed to use an index capable of defining the state of well-being of people and the social (as well the natural) environment where they live. The aim is to count with better tools to understand the actual needs of the community and the emergency fronts to intervene with priority. With the HDI, we refer to the dimension of a healthy life, knowledge and decent standard of living.

U2—Economic poverty: an essential dimension to understand the level of vulnerability is the economic poverty. This type of poverty, in fact, limits the resilience of communities, weakening the ability of people to cope with sudden changes which, it is assumed, will be increasingly frequent in the near future. Furthermore, understanding when a community is in situations of economic poverty allows us to understand how much it is possible to propose entrepreneurship initiatives in the context.

U3—Energy Poverty: one of the dimensions of poverty that must be assumed to understand the state of vulnerability is the energy poverty. In a world that consumes more and more energy, in fact, being able to count with the availability of reliable energy resources will be increasingly necessary. This means being able to count on a local and clean production, independent, as much as possible, from external resources.

U4—Strategic Alliances: the fact that the concept of "partnership" represents the objective that completes the list of 17 SDGs represents how strategic alliances are a key aspect for promoting community improvement initiatives and projects. This is even more true if we want to understand vulnerabilities in local communities, where strategic alliances can make visible the invisible demands and can attract resources for the implementation of interventions.

Focusing

F1—Digitization and Remote Sensing: in the most vulnerable communities, technology does not find a fertile environment and, often, these contexts deny technological innovations. Nonetheless, count with technological tools that allow better focusing on vulnerable communities is fundamental. Digitization and remote sensing allow a better use of resources, already scarce in vulnerable communities, providing a technological apparatus that can even be used remotely.

F2—Business Awareness: to inform and to inspire about the benefits that small business activities can have for the most vulnerable people is a key piece to implement self-sustaining interventions. Moreover, the awareness on entrepreneurial possibilities is also relevant to promote initiatives that strength community relations and lead to an improvement in the livability of a community. For these reasons, focusing on the business awareness of a local community becomes a key moment before to elaborate strategies of intervention.

F3—Social inclusion: focusing on the social relationships which are active within a community, is important since a healthy community environment becomes essential when undertaking improvement processes in a vulnerable community.

F4—Urban food system: the resilience of the production, distribution, and storage food systems is key for the easy and healthy access to food. Moreover, healthy systems create job opportunities, while encouraging and promoting healthier diets and lifestyles. For these reasons, focusing on the resilience of the urban food system becomes a key moment before to elaborate strategies of intervention.

F5—Segregation and socio-spatial justice: focusing on segregation and socio-spatial justice is central since an urban system, capable of integrating with the context and offering opportunities for connection with local services and resources, becomes a fundamental principle for strategies aimed to solve the challenges in vulnerable communities.

Strategies

S1—Temporary relief and lasting solutions: urban-architectural intervention aimed at reducing the vulnerability of a community can address two main strategies. On one hand, the need to intervene with a temporary solution that is easy to implement, so to provide the solution to an emergency, without the need for it to last beyond the initial moment of the crisis. On the other hand, the need to have an intervention that can accompany the community to gradually emerge from the condition of vulnerability.

S2—Technology as instruments of citizen participation: the possible support of technology tools is considered a very relevant strategy to facilitate discussion and emancipation of the most vulnerable communities. Technological resources must not and cannot be considered extraneous to these contexts.

S3—Holistic approach: strategies to generate effective solutions must consider phenomena from different perspectives to allow problems and opportunities to be perceived from different points of view.

S4—Integration with the formal environment: reducing vulnerability in the communities passes from the possibility of interacting in an official way with the more formal (and less vulnerable) communities present in the closest context. This strategy aims of reducing the perception and the effective segregation of vulnerable communities.

S5—Heritage and residual spaces: strategies based on the possibility of regenerating existing environments with cultural or historical value, as well as residual spaces within a community, represent an opportunity to activate social initiatives and the feeling of belonging to the community, which can reduce vulnerability levels.

S6—Opportunities for entrepreneurship: creating opportunities for people to develop local entrepreneurship initiatives is an excellent strategy to reduce the levels of vulnerability in a community. Counting with an environment that offers opportunities to start some business (albeit small), as well as spaces where to hold professional consultancy, is very important.

Based on this list of emerging topics, one of the main peculiarities of this research can be observed: challenges, understanding, focusing, and strategies highlight issues that are already addressed by the academic literature in the field of design. The peculiarity, to be underlined, here, is that these issues have never been considered together and within a process of design with vulnerable communities.

Appendix E

Project 1 "Networks and nodes"

1.1 The community is supposed to clean the river, which currently is a great source of contamination, and the new tourist corridor, which should bring visitors to the community.
1.2 Paso del Norte is currently a place with high levels of pollution due to an unconnected drainage system, which becomes a source of diseases.
1.3 Currently, the local government promotes a participatory fund for the decision about some public sources management. The project seeks for the government to look at the community again, paying attention to the distribution of resources.
1.4 In the corridor, people have the possibility to sell products made by them.
1.5 Interventions in the community (particularly in public spaces) will be accompanied by sustainable lighting, mainly for safety (currently there is an important lack of lighting).
1.6 The project aims to find an agreement with the church to create dynamics between the community and outsiders, taking advantage of the important space of the "Church House".
1.7 Digital elements to control the cars' speed and for security are supposed to be installed in the community.
1.8 Along the corridor there are opportunities for social interaction between different ages of the population. A lot of attention was paid to disabled people in wheelchairs.
1.9 Tourist corridor aims to reduce the segregation of the community and the perception of being on the other side of the city border.
1.10 There will be a corridor with green elements, where people will have the opportunity to sell products, assuming that the sale will increase over the years. Beyond this, the path could be connected in the future, with what is behind the "Peaks of the moon".
1.11 Publicize the community through the community's online presence (social media).
1.12 Various activities are expected to occur in the community (dance, sports, etc.). This will be bringing several experts to carry them out (professors, teachers, governments, civil society, etc.).
1.13 Integration internally to the neighborhood (through visually in the houses/facades) and externally with the city (through intervention of the river and corridor).
1.14 Currently there are spaces used but neglected: the baseball field is arranged to have guests from outside (tournaments, championships, etc.), the streets need interventions to reduce the speed of vehicles, and in the creeks, intervention are needed to "facilitate" the walking access to the community.
1.15 The corridor is considered as an opportunity for tourism, promoting hiking, the use of bicycles, connecting the community from outside.

Project 2 "Sense of belonging"

2.1 Through targeted activities (garbage collection, walking school bus, post-school at La Casa de la Iglesia), kids and adolescents learn how to become more responsible and to respect the place where they live.
2.2 Miss Heidi and the Church's priest explained that young boys and girls need to be involved and valued. Hence, the starting point of the process sees the young generation of Paso del Norte as the main protagonist. In particularly, the river can represent a resource for the Community of PDN but is polluted, thus its reclamation is extremely required.

2.3 The improvement of basic knowledge for everyone aims at supporting and consolidating the development of the values of sharing and mutual help in the face of a common feeling of individualism. The intention is to try to change the negative aspects of individualism and lack of sharing that are widespread in the community and to push away unhealthy temptations (drugs, alcoholism, no safety) which also reflects the bad organization of the community.
2.4 Environmental conditions can be improved by investing in the development of new green areas which can be transformed into Community Gardens.
2.5 To ensure a better organization on the social, political, and administrative level the project should be supported by the municipality and other social actors.
2.6 Citizens need to build a constructive dialogue with the municipality.
2.7 A PDN Board is fundamental to carry on the strategy in the long-term. It will be composed by the new generation and its role will be to realize the Community's will.
2.8 The role of women living in PDN has to be understood and enhanced at a social level.
2.9 Understanding the existing community's resources availability would have positive impacts for the general environment.
2.10 The process starts with kids and adolescents of the community who have the chance to improve their basic knowledge and abilities, this action affects adults who will be themselves involved in new activities.
2.11 A program of auto-construction through local material extraction is proposed to support economy and understand the land's value.
2.12 A specific Technical Group will deal with the urban quality of PDN.
2.13 Focusing on existing public spaces to organize a new area dedicated to a Local Market.
2.14 Focusing on the younger generations and getting rid of selfish behaviors.
2.15 The promotion of young people acts on the one hand on the effective improvement of the conditions of PDN, and on the other hand, inspire new feelings of responsibility and care that can evolve in the young and consequently transmitted to the older one through a bottom-up process. The discussion and exchanging of experiences help individuals to eliminate barriers and activate team-building processes.
2.16 The relationship between younger and adults is weak and needs attention. An important target is to change the diffused feeling among teenagers of not being important enough to be taken care of and valued.
2.17 Focusing on the change of perception from mere stay in a place to the feeling of belonging to that place and its importance.
2.18 Currently, streets represent a physical and social barrier by not being regularly maintained and leaving dirty. It is important focusing on this element in order to positively change flows in PDN.
2.19 The new proposed activities are oriented on taking on responsibility, taking care of the environment and each other. These activities will have a monetary retribution in order to catch interest and engagement. Establishing a circular process of exchange of both material and immaterial values aims at improving the economic aspect of residents' life.
2.20 Involving people in new gradual activities related to the social, political, economic, and environmental sphere is essential for establishing a new mentality that can reach the common good.
2.21 Recognition of all categories of people, their integration in the society, and respect to boundaries and needs.
2.22 The existing public spaces in PDN constitute a valid resource to activate social engagement.
2.23 Create a system of financial incentive when people do something for collectivity. The baseball field, the basketball court, and the playground have to be valued and exploited both in terms of human and physical capital: they constitute opportunities from an economic circular point of view, thus generating further benefits for the people in PDN.

Project 3 "Community management"

3.1 The project aims that the community could take control of the garbage management in the neighborhood.
3.2 Low quality of hygienic infrastructures, can cause health problems.
3.3 Technology is considered as a means of training the community (know how to use computers and data).
3.4 The local government is perceived as the main partner to attract actors to participate in the work.
3.5 Indexes (NUE by INEGI) is used to understand levels of schooling and income, as well as the characteristics of the dwellings.
3.6 The project aims to contribute to reducing economic poverty, through training, so to supplement the personal income.
3.7 The local government is perceived as the main partner to attract actors to participate in the work.
3.8 Training can create economic independence in the neighborhood, so as to reduce the need of daily commute far away
3.9 The project aims to offer spaces and activities which can integrate the newest part of the neighborhood, which today is not participating to the local social life.
3.10 The project aims to realize a permanent solution (hub for workshops and teaching).
3.11 The project is composed by various stages (at least, design, financing and construction) during which community is working in empowering processes.
3.12 The designers imagined the development of an app for citizen participation.
3.13 The residents understand that all their ideas need the vision and support of several different professionals.
3.14 Interventions are planned where there are public spaces (for ownership and accessibility reasons). The baseball field is defined as main intervention area.
3.15 The designed spaces aim to allow the development of activities for personal growth (entrepreneurship is just one of the aspects of personal growth).

Project 4 "Ecological corridor"

4.1 Three main goals describe the project goal: (1) focus on education of the population to improve the relationship with the natural environment to avoid negative impacts and bring positive impacts; (2) make use of nature protection (take advantage of the ecological corridor); (3) stop the destruction of the hill.
4.2 It is supposed that the community is going to work for the care of the environment.
4.3 The ecological corridor is the main mean to reach the three goals and make community take care of the environment.
4.4 People will be trained on how to better manage the garbage.
4.5 The intervention makes visible the neighborhood to the city and offers political visibility.
4.6 The Ecologic Corridor will offer economic opportunities to the community
4.7 Promotion of adobe constructions will reduce the energy consumption and the dependence of the community.
4.8 To empower the community about the advantage of taking care of the natural environment and about the construction of the ecological corridor, organizations need to be created.
4.9 The corridor will also be a promoter of small businesses, an alternative to the corridor itself.
4.10 A building for the corridor management training and assistance will be built in the community.
4.11 A project's goal is to strengthen the identity of the colony, stop perceiving new residents as strangers and a threat.
4.12 The project expects to make murals with community history along the corridor.
4.13 Study of the materials so that it does not appear threatening.

4.14 MIX: short-term training of children as guides + short, medium, and long-term community work.
4.15 It is supposed to have teaching activities and topics to support the generation of activities in the corridor.
4.16 The corridor will hallow connection with the formal city and connection with the landscape.
4.17 Since the community is relatively "young", it will allow to collect and to transmit local history;
4.18 Murals to share history and to create identity will be painted in the "urban" areas of the corridor;
4.19 The corridor is planned as an urban element which can generate business opportunities.

Project 5 "Tourist route"

5.1 The main project goal is to raise awareness in the society, about caring for the ecosystem in the area, through outdoor activities.
5.2 The project aims to improve the social environment and the way in which people coexist within the community.
5.3 Technological means are used for the promotion and enhancement of landscape and natural heritage, as well as to encourage economic activities in the area.
5.4 Political responsibilities are considered mainly for the regulation of non-deeded land.
5.5 Indexes are used as reference to give the inhabitants a better quality of life with respect to their housing, education, health, and education.
5.6 The project aims to improve the income of the residents by encouraging their businesses through digital media, as well as strategies to increase consumption on strategic days.
5.7 With the aim of improving the quality of life and reducing violence, the intervention contemplates to complete the electricity and public lighting network.
5.8 Interventions will also be focused on teaching local sellers how to improve their sales and optimize their resources.
5.9 The improvement of the baseball field aims to bring the community together and enhance the sense of belonging.
5.10 The connection of the community with the rest of the city will help to reach the project's goals.
5.11 The proposal contemplates the development of strategies and activities over time.
5.12 Capacity-building of the community, so that they are able to promote and implement strategies by themselves.
5.13 Strategies will focus on economic, social, political, tourism, and environmental improvement.
5.14 The completion of the urbanized the area (services) is one of the main interventions.
5.15 Respect, take advantage of, and improve existing areas to coexist with the spaces that are currently in place will help to reach the project's goals.
5.16 The intervention will show the inhabitants different options to develop their businesses and create their companies in an effective and lasting way.

References

1. McNeill, J.R. *The Great Acceleration an Environmental History of the Anthropocene since 1945*; Harvard University Press: Cambridge, MA, USA, 2016.
2. Batty, M. *Inventing Future Cities*; MIT Press: Cambridge, MA, USA, 2018.
3. Glaeser, E. *Triumph of the City: How Our Greatest Invention Makes Us Richer, Smarter, Greener, Healthier, and Happier*; Reprint Edizione; Penguin Books: New York, NY, USA, 2012.
4. Home, R.; Bauer, N. Researchers Working with City Administrations: Reflecting on Transdisciplinary Collaboration under Conditions of Shared Goals but Different Constraints. *Urban Ecosyst.* **2022**, *25*, 223–228. [CrossRef]
5. Foshag, K.; Aeschbach, N.; Höfle, B.; Winkler, R.; Siegmund, A.; Aeschbach, W. Viability of Public Spaces in Cities under Increasing Heat: A Transdisciplinary Approach. *Sustain. Cities Soc.* **2020**, *59*, 102215. [CrossRef]
6. Patel, Z.; Schneider, F.; Paulavets, K. Linking Local Projects With Global Processes: Learning From Transdisciplinary Collaborations in African Cities. *Front. Sustain. Cities* **2022**, *4*, 1–14. [CrossRef]
7. Mori, K.; Fujii, T.; Yamashita, T.; Mimura, Y.; Uchiyama, Y.; Hayashi, K. Visualization of a City Sustainability Index (CSI): Towards Transdisciplinary Approaches Involving Multiple Stakeholders. *Sustainability* **2015**, *7*, 12402–12424. [CrossRef]

8. Frantzeskaki, N.; Vandergert, P.; Connop, S.; Schipper, K.; Zwierzchowska, I.; Collier, M.; Lodder, M. Examining the Policy Needs for Implementing Nature-Based Solutions in Cities: Findings from City-Wide Transdisciplinary Experiences in Glasgow (UK), Genk (Belgium) and Poznań (Poland). *Land Use Policy* **2020**, *96*, 104688. [CrossRef]
9. Thiam, S.; Aziz, F.; Kushitor, S.B.; Amaka-Otchere, A.B.K.; Onyima, B.N.; Odume, O.N. Analyzing the Contributions of Transdisciplinary Research to the Global Sustainability Agenda in African Cities. *Sustain. Sci.* **2021**, *16*, 1923–1944. [CrossRef]
10. Gutkind, E.A. *The Expanding Environment: The End of Cities-the Rise of Communities*; Freedom Press: London, UK, 1953.
11. Jackson, T. *Prosperity without Growth: Economics for a Finite Planet*; Earthscan: London, UK; New York, NY, USA, 2009.
12. Giorgi, E.; Cattaneo, T.; Flores Herrera, A.M.; del Aceves Tarango, V.S. *Design for Vulnerable Communities*; The Urban Book Series; Springer: Cham, Switzerland, 2022.
13. Paul, S.K. Vulnerability Concepts and Its Application in Various Fields: A Review on Geographical Perspective. *J. Life Earth Sci.* **2013**, *8*, 63–81. [CrossRef]
14. Eakin, H.; Luers, A.L. Assessing the Vulnerability of Social-Environmental Systems. *Annu. Rev. Environ. Resour.* **2006**, *31*, 365–394. [CrossRef]
15. Wolf, S.; Hinkel, J.; Hallier, M.; Bisaro, A.; Lincke, D.; Ionescu, C.; Klein, R.J.T. Clarifying Vulnerability Definitions and Assessments Using Formalisation. *Int. J. Clim. Chang. Strateg. Manag.* **2013**, *5*, 54–70. [CrossRef]
16. Huq, E.; Shoeb, A.Z.M.; Hossain, M.A.; Fahad, S.; Kamruzzaman, M.M.; Javed, A.; Saleem, N.; Adnan, K.M.M.; Sarker, S.A.; Ali, M.Y.; et al. Measuring Vulnerability to Environmental Hazards: Qualitative to Quantitative. In *Environment, Climate, Plant and Vegetation Growth*; Fahad, S., Hasanuzzaman, M., Alam, M., Ullah, H., Saeed, M., Ali Khan, I., Adnan, M., Eds.; Springer International Publishing: Cham, Switzerland, 2020; pp. 421–452. [CrossRef]
17. Adger, W.N. Vulnerability. *Glob. Environ. Chang.* **2006**, *16*, 268–281. [CrossRef]
18. Cattaneo, T.; Giorgi, E.; Herrera, A.M.F.; del Socorro Aceves Tarango, V. Introduction on Design for Vulnerable Communities. In *Design for Vulnerable Communities*; Giorgi, E., Cattaneo, T., Flores Herrera, A.M., del Aceves Tarango, V.S., Eds.; The Urban Book Series; Springer International Publishing: Cham, Switzerland, 2022; pp. 1–17. [CrossRef]
19. Salas, J.; Yepes, V. Urban Vulnerability Assessment: Advances from the Strategic Planning Outlook. *J. Clean. Prod.* **2018**, *179*, 544–558. [CrossRef]
20. Anurudran, A.; Yared, L.; Comrie, C.; Harrison, K.; Burke, T. Domestic Violence amid COVID-19. *Int. J. Gynecol. Obstet.* **2020**, *150*, 255–256. [CrossRef]
21. Giorgi, E.; Martín López, L.; Garnica-Monroy, R.; Krstikj, A.; Cobreros, C.; Montoya, M.A. Co-Housing Response to Social Isolation of COVID-19 Outbreak, with a Focus on Gender Implications. *Sustainability* **2021**, *13*, 7203. [CrossRef]
22. Aven, T. On Some Recent Definitions and Analysis Frameworks for Risk, Vulnerability, and Resilience. *Risk Anal.* **2011**, *31*, 515–522. [CrossRef]
23. Polsky, C.; Eakin, H. Global Change Vulnerability Assessments: Definitions, Challenges, and Opportunities. In *The Oxford Handbook of Climate Change and Society*; Oxford University Press: Oxford, UK, 2012. [CrossRef]
24. Warburton, D. (Ed.) *Community and Sustainable Development: Participation in the Future*; Routledge: London, UK, 2013. [CrossRef]
25. Ugwu, A.N.; Aruma, E.O. Community participation as a tool for the promotion of sustainable community development. *Int. J. Community Coop. Stud.* **2019**, *7*, 1–10.
26. Santhanam, M.L. Community Participation for Sustainable Development. *Indian J. Public Adm.* **1993**, *39*, 413–423. [CrossRef]
27. Gutiérrez, K.D. 2011 AERA Presidential Address: Designing Resilient Ecologies: Social Design Experiments and a New Social Imagination. *Educ. Res.* **2016**, *45*, 187–196. [CrossRef]
28. Hagen, J.J. Queering Women, Peace and Security. *Int. Aff.* **2016**, *92*, 313–332. [CrossRef]
29. Oreni, D.; Brumana, R.; Torre, S.D.; Banfi, F. Survey, HBIM and Conservation Plan of a Monumental Building Damaged by Earthquake. *Int. Arch. Photogramm. Remote Sens. Spat. Inf. Sci.* **2017**, *42*, 337–342. [CrossRef]
30. Newman, G.; Shi, T.; Yao, Z.; Li, D.; Sansom, G.; Kirsch, K.; Casillas, G.; Horney, J. Citizen Science-Informed Community Master Planning: Land Use and Built Environment Changes to Increase Flood Resilience and Decrease Contaminant Exposure. *Int. J. Environ. Res. Public Health* **2020**, *17*, 486. [CrossRef] [PubMed]
31. van Lier, J.R.; Harasti, D.; Laird, R.; Noble, M.M.; Fulton, C.J. Importance of Soft Canopy Structure for Labrid Fish Communities in Estuarine Mesohabitats. *Mar. Biol.* **2017**, *164*, 5. [CrossRef]
32. Driver, A.; Mehdizadeh, C.; Bara-Garcia, S.; Bodenreider, C.; Lewis, J.; Wilson, S. Utilization of the Maryland Environmental Justice Screening Tool: A Bladensburg, Maryland Case Study. *Int. J. Environ. Res. Public Health* **2019**, *16*, 348. [CrossRef]
33. Fischer, H.W. Policy Innovations for Pro-Poor Climate Support: Social Protection, Small-Scale Infrastructure, and Active Citizenship under India's MGNREGA. *Clim. Dev.* **2020**, *12*, 689–702. [CrossRef]
34. Núñez Collado, J.R.; Wang, H.-H. Slum Upgrading and Climate Change Adaptation and Mitigation: Lessons from Latin America. *Cities* **2020**, *104*, 102791. [CrossRef]
35. Lebel, L.; Salamanca, A.; Kallayanamitra, C. The Governance of Adaptation Financing: Pursuing Legitimacy at Multiple Levels. *Int. J. Glob. Warm.* **2017**, *11*, 226–245. [CrossRef]
36. File, D.J.M.; Derbile, E.K. Sunshine, Temperature and Wind: Community Risk Assessment of Climate Change, Indigenous Knowledge and Climate Change Adaptation Planning in Ghana. *Int. J. Clim. Chang. Strateg. Manag.* **2020**, *12*, 22–38. [CrossRef]

37. Merino, G. Poverty and Design, an Economics and Policy Perspective. In *Design for Vulnerable Communities*; Giorgi, E., Cattaneo, T., Flores Herrera, A.M., del Aceves Tarango, V.S., Eds.; The Urban Book Series; Springer International Publishing: Cham, Switzerland, 2022; pp. 45–64. [CrossRef]
38. Harari, Y.N. *Sapiens: A Brief History of Humankind*; Harper: New York, NY, USA, 2015.
39. Marcu, A.; Vangenechten, D.; Org, I. Managing a Sustainable Transition to a Low-Carbon Society: The Socio-Economic Impacts of Mitigation Policies. *Geneva Int. Cent. Trade Sustain. Dev.* **2018**, *12*, 1.
40. Lucatello, S. Climate Resilient Development Pathways in the US-Mexico Border Region: The Case of the El Paso Del Norte Metropolitan Area. In *Design for Vulnerable Communities*; Giorgi, E., Cattaneo, T., Flores Herrera, A.M., del Aceves Tarango, V.S., Eds.; The Urban Book Series; Springer International Publishing: Cham, Switzerland, 2022; pp. 361–375. [CrossRef]
41. Markkanen, S.; Anger-Kraavi, A. Social Impacts of Climate Change Mitigation Policies and Their Implications for Inequality. *Clim. Policy* **2019**, *19*, 827–844. [CrossRef]
42. Petrini, M.A.; Rocha, J.V.; Brown, J.C. Mismatches between Mill-Cultivated Sugarcane and Smallholding Farming in Brazil: Environmental and Socioeconomic Impacts. *J. Rural Stud.* **2017**, *50*, 218–227. [CrossRef]
43. Hallegatte, S.; Rozenberg, J. Climate Change through a Poverty Lens. *Nat. Clim. Chang.* **2017**, *7*, 250–256. [CrossRef]
44. Climate Change and Health. Available online: https://www.who.int/news-room/fact-sheets/detail/climate-change-and-health (accessed on 1 May 2022).
45. Frumkin, H.; Hess, J.; Luber, G.; Malilay, J.; McGeehin, M. Climate Change: The Public Health Response. *Am. J. Public Health* **2008**, *98*, 435–445. [CrossRef] [PubMed]
46. McMichael, C.; Barnett, J.; McMichael, A.J. An Ill Wind? *Climate Change, Migration, and Health. Environ. Health Perspect.* **2012**, *120*, 646–654. [CrossRef] [PubMed]
47. von Uexkull, N.; Buhaug, H. Security Implications of Climate Change: A Decade of Scientific Progress. *J. Peace Res.* **2021**, *58*, 3–17. [CrossRef]
48. Grewal, D.; Hulland, J.; Kopalle, P.K.; Karahanna, E. The Future of Technology and Marketing: A Multidisciplinary Perspective. *J. Acad. Mark. Sci.* **2020**, *48*, 1–8. [CrossRef]
49. Agarwal, R.; Dugas, M.; Gao, G.; Kannan, P.K. Emerging Technologies and Analytics for a New Era of Value-Centered Marketing in Healthcare. *J. Acad. Mark. Sci.* **2020**, *48*, 9–23. [CrossRef]
50. Molina, C. Towards Conscious Design and Urban Planning: Inspiration from Consciousness in Business. In *Design for Vulnerable Communities*; Giorgi, E., Cattaneo, T., Flores Herrera, A.M., del Aceves Tarango, V.S., Eds.; The Urban Book Series; Springer International Publishing: Cham, Switzerland, 2022; pp. 103–115. [CrossRef]
51. Zhu, X.; Leuba dit Galland, P. Thinking in Systems: Sustainability Cognition for Design Communities. In *Design for Vulnerable Communities*; Giorgi, E., Cattaneo, T., Flores Herrera, A.M., del Aceves Tarango, V.S., Eds.; The Urban Book Series; Springer International Publishing: Cham, Switzerland, 2022; pp. 91–102. [CrossRef]
52. Malcolm, A. Thinking Socially: Anthropological Approaches to Contemporary Research. In *Design for Vulnerable Communities*; Giorgi, E., Cattaneo, T., Flores Herrera, A.M., del Aceves Tarango, V.S., Eds.; The Urban Book Series; Springer International Publishing: Cham, Switzerland, 2022; pp. 83–90. [CrossRef]
53. Ignaccolo, C.; Zhai, Y. Urban Form and Social Vulnerability in Shanghai: A Comparative Study of Hongkou District Before and After the 1990s Urban Renewal. In *Design for Vulnerable Communities*; Giorgi, E., Cattaneo, T., Flores Herrera, A.M., del Aceves Tarango, V.S., Eds.; The Urban Book Series; Springer International Publishing: Cham, Switzerland, 2022; pp. 225–243. [CrossRef]
54. Verdini, G.; Dean, C. Climate Urbanism in the Post-Pandemic World: Mapping Vulnerabilities and Exploring Community Activism in East London. In *Design for Vulnerable Communities*; Giorgi, E., Cattaneo, T., Flores Herrera, A.M., del Aceves Tarango, V.S., Eds.; The Urban Book Series; Springer International Publishing: Cham, Switzerland, 2022; pp. 245–262. [CrossRef]
55. Ni, M. Digital Participation for Inclusive Growth: A Case Study of Singapore's Collaborative Digital Governance Model. In *Design for Vulnerable Communities*; Giorgi, E., Cattaneo, T., Flores Herrera, A.M., del Aceves Tarango, V.S., Eds.; The Urban Book Series; Springer International Publishing: Cham, Switzerland, 2022; pp. 323–337. [CrossRef]
56. Diaz-Barriga, V.B.; Barnhart, A. Sustainable Energy Through Design: An Approach to Alleviate Energy Poverty in Vulnerable Communities on the US–Mexico Border Region. In *Design for Vulnerable Communities*; Giorgi, E., Cattaneo, T., Flores Herrera, A.M., del Aceves Tarango, V.S., Eds.; The Urban Book Series; Springer International Publishing: Cham, Switzerland, 2022; pp. 423–448. [CrossRef]
57. Krstikj, A.; Lukoseviciute, G.; Boyes, C.; Contreras Ruiz Esparza, M.G. Nutritious Landscapes: The Food Environments in the Metropolitan Peripheries of Mexico. In *Design for Vulnerable Communities*; Giorgi, E., Cattaneo, T., Flores Herrera, A.M., del Aceves Tarango, V.S., Eds.; The Urban Book Series; Springer International Publishing: Cham, Switzerland, 2022; pp. 377–394. [CrossRef]
58. Maya, M.; Cobreros, C.; Ontiveros, E.; Biondi, S. Community collaboration for product design (co-co design): An academic alternative for social innovation. In *DS 95: Proceedings of the 21st International Conference on Engineering and Product Design Education (E&PDE 2019), University of Strathclyde, Glasgow, UK, 12–13 September 2019*; University of Strathclyde: Glasgow, UK, 2019. [CrossRef]
59. Treviño Sherk, J.; Cobreros Rodriguez, C. Rural democratic design: Participatory design and service learning strategies in sustainable development to promote civic mindedness in community development. In *DS 95: Proceedings of the 21st International Conference on Engineering and Product Design Education (E&PDE 2019), University of Strathclyde, Glasgow, UK, 12–13 September 2019*; University of Strathclyde: Glasgow, UK, 2019. [CrossRef]

60. Papanek, V. *Design for the Real World: Human Ecology and Social Change*; Bantam Books: New York, NY, USA, 1973.
61. Besselaar, P.V.D.; Heimeriks, G. Disciplinary, Multidisciplinary, Interdisciplinary: Concepts and Indicators. In Proceedings of the 8th conference on Scientometrics and Informetrics—ISSI2001, Sydney, Australia, 16–20 July 2001; Davis, M., Wilson, C.S., Eds.; UNSW: Sydney, Australia, 2001; pp. 705–716.
62. Thompson Klein, J. *Interdisciplinarity. History, Theory and Practice*; Wayne State University Press: Detroit, MI, USA, 1991.
63. Choi, B.C.K.; Pak, A.W.P. Multidisciplinarity, Interdisciplinarity and Transdisciplinarity in Health Research, Services, Education and Policy: 1. Definitions, Objectives, and Evidence of Effectiveness. *Clin. Investig. Med.* **2006**, *29*, 351–364.
64. Cattaneo, T.; Giorgi, E.; Ni, M. Landscape, Architecture and Environmental Regeneration: A Research by Design Approach for Inclusive Tourism in a Rural Village in China. *Sustainability* **2019**, *11*, 128. [CrossRef]
65. Van Ouwerkerk, M.; Rosemann, J. *Research by Design: International Conference Faculty of Architecture Delft University of Technology in Co-Operation with the EAAE/AEEA 1–3 November 2000: Proceedings A*; Delft University Press: Delft, The Netherlands, 2001.
66. Hauberg, J. *Research by Design—A Research Strategy*; AE Revista Lusófona de Architectura e Educacao: Lisboa, Portugal, 2011; pp. 46–56.
67. Roggema, R. Research by Design: Proposition for a Methodological Approach. *Urban Sci.* **2017**, *1*, 2. [CrossRef]
68. Nassauer, J.I.; Opdam, P. Design in Science: Extending the Landscape Ecology Paradigm. *Landsc. Ecol.* **2008**, *23*, 633–644. [CrossRef]
69. Schoonderbeek, M. A Theory of "Design by Research"; Mapping Experimentation in Architecture and Architectural Design. *Ardeth Mag. Power Proj.* **2017**, *1*, 63–79. [CrossRef]
70. Design for Vulnerables. Designforvulnerables. Available online: https://www.designforvulnerables.com/ (accessed on 25 April 2022).
71. Chihuahua: Economía, Empleo, Equidad, Calidad de Vida, Educación, Salud Y Seguridad Pública. Data México. Available online: https://datamexico.org/es/profile/geo/chihuahua-ch (accessed on 28 June 2022).
72. Paso Del Norte | Design for Vulnerables. Designforvulnerables. Available online: https://www.designforvulnerables.com/paso-del-norte (accessed on 28 June 2022).
73. Verbeke, J. This Is Research by Design. In *Design Research in Architecture*; Fraser, M., Ed.; Ashgate: Farnham, UK, 2013; pp. 137–159.
74. Aish, R. Human Computer Interaction Systems and Educational Strategies to Support Design Participation. In *aae2016 International Peer-Reviewed Conference on "Research Based Education"*; UCL Publisher: London, UK, 2016; p. 468.
75. Vines, J.; McNaney, R.; Clarke, R.; Lindsay, S.; McCarthy, J.; Howard, S.; Romero, M.; Wallace, J. Designing For- and with-Vulnerable People. In *CHI '13 Extended Abstracts on Human Factors in Computing Systems on—CHI EA '13*; ACM Press: Paris, France, 2013; p. 3231. [CrossRef]
76. "Intuition Must Be Grounded to the Site And Context": In Conversation with Oscar Ko of Interval Architects. Available online: https://www.archdaily.com/914833/intuition-must-be-grounded-to-the-site-and-context-in-conversation-with-oscar-ko-of-interval-architects (accessed on 27 June 2022).
77. Cole, R.J. Transitioning from Green to Regenerative Design. *Build. Res. Inf.* **2012**, *40*, 39–53. [CrossRef]
78. Zhang, X.; Skitmore, M.; De Jong, M.; Huisingh, D.; Gray, M. Regenerative Sustainability for the Built Environment—from Vision to Reality: An Introductory Chapter. *J. Clean. Prod.* **2015**, *109*, 1–10. [CrossRef]
79. Sianipar, C.P.M.; Dowaki, K.; Yudoko, G. Technological Solution for Vulnerable Communities: How Does Its Approach Matter? *IOP Conf. Ser. Mater. Sci. Eng.* **2014**, *58*, 012022. [CrossRef]
80. Leśniak, A.; Górka, M.; Skrzypczak, I. Barriers to BIM Implementation in Architecture, Construction, and Engineering Projects—The Polish Study. *Energies* **2021**, *14*, 2090. [CrossRef]
81. Chan, D.W.M.; Olawumi, T.O.; Ho, A.M.L. Perceived Benefits of and Barriers to Building Information Modelling (BIM) Implementation in Construction: The Case of Hong Kong. *J. Build. Eng.* **2019**, *25*, 100764. [CrossRef]
82. Oke, A.E.; Arowoiya, V.A. Critical Barriers to Augmented Reality Technology Adoption in Developing Countries: A Case Study of Nigeria. *J. Eng. Des. Technol.* **2021**, *20*, 1320–1333. [CrossRef]
83. Oxman, N. Age of Entanglement. *J. Des. Sci.* **2016**. [CrossRef]
84. Friedman, K. Theory Construction in Design Research: Criteria: Approaches, and Methods. *Des. Stud.* **2003**, *24*, 507–522. [CrossRef]
85. Megahed, Y. On Research by Design. *ARQ Archit. Res. Q.* **2017**, *21*, 338–343. [CrossRef]
86. Salas, J.; Yepes, V. MS-ReRO and D-ROSE Methods: Assessing Relational Uncertainty and Evaluating Scenarios' Risks and Opportunities on Multi-Scale Infrastructure Systems. *J. Clean. Prod.* **2019**, *216*, 607–623. [CrossRef]
87. Hall, J.; Keller, R.; Hackbarth, A.; Mijere, C.; McInerney, D. Robust Climate Policies Under Uncertainty: A Comparison of Robust Decision Making and Info-Gap Methods. *Risk Anal.* **2012**, *32*, 1657–1672. [CrossRef] [PubMed]
88. COP23: Conferencia de la ONU Sobre El Cambio Climático de 2017. Available online: https://www.un.org/sustainabledevelopment/es/cop23-conferencia-de-la-onu-sobre-el-cambio-climatico-de-2017/ (accessed on 15 August 2022).

89. Giorgi, E. How Technology Devices Can Help or Harm Vulnerable Communities in Technocene. Issues for Designers, Architects, and Policy Makers. In *Design for Vulnerable Communities*; Giorgi, E., Cattaneo, T., Flores Herrera, A.M., del Aceves Tarango, V.S., Eds.; The Urban Book Series; Springer International Publishing: Cham, Switzerland, 2022; pp. 21–43. [CrossRef]
90. de Cote, E.P.M.L.M.; Flores Herrera, A.M.; Giorgi, E.; Cattaneo, T. Augmented Reality (AR) and Virtual Reality (VR) as Tools to Empower Vulnerable Communities: Opportunities and Challenges for Designers. In *Design for Vulnerable Communities*; Giorgi, E., Cattaneo, T., Flores Herrera, A.M., del Aceves Tarango, V.S., Eds.; The Urban Book Series; Springer International Publishing: Cham, Switzerland, 2022; pp. 307–321. [CrossRef]

buildings

MDPI

Article

A Parametric Framework to Assess Generative Urban Design Proposals for Transit-Oriented Development

Xiaoran Huang [1,2,*,†], Wei Yuan [3,†], Marcus White [2] and Nano Langenheim [4]

1 School of Architecture and Art, North China University of Technology, Beijing 100144, China
2 Centre for Design Innovation, Swinburne University of Technology, Hawthorn, VIC 3122, Australia
3 Edinburgh School of Architecture and Landscape Architecture, Edinburgh College of Art, The University of Edinburgh, Edinburgh EH1 1JZ, UK
4 Melbourne School of Design, University of Melbourne, Masson Rd, Parkville, VIC 3010, Australia
* Correspondence: xiaoran.huang@ncut.edu.cn; Tel.: +86-88-803-399
† These authors contributed equally to this work.

Abstract: Urban design has been valuable in bringing the principles of transit-oriented development (TOD) into reality. However, a majority of recommendations summarized by scholars for promoting TODs through urban design have failed to promote the progress of the urban design. The main reason for this issue is the long-standing tradition of design decision-making based on designers' experience and the lack of quantitative assessment feedback on design schemes. With the development of big data and artificial intelligence, optimisation-based generative design has been explored to overcome the limitations of experience-based urban design approaches. However, the techniques and workflows are still not mature enough for designers to adopt. In response to these challenges, this study proposes a framework that integrates the generative design method and data-driven decision-making approach for urban design solutions that better implement the basic principles of TODs. Based on the urban design intelligence for TODs, this framework uses parametric tools and models to evaluate the generative urban design proposals, providing timely feedback to support the design decisions. The framework is applied to a case study to examine the feasibility. It is demonstrated that this approach succeeds in selecting optimal TOD design solutions. The role of designers' decision-making in generative urban design, as well as the importance of quantitative and qualitative assessment in experience-based decision-making, are highlighted.

Keywords: generative urban design; evidence-based design decision-making; activity-based model; transit-oriented development; walkability; amenity accessibility

Citation: Huang, X.; Yuan, W.; White, M.; Langenheim, N. A Parametric Framework to Assess Generative Urban Design Proposals for Transit-Oriented Development. *Buildings* **2022**, *12*, 1971. https://doi.org/10.3390/buildings12111971

Academic Editors: Liyin Shen, Jorge Ochoa and Haijun Bao

Received: 4 October 2022
Accepted: 10 November 2022
Published: 14 November 2022

1. Introduction

Transit-oriented development (TOD) is a planning strategy that promotes non-motorized travel modes through mixed-use, high-density, and walkable neighborhoods within walking distance of transportation stations. It is widely recognized as an essential paradigm for fostering sustainable urban development since it contributes to reducing air pollution and regional congestion, boosting economic development, and improving urban vitality [1,2]. On the one hand, TOD can reduce residents' demands for private cars, thereby alleviating traffic congestion and reducing greenhouse gas emissions. Previous studies have established that residents of transit-oriented neighborhoods are more likely to travel by public transportation instead of driving and take more leisurely walks than residents of car-oriented neighborhoods [3]. TOD projects in many cities have contributed significantly to local GHG reduction goals. As an example, in the Chicago Metropolitan Region, the GHG emission of the average household in the neighborhoods near the transport station is reduced by 43 percent compared with non-TOD areas. According to SDG goals, combating climate change is currently an important task for all countries in the world. In this context, TOD should be greatly promoted to stop global warming. On the other hand, by reducing transportation costs and increasing employment opportunities, TOD can promote a robust regional economy. A number of studies have indicated that local taxes benefit from TOD through increasing land prices and sales tax revenues from restaurants and retailers [1,2]. In addition to promoting active transportation modes and facilitating regional economic development, TOD has the potential to bring vitality to communities. The mixed-land uses in TODs provide favorable conditions for various social activities and interactions [4]. It has been found that people living in TODs have significantly higher levels of connection with their neighbors than in other communities [5]. The performance of TODs is predicated on four major principles: (1) walkability—providing a pleasant, continuous, networked pedestrian environment along with a wide range of experiences and amenities; (2) transit accessibility—ensuring close proximity in distance or time for residents and workers to reach transit facilities; (3) density—optimizing employment and residential densities along transit corridors or station areas to promote walking and transit use; (4) diversity—providing access to retail, commercial, and civic services, employment, and recreational facilities without needing to travel by automobile [6,7]. A well-performed urban design can be a key mechanism for transforming these guidelines into successful cases. Jacobson and Forsyth [8] enumerated twelve aspects of good urban design initiatives for TODs (Table 1). These twelve elements are derived from the literature review and understood in depth through case studies. Of all the aspects, five are highlighted regarding place-making. First of all, designing on a human scale is fundamental to creating a pedestrian-friendly environment. According to environmental psychology, people are born with the perception of their surroundings. The characteristics of the built environment (such as the sense of enclosure, sky view factor, etc.) play a major role in the comfort that people feel in the space, and the comforts of the walking environment are closely related to residents' travel demand [9,10]. For instance, the atmosphere created by excessively tall buildings with narrow streets tends to inhibit residents from moving around the streets. With this in mind, the walkability of residents can be facilitated by controlling the scale of buildings and streets. The ratio of building height to street width in TODs is supposed to be designed to improve the pedestrian experience. Second, public spaces emerge in the case studies as key components of TODs [10]. Open spaces not only provide opportunities for residents to interact and exercise, but also allow for various events. As suggested by case studies, the combination of transit stops and well-designed open spaces can improve the recognition of the TODs and increase transit ridership [8]. Third, pedestrian safety serves as an important factor for people to embrace the public spaces in TODs. Previous research has established that real and perceived traffic safety is closely related to residents' walking behavior to transport [11]. In terms of urban design solutions in TOD, security is a consideration for the way the driveways and sidewalks are joined. To ensure people walk safely in transit-oriented neighborhoods, places such as parks require a ban on vehicle traffic [12]. Fourth, the variety of land use, visual experience and social aspects are all essential aspects in the design of public spaces. TODs need sufficient public spaces for walking and cycling, and also spaces to promote interaction among various social groups. It is generally accepted in urban design that the diversity in visual experiences creates a sense of place, which gives open spaces distinct characteristics, and therefore, enhances their attractiveness to residents. These have led to more people congregating in open spaces with more events taking place. Inviting and lively public spaces in TOD areas will, in turn, attract more residents to move in and bring about more transit ridership [2]. Fifth, street connections are essential for the creation of pedestrian movements [13]. Well-organized street patterns enable pedestrians and cyclists to move continuously in various ways [8]. Elaborate footpaths and cycle paths are the basis for residents to approach transit facilities. Subsequently, Ogra and Ndebele [14] generalized six variables that are vital for reaching the goals of the TODs, which are design, diversity, density, distance, destination, and demand management. In terms of the built environment design, it is pinpointed that providing various amenities is the key to walkable transit-oriented neighborhoods. According to previous studies, the diverse range of amenities can provide residents with abundant activities and thus stimulates walking and cycling trips [15,16]. In addition, all kinds of amenities make walking less boring and bring joy to pedestrians [12].

Table 1. The summary of twelve aspects of good urban design initiatives for TODs.

Topics	Aspects	Descriptions
process	Time	TOD design should take into account changes over time and future possibilities.
	Engagement with public	The visions of different stakeholders should be considered in the whole design process.
	Programming	Arrange events and activities for the public in open spaces.
	Maintenance	Manage the budget to ensure investment in maintenance and landscaping.
places	Scale	Design at a human scale to create a comfortable walking environment.
	Public spaces for human use	Create public space for pedestrian activities
	Safety	Create safe walking environments and public spaces.
	Variety and complexity	Pay attention to the variety of land use, visual experience, and social aspects.
	Connections	Connecting places to create good walking and cycling experiences (including building and outdoor connections, sidewalk connections, cycling path connections, etc.)
facilities	Pedestrian facilities	Design safe and vibrant sidewalks
	Transit	Connect transportation facilities and the surrounding environment
	Car movement and parking	Ensure a safe and comfortable pedestrian environment. Adjust the direction and speed of cars through urban design. Parking spaces should be designed to meet the demands while not impeding walking.

Based on the four principles, the above aspects (human scale, public spaces, safety, variety of visual experience, and amenity diversity) regarding urban design for TODs provide valuable suggestions for urban designers [17]. Nevertheless, useful advice plays an insignificant role in guiding potential urban design improvements. Few design initiatives are given quantitative or qualitative evaluations, which can result in a lack of evidence and feedback to support design decisions. Starting with good intentions but ending with poor design execution can result in no improvement or even harm to the surrounding environment [18]. Thinking further about this particular issue, it roots in a long tradition of the experience-based design workflow, i.e., designers use their own experience or personal preferences to determine the design solutions. In the majority of countries, the evidence-based design approach is not yet widespread. Therefore, some schemes are limited by the designers' subjective opinions or clients' requirements, and often fail to be effective TOD proposals. In recent years, parametric and generative design has received considerable attention, which explores potential solutions to decision-making issues in the field of architecture, urban design, and urban planning [19,20]. Using big data and algorithms, these approaches can yield unlimited possible solutions that are beyond one's imagination, with automated optimization solutions based on predefined objectives [21–26]. Compared with the traditional decision-making approach, they are advantaged in overcoming the limitation of individual thoughts to inform more feasible alternatives, and are able to generate data-based feedback for each solution. To date, scholars have explored the potential of generative urban design in the light of various objectives. The works related to TODs centered around design generation and optimization, based on walkability or/and amenity distribution [21,24,27,28]. Using a walk score as an indicator, the network optimization model created by Tarek and Christoph [21] provided a promising insight for later studies. They used genetic algorithms (the natural selection-based approaches to solve both constrained and unconstrained optimization issues) to optimize the initially generated street network design and obtained a series of viable options. However, this approach was later criticized for lacking consideration of the impact of amenities on the street network. A new workflow to create street networks and amenity distribution schemes was developed by Yang et al. [17], which takes a good account of the interplay between amenities and networks and the adaptability of specific contexts. While the weakness is that they fail to provide information on building configurations that can be influenced by network layouts, which is inappropriate to be considered separately in urban design. Lima [24] et al. leveraged multiple optimization algorithms to create urban networks in terms of transit accessibility and infrastructure cost. Unfortunately, this approach idealises the local context, and its ability to solve real-world problems is uncertain. More importantly, the quantitative indicators still need to be complemented by qualitative dimensions [29]. This is because some solutions meet the quantitative metrics well, but are not preferred by residents due to the weakness in qualitative features (e.g., urban design quality, maintenance of historical sites, etc.) On account of the complexity of the urban system, design decisions cannot yet entirely rely on algorithms. Designers still have the responsibility to perform qualitative analysis and make the final decision. In response to these concerns, this paper proposes an original framework to evaluate and interpret generative urban design proposals for TODs. This is the first comprehensive framework that transforms urban design principles for TOD into an evaluation methodology that utilizes both data feedback and experts' experience to guide designers in their decision-making. It is later applied to a case study in a TOD area in the city of Glen Eira, Melbourne, to validate its capacity to address real-world issues.

2. Data and Method

2.1. Assessment Indicators and Methods

Given its enlightening and objective-based optimization capabilities, the generative urban design method is utilized in the study to propose different solutions for TOD. A t the core of this study is the creation of an evaluation framework for these generative urban design proposals. On the basis of the good urban design recommendations summarized by Jacobson, Forsyth, Ogra, and Ndebele, the evaluation method is developed. For some aspects, indicators can be set up for quantitative assessment. (1) It is commonly recognized that the ratio of building height to street width has a strong relationship with how people feel in urban space. Therefore, it is chosen as the assessment indicator in the framework to reflect the comfort level of residents moving around in public spaces. As suggested by scholars, the ideal height-to-width ratios for public spaces are between 1:1 to 1:3 [30–32]. The ratios of design proposals that fall within this interval range are identified as the optimal ratios. (2) A walk score is a reliable metric of walkability recognized by many experts [33]. While most walkability metrics apply to a region, the walk score quantifies both the walkability of an area and the walkability of a housing unit. Visualizing the walkability of each housing unit in a TOD area is vital for evaluating design strategies. For example, different street network designs may result in the same regional walkability results, but contribute differently to the walkability results of each building block. Understanding the variation in walkability between individual units can help designers make trade-offs in their solutions. The Walk Score algorithm, which ranges from 0 to 100 scores, uses the distance decay function (Equation (1)) to rate locations based on the minimum distance to amenities in each category [34,35]. A higher score for a location means a more walkable level. (3) TODs encourage a wide variety of amenities. However, it is not the case that the greater the variety and number of amenities, the better. When the demand for amenities in an area exceeds the supply, it would be a loss for investors. The Amenity score is a metric that seeks to quantify the disparity between the supply and demand of various amenity types in an area, which can help the decision-makers to determine the right number and type of amenities. An Amenity score close to zero means that the supply of amenities in the study area is close to the demand. A value below zero for a certain amenity type means that it is not well configured and is in short supply. The opposite is true for amenity scores greater than zero [16]. (4) Two auxiliary metrics (Amenity Hits and street hits) provide information on people's activities in TOD areas, which help designers reflect on their choices of amenity locations and the forms of the street networks. The indicator of Amenity Hits sums up the total number of residents visiting a certain amenity across all trips. The metric of Street Hits measures the total number of people using certain street segments on all trips. For each amenity or street segment, a higher score indicates a larger number of users. By further visualizing these two indicators, urban designers can intuitively understand the activeness of different parts of the study area in terms of amenities and streets, and thus adjust their design solutions.

$$\text{Decay (x)} = -17.15x^5 + 89.45x^4 - 126.37x^3 + 4.639x^2 + 7.58x + 99.5 \quad (1)$$

Due to the complexity of urban design, not all the issues can be analyzed relying on indicators and evaluation criteria. Qualitative analysis is suggested for the following dimensions. (1) Public spaces are often designed to strike a balance between aesthetics, the scheduled activities to be accommodated, local regulations, and other aspects [36]. There is no consistent standard for the size and shape of public spaces. The reliable method for assessing the quality of public spaces is to use the public space index (PSI) [37]. This index involves a combination of more than forty factors in terms of inclusiveness, meaningful activities, comfort, safety, and pleasurability. Although this method is well-established, it takes months, or even years, for the evaluator to engage in observations. It is not a wise choice for urban designers due to the lack of timely and effective design feedback. What can be confirmed is that it is more desirable to have open space in TOD areas than not. For the specific size and form of the public space, urban designers are advised to make decisions based on 3D models and their own experiences. (2) The visual experience in public spaces is also a difficult element to quantify. A good way to analyze the visual experience in urban spaces is through the use of isovist [38]. The isovist is the area or volume of space visible from a given point in space, which intuitively reflects the visual–spatial qualities in the built environment [39]. According to Batty [40], factors such as area, perimeter, and the average distance of a series of isovists at different locations on a walking path can reflect changes in visual experience. In addition, 3D models and renderings are recommended to aid the analysis process. In light of this, the evaluation framework utilizes shapes and areas of isovist to assist designers in understanding the visual experiences in the existing built environment and their design proposals. Specifically, the shape and area of the isovist along a walking path are measured for the analysis of visual changes in public spaces. Previous literature has demonstrated the methodology of DecodingSpaces toolbox to be useful for isovist measurements [41,42].

2.2. Computational Tools and Overall Framework

Rhinoceros3D-Grasshopper (GH) is chosen as the platform to conduct the assessment process. Rhinoceros3D software and its inherited parametric design platform Grasshopper can be used by urban designers to create three-dimensional city models, visualizing simulations and analytic solutions in real-time. Compared with other 3D modeling software, Rhinoceros3D has its advantages in terms of data visualization and efficient parametric workflow. The parametric evaluation framework in this study relies heavily on 3D models and the visualization of spatial data. Taking street network design, for example, it has an impact on both visual diversity and regional walkability. City designers need to analyze the diversity of visual changes based on a three-dimensional spatial environment, and also need to get data feedback on walkability. These requirements make the Rhinoceros3D-Grasshopper (GH) platform a suitable choice. The following two plug-ins are used in the evaluation and generative process: the Urbano and the DeCodingspaces toolboxes. The Urbano tool is a useful analytical tool that provides measurable design feedback in terms of walkability and the activeness of amenities and streets. It utilizes data input from designers to simulate human activity in the city and evaluate design scenarios with built-in algorithms and metrics [16,43]. It is worth being used in this study because of its well-established workflow and compatibility with 3D models. The DeCodingspacestoolbox contains a variety of analytical and generative elements, which provides technical support for the generative design process. According to the previous literature, the DeCodingspaces toolbox is more functional and easier to use than other computationally generated methods [25,44–46]. The tool has the potential to become widespread, as urban designers and planners can operate it with a simple understanding of the data structure and the meaning of the parameters. Hence it serves as the obvious choice for this study. The overall framework can be divided into three steps: context modeling and assessment, computational generation of urban design proposals, and quantitative assessment and qualitative analysis of generative design proposals. Each step (including input parameters and operation methods) will be detailed in the following sections.

2.3. Context Modeling and Assessment

To inform the subsequent generative design solutions, the existing built environment needs to be modeled and evaluated. By measuring aspects such as the walk score and amenity score of the built environment, designers can realize the issues that need to be improved. The method of context modeling and assessment consists of three parts (Figure 1): context modeling, active mobility simulation, and context assessment. These three aspects are proposed based on the Urbano workflow [16,47]. According to the workflow, two models (the contextual model and activity-based model) and four metrics (walk score, amenity score, street hits, and amenity hits) are required to this end. The contextual model refers to the model of the existing built environment in Rhinoceros3D, which serves as the physical basis of the assessment process. The activity-based model is a model that estimates people's activity trips according to different design scenarios in an area. It is a concept proposed by Joe et al. [15], which later becomes the theoretical foundation of the mobility simulation process in the Urbano workflow. The four metrics are used to quantify the results of active mobility simulation. All three aspects, with their components, will be introduced in detail in the following subsections. Table 2 illustrates the details of input parameters in these three aspects.

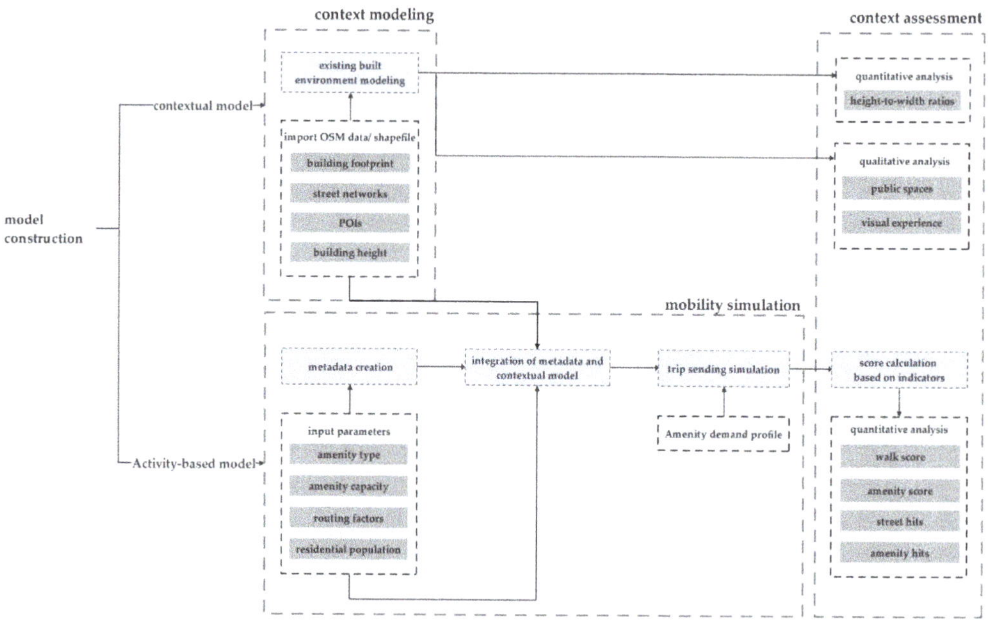

Figure 1. The workflow of context modeling and assessment.

Table 2. The details of input parameters of context modeling and assessment.

Parameters	Data type	When to Select	Data Source	Reference
Building footprint	OSM/ shapefile	Must be selected when creating a contextual model.	OSM: from OpenStreetMap website; Shapefile: from governments, developers, etc.	[16,43]
Street networks	OSM/ shapefile	Must be selected when creating a contextual model.	OSM: from OpenStreetMap website; Shapefile: from governments, developers, etc.	[16,43]
POIs	OSM/ shapefile	Must be selected when creating a contextual model.	OSM: from OpenStreetMap website; Shapefile: from governments, developers, etc.	[16,43,47]
Building height	OSM/ shapefile	Must be selected when creating a contextual model.	OSM: from OpenStreetMap website; Shapefile: from governments, developers, etc.	[16,43]
Amenity type	metadata	Must be selected for mobility simulation.	It can be customized by the designer or extracted from the OSM data.	[16,43]
Amenity capacity	metadata	Optional for mobility simulation.	It can be customized by the designer or derived from the Urbano database.	[16,27]
Routing factors	metadata	Optional for mobility simulation. Use it only when the bike score calculation is needed.	It can be customized by the designer	[16,27]
Residential population	metadata	Optional for mobility simulation.	It can be customized by the designer or calculated by Urbano components.	[16]
Amenity demand profile	CSV	Must be selected for mobility simulation.	It can be an be customized by the designer or derived from the Urbano database.	[16,43]

2.3.1. Context Modeling

There are three kinds of data that serve as the basis for modeling existing built environments: building footprints, street networks, and point of interest (POI), which can be either OSM data or shapefiles. POI refers to the place where an amenity is located. The building footprint shapefiles are available for download on the official government websites in many countries (such as the city of Melbourne and the city of New York). For establishing street networks and POI models, it is common to use OSM data since it is open to the public and available from the OpenStreetMap website (https://www.openstreetmap.org accessed on 10 August 2022). However, it is worth noting that the quality of POI data from the OSM website is not high, with fewer POI entries than other shapefile sources such as Google Maps [43]. The use of OSM data for POIs may lead to errors in the research. Therefore, it is suggested to use shapefiles in terms of POIs modeling. The three types of data can be parsed via the Urbano component and transformed into geometric shapes in Rhino [16].

2.3.2. Mobility Simulation

Mobility simulation enables the designer to understand the impact of their design solutions on residents' active mobility. It is fundamental to the subsequent evaluation process regarding walkability and amenity diversity, which are essential aspects of good TOD design. The mobility simulation comprises three parts, i.e., the metadata creation, the integration of metadata and contextual model, and the trip-sending simulation. Metadata creation prepares the necessary data for the trip-sending simulation. The parameters that must be included are Building height, Amenity type, and Amenity demand profile (ADP). Building height and Amenity type are metadata, which can be either customized by designers or extracted from OSM data. The metadata is supposed to be appended to geometric data and provide additional information, which requires the integration of metadata and contextual model. When the building geometry and Building height are combined, the population contained in the building can be calculated by the Urbano component. When Amenity type and POIs are combined, spatial points with amenity information are generated. ADP is an estimation of the proportion of residents participating in different activities in the study area, which is the driver of the trip-sending process [16]. The ADP data represents the weight of different activities or the activeness of different amenities in the area, which can be customized by designers or obtained directly from the Urbano dataset. The specific method can be referred to [43]. In light of the activity-based model [15], the trip-sending process in Urbano workflow can be explained in three parts—trip generation, trip distribution, mode choice, and route assignment (Figure 2). In this process, residential buildings are defined as the starting points, and amenities are as the destinations. For each building, (a) The population is divided according to the ADP to derive the number of people involved in different activities. (b) Those who are divided will be matched with the corresponding amenities within a walkable distance. Depending on the chosen mode of travel (e.g., by nearest destination and by amenity capacity), residents are allocated to amenities in different ways. (c) The routes are formed based on the starting point and destinations. As a result, visitors per amenity and per street segment can be calculated as amenity hits and street hits. The mobility simulations for all buildings in the area can be used to analyze regional mobility.

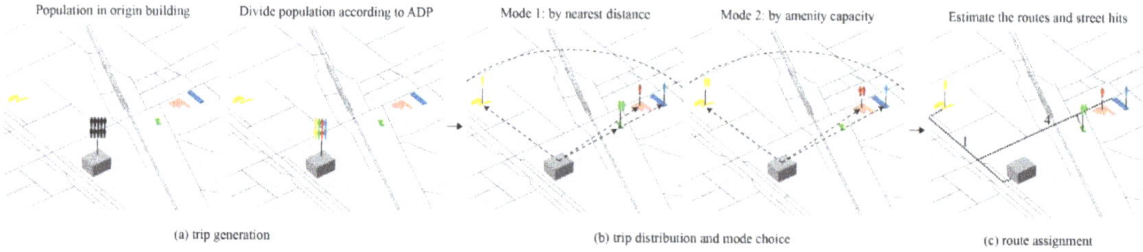

Figure 2. Trip-sending simulation process for each building.

2.3.3. Context Assessment

A context assessment can help urban designers identify problems of the existing condition, which serves as a reference for the subsequent generative design evaluation. The assessment involves five metrics (height-to-width ratios, walk score, amenity score, amenity hits, and street hits) and two qualitative aspects (public spaces and visual experience). The mobility simulation lays the foundation for the calculation of the walk score and amenity score via Urbano components [16]. Based on the walk score methodology, the walk score for each activity trip in the mobility simulation can be measured. Amenity scores, on the other hand, can be derived from Amenity hits according to Equation (2) (where A stands for Amenity score, H stands for Amenity hits, and C stands for Amenity capacity). Other metrics and evaluation methods can be referred to in Section 2.1.

$$A = H/C - 1 \tag{2}$$

2.4. Computational Generation of Urban Design Proposals

After selecting the site based on the contextual model, parameters can be set for generative urban design solutions. Among various ways for computational generation of urban design proposals, this study follows the method proposed by Koenig et al. [45] via the DeCodingspaces toolbox. Unlike other generative design approaches, this method is not limited to the separate production of building schemes or street network solutions, but can generate street networks, plots, parcels, and buildings in sequence, forming a well-function system [25,45]. The consistency of multiple elements is crucial in urban design. The generative design process comprises five steps: street network generation, block generation, parcel generation, building generation, and amenity generation. The parameters used in each step with related information are listed in Table 3. Together, these parameters control the forms of streets, plots, and buildings.

Table 3. The information of input parameters in generative urban design process.

Parameters	Explanation	Required/Optional	Step	Reference
B	Boundary to generate street networks	required	Street network generation	[45]
IS	Street segments as the starting points for generation	optional	Street network generation	[45]
MDist	The shortest distance between the start and end of a street segment	required	Street network generation	[44,45]
RA	Random angle defining the direction of the street segments	required	Street network generation	[44,45]
TD	Tree depth for controlling branch levels of tree structures to define the size of street networks	required	Street network generation	[44,45]
MA	Maximum number of arms for crossroads	required	Street network generation	[45]
RndS	Random seed number for choosing the generative street network pattern	optional	Street network generation	[45]
BA	Buildable area on each parcel	required	Street network generation	[45]
BT	Building types (including block building, row building, and free-standing)	required	building generation	[45,48]
Blen	The length of the building	required	building generation	[45]
Bdep	The depth of the building	required	building generation	[45]
FAR	Floor area ratio. It determines the building height when the building footprint is defined	optional	building generation	[45]
Orientation	Building setback from the street	optional	building generation	[45]

Figure 3 shows the grasshopper components used in the computational generation process. The street network generation rests on a particular data structure—the instruction tree [45]. It has advantages in substituting sophisticated street networks with simple tree structures connected by nodes, which makes it easier for computing and mutating. The instruction trees determine the structure of the street networks and are mainly controlled by the parameters MDist, RA, TD, and MA [44]. Therefore, to generate street networks, these three parameters are required for the street network generator component (Figure 3a). In addition, parameter B is required to define the boundary of the street network. The output L returns a series of line segments representing the street network (Figure 4a). For the block generation (Figure 3b), the extract polygons component transforms street networks into their dual-directed graphs [44]. The output P creates polygons representing street blocks (Figure 4b). The parcel generation is based on the slicing tree structure [49], according to which the street blocks are divided into smaller polygons (parcels). The parcel component takes street block polygons as input (Figure 3c) and output Pcl as parcel polygons (Figure 4c). The building generation is based on simple calculations and extrusions, which consist of two steps. First, the buildable component takes the polygons of parcels and blocks as input to calculate BA as the buildable area in each parcel (Figure 3c). Second, the building component utilizes BA and parcel polygons to generate Ftpt (building footprint) and

BH (building height) (Figure 3d). In this process, the parameters BT, Blen, and Bdep are required to control the building forms. The output Ftpt can be further extruded as building blocks via Extr component. All the optional parameters involved in the generative design process are used to refine the results.

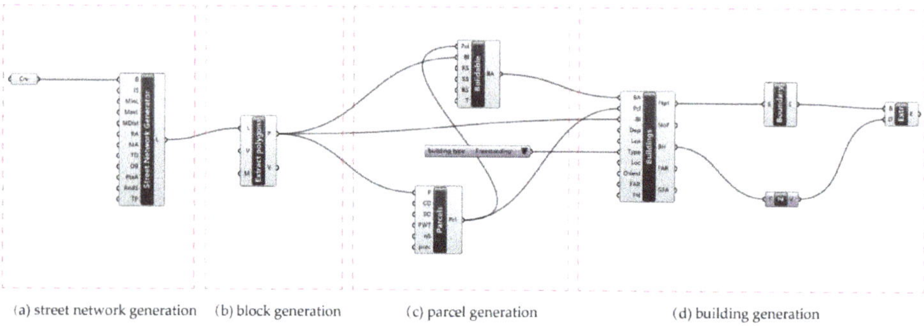

Figure 3. The grasshopper components used in computational generation process.

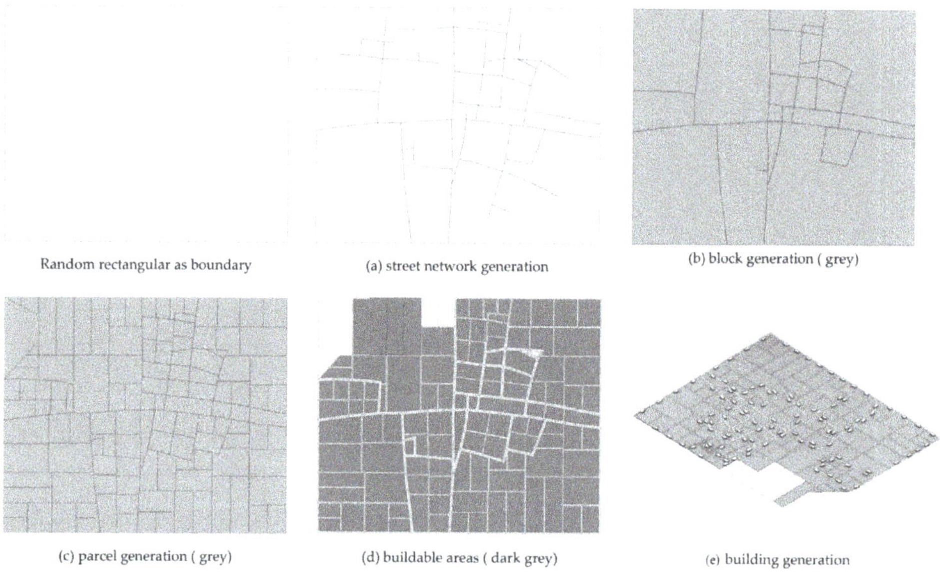

Figure 4. The results of each step in the generative design process (with random rectangle as boundary and default input parameters).

The amenity generation is the basis for assessing the walkability of generative solutions. It is required that urban designers determine the type and number of amenities in their proposals depending on the client's requirements or the zoning regulations. Information on the type and number of amenities needs to be added to generative design schemes in the form of metadata. The method can be referred to as the metadata creation in Section 2.3.1.

2.5. *Quantitative Assessment and Qualitative Analysis of Generative Design Proposals*

The quantitative assessment and qualitative analysis of generative design proposals are rooted in the evaluation methods proposed in Section 2.1. The quantitative assessment includes the measurement of height-to-width ratios, walk score, and amenity score. The walk score and amenity score calculation are based on mobility simulation, the method of which can be referred to in Sections 2.3.2 and 2.3.3. For qualitative analysis, the visual experience analysis and public space analysis are involved. The workflow for quantitative assessment and qualitative analysis of generative design proposals is illustrated in Figure 5.

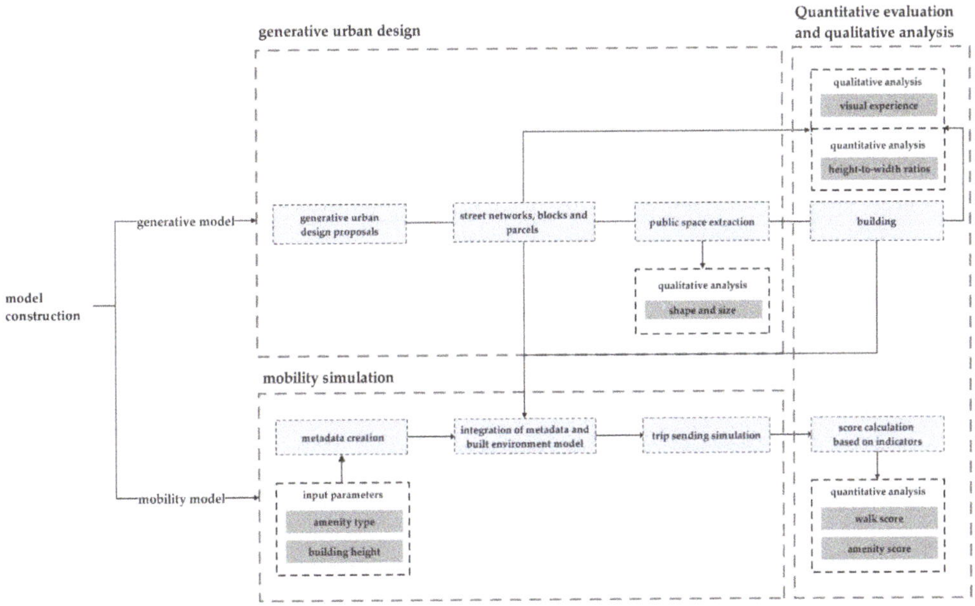

Figure 5. The workflow for quantitative assessment and qualitative analysis of generative design proposals.

3. Case Study

3.1. Assessment of the Study Area

Carnegie is a major activity center in the City of Glen Eira, an inner suburb precinct located in Melbourne, Victoria. Due to the rapid growth of the population, the local government started a new planning process that aims to accommodate the growing population, while promoting new and sustainable development. One of the vital decisions was to direct population growth to areas near public transportation, and to transform these areas into mix-used, high-density, and walkable neighborhoods. The area within 1/4 miles of Carnegie station is selected as the study area, and an urban renewal site is identified as the site for the computational generation of design proposals (Figure 6).

First, the walkability of the study area is examined. The average walk score in the study area is calculated as 57.3, which indicates that there is still much room for improvement in local walkability. As can be seen from Figure 3, amenities in the area are clustered along the central axis, and the number gradually decreases as the distance from the station increases. Poor road connections in the northwest may affect accessibility to amenities. The hypothesis is, therefore, formulated that poor street connectivity and the uneven distribution pattern of amenities account for the unsatisfactory low walk score. Second, the average amenity scores, amenity hits, and street hits in the study area are calculated. Figure 7a shows the average amenity scores of the study area by amenity type. It can be found that the score of each amenity type is greater than zero. This reveals that the number of these six types of amenities available in the area is already sufficient to meet the needs of the residents. Therefore, there is no need to add more counterparts of the same type to the renewal site. Figure 7b visualizes the street hits and amenity hits in the study area. The darker the color, the higher the activeness of the street segments or amenities. It can be noticed that the renewal site features low street vitality and amenity occupancy, further validating the previous assumptions on walkability. This informs the designers to enhance street connectivity within the site.

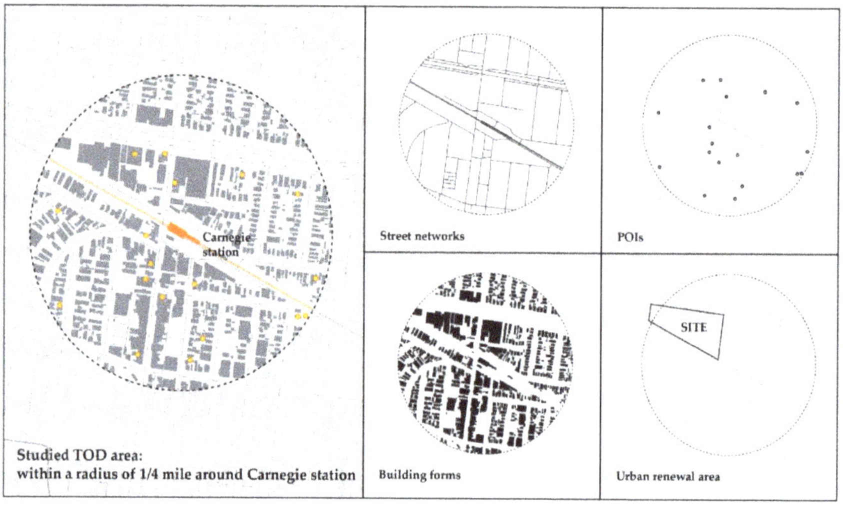

Figure 6. Profile of the study area.

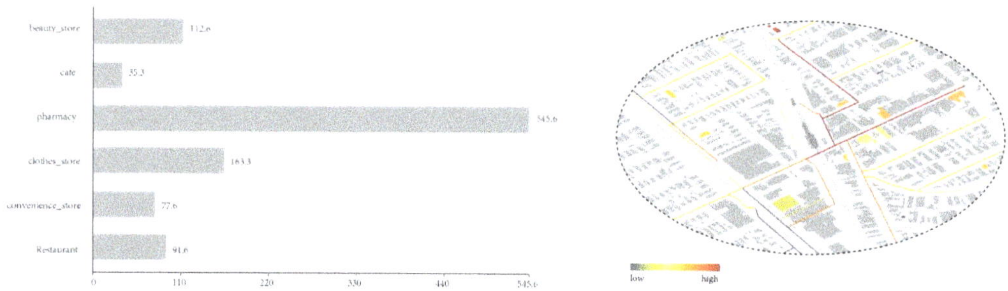

(**a**) (**b**)

Figure 7. (**a**) Average amenity scores of the study area by amenity type; (**b**) The activeness of streets and amenities in the study area.

According to the principles of good urban design in TODs, public spaces, such as streets and parks, need to be designed to increase their attractiveness to residents through a diversity of visual experiences. To explore the visual experiences of the existing built environment, a street segment adjacent to the renewal site is selected, with the shape and area of isovists being measured (Figure 8). It can be seen that there is a significant visual change from point A to B, with the view gradually opening up. This indicates that the present public space is visually attractive.

Further, the height-to-street width ratios (H/W) of the street-facing buildings in the renewal site are measured and recorded in Figure 9. All of these ratios are in the range of 1:1 to 1:3, indicating that the current public space is considered comfortable for pedestrians and has a sense of enclosure.

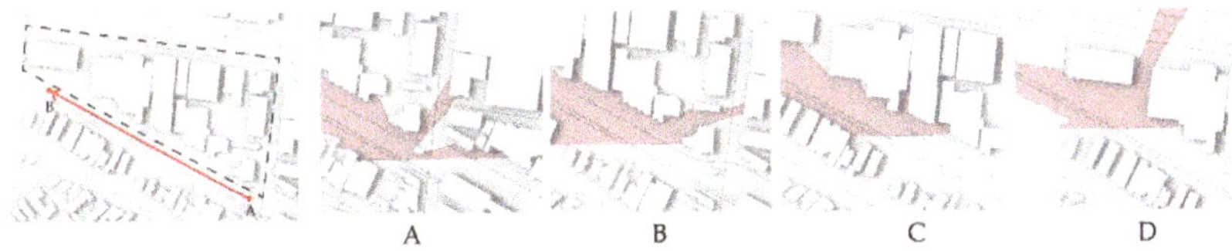

(a) The shape of isovists from point A to B

(b) the area of isovists from point A to B

Figure 8. Visual experience analysis of the renewal site.

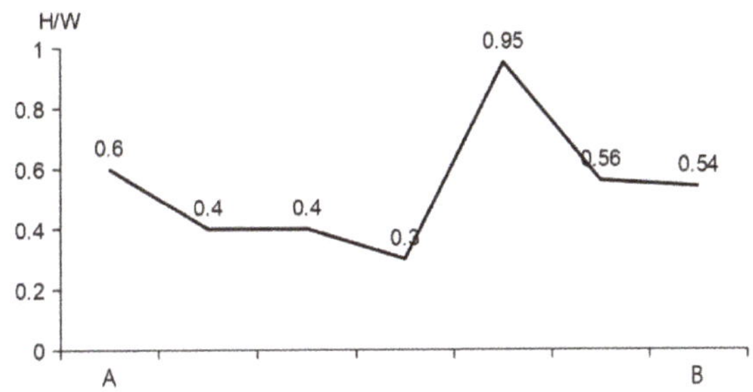

Figure 9. The height-to-street width ratios of the street-facing buildings in the renewal site (The x-axis represents, from left to right, the height-to-width ratio of the buildings passing from point A to B).

3.2. Generative Urban Design Proposals

The context assessment of the renewal site informs the creation and selection process of generative design solutions. According to the assessment results, the main issue of the renewal site is the underutilization of amenities and streets. This can be improved by increasing the number and type of amenities and changing the form of the road network. Regarding amenities, providing residents with a wealth of activities is not only a requirement of the TOD principles but also a practical necessity in Carnegie. According to the government report of Glen Eira activity centers [50], the survey on local amenities shows that 72 percent of residents want new retails and say they are overwhelmed by too many restaurants. Three types of amenities (butchers, newsagents, and bookstores) are most in demand by residents—accounting for 50 percent of the total population. Therefore, these three types are added to the generative schemes. After 25 iteration experiments, a total of 150 schemes are generated, of which ten representative schemes are selected. Compared with the original state, new design solutions need to enhance the walkability of the area with amenities that better meet the needs of the residents. As a result, design solutions with higher average walk scores and lower amenity scores are chosen. From these design alternatives, the experts select ten satisfactory options that can be further developed in terms of building forms, street patterns, and interesting public spaces. The input parameters of ten representative urban design proposals are recorded in Table 4.

Table 4. Input parameters of 10 representative urban design proposals.

Input Parameters	Proposal 1	Proposal 2	Proposal 3	Proposal 4	Proposal 5
MDist	50	50	50	30	30
MA	4	4	4	4	4
RA	10	10	10	10	10
TD	5	5	5	5	5
RndS	2	1	5	5	6
BT	bl	bl	bl	bl	bl
Blen	80	80	80	80	80
Bdep	default = 15	default = 15	default = 15	default = 15	default = 15
FAR	3	3	5	5	5
Orientation	3.14	3.14	3.14	3.14	3.14
Input parameters	**Proposal 6**	**Proposal 7**	**Proposal 8**	**Proposal 9**	**Proposal 10**
MDist	20	20	20	20	20
MA	4	4	4	4	4
RA	10	10	10	10	10
TD	5	5	5	5	5
RndS	3	5	2	2	6
BT	bl	rw	bl	rw	bl
Blen	80	default = 25	80	default = 25	80
Bdep	default = 15	default = 15	default = 15	default = 15	default = 15
FAR	3	3	3	3	3
Orientation	3.14	3.14	3.14	3.14	3.14

"bl" for block building. "rw" for row building.

4. Results and Discussion

To understand the role of generative urban design in facilitating transit-oriented development, this evaluation framework examines design solutions from the following five perspectives.

4.1. *Walkability Assessment*

This framework both quantifies the average walk score of the study area and visualizes the walk score of the housing units within the area (Figure 10). The average walk score represents the walkability of the studied TOD area, which allows designers to understand the impact of their solutions on the entire region. Of the ten scenarios, proposal 1 (average walk score = 95.8) and proposal 7 (average walk score = 95.1) provide the greatest enhancements to regional walkability. The walk score of the housing units, on the other hand, emphasizes the equity of walkability in the region. Even in areas with high walkability, there may exist households with poor walkability. While the overall walkability of the study area in Proposal 1 is higher, the variation is smaller in Proposal 7. This requires urban designers and urban planners to make trade-offs and think about improvements.

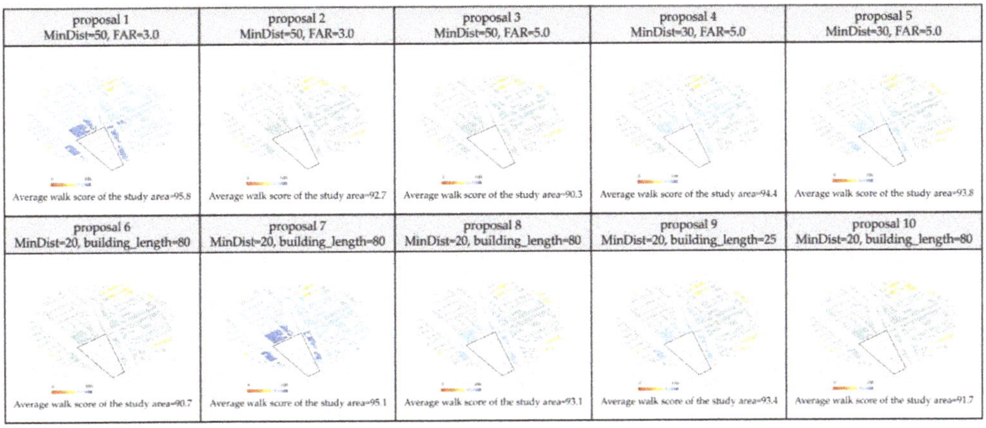

Figure 10. Walk scores of 10 representative urban design proposals.

4.2. Amenity Assessment

According to the results of the amenity assessment (Table 5), Proposal 8 has the smallest amenity score among all options, meaning that it has the most reasonable configuration of amenities. The ten design scenarios are generated based on the same type (butchers, newsagents, and bookstores) and number (a total of five) of amenities, but yield different amenity scores. A possible explanation for this is the building density, location of amenities, and street network patterns vary in these design scenarios. In light of the trip-sending simulation process, the building-level population and the degree of connectivity of the street network determine the number of visitors to each amenity. In Urbano's algorithm, the building height is a determinant of the building-level population. The amenity assessment enables designers to understand how different aspects of their design (building height, location of amenities, and road network patterns) can impact the relationship between supply and demand for local amenities.

Table 5. Average amenity scores of 10 representative urban design proposals.

	Proposal 1	**Proposal 2**	**Proposal 3**	**Proposal 4**	**Proposal 5**
Average amenity scores	50.1	48.1	76.7	68.3	59.3
	Proposal 6	Proposal 7	Proposal 8	Proposal 9	Proposal 10
Average amenity scores	50.2	62.5	38.6	41.3	52.1

4.3. Height-to-Street Width Ratio Assessment

Figure 11 shows the height-to-street width ratios of buildings in 10 representative urban design proposals. It can be found that the ratio is more than 1:1 for all proposals except Proposals 1, 6, and 9, where H/W is basically between 1:1 and 1:3. This can be explained in two aspects. The first is that TOD promotes an increase in building density (floor area ratio). This is directly reflected in an increase in building heights. Secondly, the DecodingSpaces workflow leads to the uncertainty of the building heights, since it is difficult for designers to manually assign building height values when a large number of buildings are generated automatically. According to the algorithm of computational design generation, the building height is determined by the FAR value and building footprint. The building footprint is influenced by the buildable area in each plot, which has a tendency to be random. This reflects that the generative design is not yet ideal in terms of height control for building mass generation. Based on the results of the height-to-street width ratio assessment, it can be inferred that H/W tends to be desirable when the FAR is less than or equal to 3 in the TOD design.

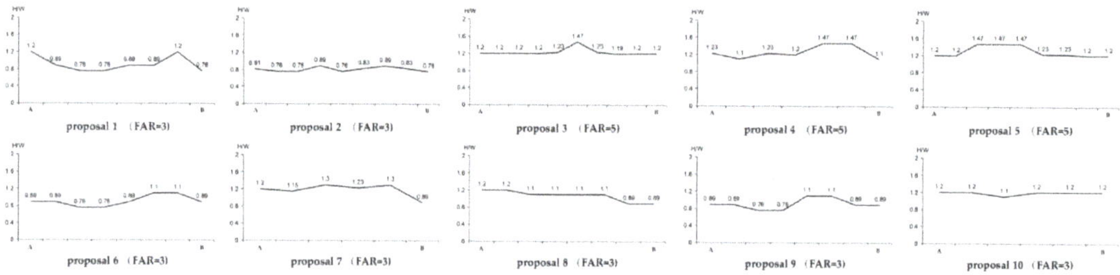

Figure 11. Height-to-street width ratios of buildings in 10 representative urban design proposals (The x-axis represents, from left to right, the height-to-width ratio of the buildings passing from point A to B).

4.4. *Visual Experience Analysis*

The visual experience is difficult to measure directly through metrics, so the evaluation framework incorporates qualitative analysis regarding residents' visual experiences, which is to use the variation in isovist areas to help urban designers understand the impact of their solutions on the visual experience of residents as they walk in public spaces. The same path as the context assessment (from point A to B) is selected for analysis. Figure 12 shows a variety of visual experiences of ten representative design proposals, which can be mainly divided into two categories—the field of vision that gradually becomes smaller (Proposal 2,5,6,7,8,9,10), and the field of vision with few changes (Proposal 1,3,4,5). There are no good or bad criteria for evaluating the changes in visual experience. Designers can make trade-offs depending on the atmosphere they want to create in the public spaces.

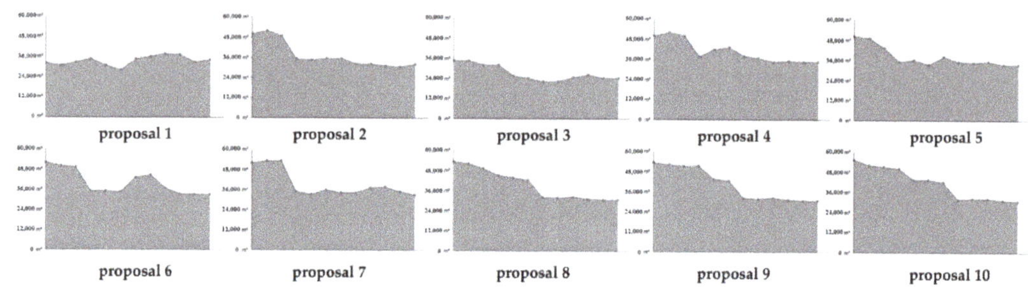

Figure 12. The area of isovist from point A to B in 10 representative urban design proposals.

4.5. *Public Space Analysis*

As suggested in the assessment methods (Section 2.1), there is no specific standard for deciding the size and shape of public space. It depends on many factors, such as citizen preferences, local context, aesthetics, etc [38]. The 3D model can be used as a tool to assist the designers in decision-making. For the selection of public spaces in these ten proposals (Figure 13), the experts have given some suggestions. First, since the renovation site contains a variety of retail stores, the large public spaces near the street can be more attractive to visitors than scattered small public spaces. In addition, the public spaces that are located on the main axis can create a certain sense of sequence. Therefore, the public spaces in Proposals 3 and 8 are considered to be suitable choices.

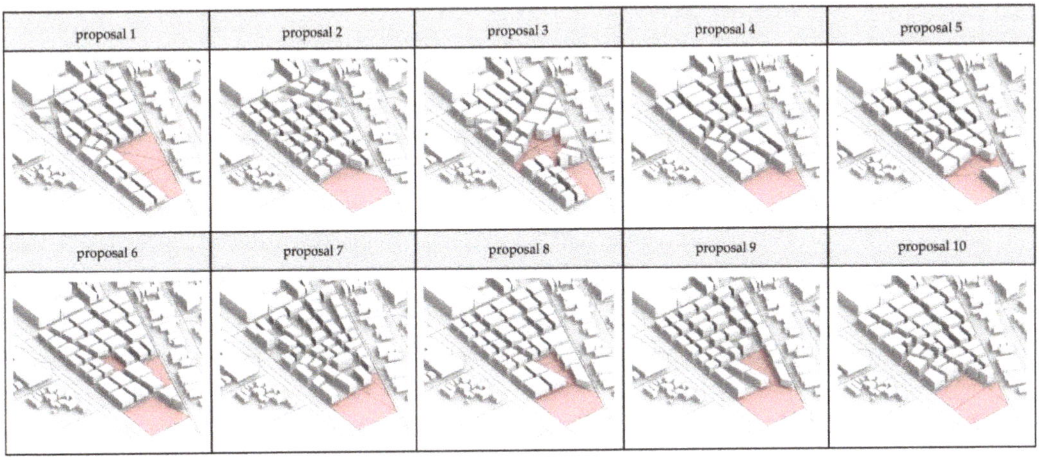

Figure 13. The public spaces in 10 representative urban design proposals.

4.6. Comprehensive Analysis

Taking into account the five aspects of the evaluation framework, Proposal 1 seems to be the optimal choice. However, this by no means indicates that it is flawless. Almost all the generative scenarios produced irregular building forms and undesirable building sizes in 25 iterations, which requires the designers to make further adjustments. The deficit suggests that although the smart algorithm is informative and powerful during the conceptual design stage, the intervention and engagement of experienced designers should not be overlooked. It also verifies two arguments made earlier in this paper: when considering generative urban design, one cannot focus on the road network alone and ignore other essential factors, such as the building layouts, and one cannot rely entirely on algorithms for design generation.

4.7. Strengths and Limitations of the Evaluation Framework

To the best of our knowledge, this is the first comprehensive framework that translates urban design recommendations for TOD into an evaluation methodology that utilizes both data feedback and experts' experience to guide designers in their selection of options. Affirmatively, a relatively satisfactory proposal can be selected using this framework. The advantages of this framework are demonstrated in two aspects. Firstly, the computational design generation has been notoriously hard to interpret [25], which hindered its application in real-world problems. This framework contributes to the interpretability of computational generative urban design by providing useful explanations of generative design solutions (in terms of walkability, amenity accessibility, open space creation, visual experience, and hight-to-width ratio) to help designers understand their potential in TOD design. Secondly, the shortcomings of the optimization methods in the generative urban design proposed by previous studies are enhanced by the qualitative analysis methods and the intervention of experts' experience. At the same time, the framework avoids the disadvantages of completely subjective decisions by designers (with no optimization objectives and decision criteria).

However, this assessment framework still has some areas that could be improved. On the one hand, safety as an important aspect of TOD design is not included in this framework due to the lack of a suitable evaluation method. On the other hand, because of the introduction of qualitative analysis in the framework, the various dimensions cannot be weighed in the assessment process by simply applying weights or other methods. Further research could usefully explore in terms of these two limitations.

5. Conclusions

Good urban design can play an important role in promoting TOD, and the enlightening and objective-based optimization capabilities of computational urban design bring new opportunities for city designers to realize good urban design. To help them better understand the role of generative urban design in TOD, this study proposes a novel evaluation framework that aims to assess and explain the use of generative design in TOD. The findings of the evaluation process emerge from five aspects. With regard to the walkability assessment, the walk score metric succeeds in allowing designers to filter out the generative design options that contribute the most to the walkability of a TOD area. However, considering the equity of walkability, designers and planners need to make further trade-offs. The amenity assessment clarifies that building heights, street network patterns, and amenity locations in generative design can influence the supply and demand for amenities in TOD areas. The height-to-street width ratio assessment points out the defects of generative design, i.e., the randomness of building generation and the difficulty of controlling building heights. For visual experience analysis, it is concluded that the impact of generative design on people's visual experience is difficult to quantify and there is no fixed standard. The designer's experience needs to be involved in the analysis. Regarding public space analysis, it is suggested in the literature that the shape and size of public spaces are determined by a variety of factors. Taking expert advice is the most effective way to make decisions in public space design. By combining the results of the five evaluations, a suitable design solution can be derived. In general, the evidence from this study strengthens the idea that neither experts' judgment (e.g., qualitative analysis, manipulation of architectural form and scale) nor quantitative metrics can be absent in the evaluation process of generative urban design solutions.

The contribution of this study is two-fold. First of all, the study proposes the first comprehensive framework that transforms TOD urban design guidelines into an evaluation approach to assist designers in making decisions. Second, by offering helpful explanations of generative design solutions, the study contributes to the interpretability of computational generative urban design and enables designers to recognize the potential of these solutions in TOD design. Nevertheless, there is room for improvement in this framework. It could benefit from further exploration of integrating the safety evaluation into the assessment framework, as well as balancing quantitative and qualitative evaluations. In addition, the method for analyzing the size and shape of public space can be further improved.

Author Contributions: Conceptualization, W.Y. and X.H.; methodology, W.Y. and X.H.; software, W.Y.; validation, W.Y. and X.H.; formal analysis, W.Y.; investigation, W.Y. and X.H.; resources, X.H., M.W. and N.L.; data curation, W.Y. and X.H.; writing—original draft preparation, W.Y. and X.H.; writing—review and editing, M.W. and N.L.; visualization, W.Y.; supervision, X.H.; project administration, X.H., M.W. and N.L.; and funding acquisition, X.H. and M.W. All authors have read and agreed to the published version of the manuscript.

Funding: This project is funded by the National Natural Science Foundation of China (NSFC) [52208039], the National key R&D program "Science and Technology Winter Olympics" key project "Evacuation system and support technology for assisting physically challenged communities" [2020YFF0304900], the Beijing High-level Overseas Talents Support Funding, R&D Program of Beijing Municipal Education Commission (KM202210009008), the NCUT Young Scholar Development Project, and the Australian Research Council Linkage Project [LP190100089].

Data Availability Statement: The datasets of POI, street network, and building information used in this project are provided by Australian Urban Research Infrastructure Network (AURIN), OpentreestMap, and PSMA Australia (accessed on 10 August 2022).

Conflicts of Interest: The authors declare no conflict of interest.

References

1. Thomas, R.; Bertolini, L. *Transit-Oriented Development: Learning from International Case Studies;* Springer International Publishing: Cham, Switzerland, 2020. Available online: http://link.springer.com/10.1007/978-3-030-48470-5 (accessed on 13 June 2022).
2. Ibraeva, A.; de Correia, G.H.A.; Silva, C.; Antunes, A.P. Transit-oriented development: A review of research achievements and challenges. *Transp. Res. Part A Policy Pract.* **2020**, *132*, 110–130. [CrossRef]
3. Cervero, R.; Radisch, C. Travel choices in pedestrian versus automobile oriented neighborhoods. *Transp. Policy* **1996**, *3*, 127–141. [CrossRef]
4. Currie, G.; Stanley, J. Investigating links between social capital and public transport. *Transp. Rev.* **2008**, *28*, 529–547. [CrossRef]
5. Kamruzzaman, M.; Wood, L.; Hine, J.; Currie, G.; Giles-Corti, B.; Turrell, G. Patterns of social capital associated with transit oriented development. *J. Transp. Geogr.* **2014**, *35*, 144–155. [CrossRef]
6. Calthorpe, P.; Fulton, W.; Fulton, W.B. *The Regional City;* Island Press: Washington, DC, USA, 2001; 298p.
7. Suzuki, H.; Cervero, R.; Iuchi, K. *Transforming Cities with Transit: Transit and Land-Use Integration for Sustainable Urban Development;* World Bank Publications: Washington, DC, USA, 2013; 233p.
8. Jacobson, J.; Forsyth, A. Seven American TODs: Good Practices for Urban Design in Transit-Oriented Development Projects. JTLU. 2008. Available online: https://www.jtlu.org/index.php/jtlu/article/view/67 (accessed on 18 September 2022).
9. Lynch, K. *A Theory of Good City Form;* MIT Press: Cambridge, MA, USA, 1981; 514p.
10. Dittmar, H.; Ohland, G. *The New Transit Town;* Island Press: Washington, DC, USA, 2012.
11. Owen, N.; Humpel, N.; Leslie, E.; Bauman, A.; Sallis, J.F. Understanding environmental influences on walking: Review and research agenda. *Am. J. Prev. Med.* **2004**, *27*, 67–76. [CrossRef] [PubMed]
12. Gehl, J. *Cities for People*; Island Press: Washington, DC, USA, 2013.
13. Forsyth, A. What is a walkable place? The walkability debate in urban design. *Urban Des Int.* **2015**, *20*, 274–292. [CrossRef]
14. Ogra, A.; Ndebele, R. PDF Document of The Role of 6Ds: Density, Diversity, Design, Destination, Distance, and Demand Management in Transit Oriented Development (TOD). 2014. Available online: https://ujcontent.uj.ac.za/vital/%20access/manager/Repository/uj:5017/CONTENT1 (accessed on 12 August 2022).
15. Castiglione, J.; Bradley, M.; Gliebe, J. *Activity-Based Travel Demand Models: A Primer;* Transportation Research Board: Washington, DC, USA, 2015.
16. Szczepura-McLean, C. URBANO: A Computational Tool-Kit for Integrated Urban Design. New York. 31 December 2019, p. 23. Available online: https://ecommons.cornell.edu/handle/1813/102682 (accessed on 18 September 2022).
17. Gutiérrez, J.; Cardozo, O.D.; García-Palomares, J.C. Transit ridership forecasting at station level: An approach based on distance-decay weighted regression. *J. Transp. Geogr.* **2011**, *19*, 1081–1092. [CrossRef]
18. Setiawan, B. Towards the new urban agenda of safe cities: Urban crimes in four Indonesian cities. *IOP Conf. Ser. Earth Environ. Sci.* **2017**, *99*, 012037. [CrossRef]
19. Nagy, D.; Villaggi, L.; Benjamin, D. Generative Urban Design: Integrating Financial and Energy Goals for Automated Neighborhood Layout. In Proceedings of the 2018 Symposium on Simulation for Architecture and Urban Design (SimAUD 2018), Delft, The Netherlands, 5–7 June 2018; Society for Modeling and Simulation International (SCS): Delft, The Netherlands, 2018. Available online: https://dl.acm.org/citation.cfm?id=3289775 (accessed on 16 September 2022).
20. Qeisi, S.A.; Al-Alwan, H. Generative Urban Design Concepts and Methods: A Research Review. *IOP Conf. Ser. Mater. Sci. Eng.* **2021**, *1090*, 012085. [CrossRef]
21. Rakha, T. Generative Urban Modeling: A Design Work Flow for Walkability-Optimized Cities. In Proceedings of the Fifth National Conference of IBPSA-USA (SimBuild 2012), Madison, Wisconsin, 1–3 August 2012; pp. 255–262.
22. Hidalgo, C.A.; Castañer, E.; Sevtsuk, A. The amenity mix of urban neighborhoods. *Habitat Int.* **2020**, *106*, 102205. [CrossRef]
23. Trubka, R.; Glackin, S.; Lade, O.; Pettit, C. A web-based 3D visualisation and assessment system for urban precinct scenario modelling. *ISPRS J. Photogramm. Remote Sens.* **2016**, *117*, 175–186. [CrossRef]
24. Lima, F.; Brown, N.; Duarte, J. Urban Design Optimization: Generative Approaches towards Urban Fabrics with Improved Transit Accessibility and Walkability-Generative Approaches towards Urban Fabrics with Improved Transit Accessibility and Walkability. In Proceedings of the 2021 Computer-Aided Architectural Design Research in Asia (CAADRIA 2021), Hongkong, China, 29 March–1 April 2021; CAADRIA: Hongkong, China, 2021; pp. 719–728. Available online: http://papers.cumincad.org/cgi-bin/works/paper/caadria2021_055 (accessed on 27 June 2022). [CrossRef]
25. Miao, Y.; Koenig, R.; Knecht, K. The Development of Optimization Methods in Generative Urban Design: A Review. In Proceedings of the Symposium on Simulation for Architecture and Urban Design (SimAUD 2020), Online, 25–27 May 2020; pp. 247–254.
26. Shach-Pinsly, D.; Bindreiter, S.; Porat, I.; Sussman, S.; Forster, J.; Rinnerthaler, M. Multiparametric Analysis of Urban Environmental Quality for Estimating Neighborhood Renewal Alternatives. *UP* **2021**, *6*, 172–188. [CrossRef]
27. Yang, Y.; Samaranayake, S.; Dogan, T. An Adaptive Workflow to Generate Street Network and Amenity Allocation for Walkable Neighborhood Design. In Proceedings of the Symposium on Simulation for Architecture and Urban Design (SimAUD 2020), Online, 25–27 May 2020; pp. 195–202. [CrossRef]
28. Ortega, E.; MartÍN, B.; LÓPez-Lambas, M.E.; Soria-Lara, J.A. Evaluating the impact of urban design scenarios on walking accessibility: The case of the Madrid 'Centro'district. *Sustain. Cities Soc.* **2021**, *74*, 103156. [CrossRef]

29. Goodspeed, R. *Scenario Planning for Cities and Regions: Managing and Envisioning Uncertain Futures*; Lincoln Institute of Land Policy: Cambridge, MA, USA, 2020.
30. Lynch, K.; Hack, G. *Site Planning*; MIT Press: Cambridge, MA, USA, 1984.
31. Alexander, C. *A Pattern Language: Towns, Buildings, Construction*; Oxford University Press: Oxford, UK, 1977.
32. Moughtin, C. *Urban Design: Street and Square*; Routledge: London, UK, 2007.
33. Carr, L.J.; Dunsiger, S.I.; Marcus, B.H. Validation of Walk Score for estimating access to walkable amenities. *Br. J. Sport. Med.* **2011**, *45*, 1144–1148. [CrossRef] [PubMed]
34. Hall, C.M.; Ram, Y. Walk score®and its potential contribution to the study of active transport and walkability: A critical and systematic review. *Transp. Res. Part D Transp. Environ.* **2018**, *61*, 310–324. [CrossRef]
35. Walk Score Methodology. Walk Score. Available online: https://www.walkscore.com/methodology.shtml (accessed on 19 September 2022).
36. Madanipour, A. *Whose Public Space? International Case Studies in Urban Design and Development*; Routledge: London, UK, 2013.
37. Mehta, V. Evaluating Public Space. *J. Urban Des.* **2014**, *19*, 53–88. [CrossRef]
38. Turner, A. Analysing the Visual Dynamics of Spatial Morphology. *Environ. Plann B Plann Des.* **2003**, *30*, 657–676. [CrossRef]
39. Schneider, S.; König, R.; Weimar, B.U. Exploring the Generative Potential of Isovist Fields. In Proceedings of the Computer Aided Architectural Design in Europe (eCAADe 2012), Prague, Czech, 12–14 September 2012; pp. 355–364.
40. Batty, M. Exploring Isovist Fields: Space and Shape in Architectural and Urban Morphology. *Environ. Plan. B Plan. Des.* **2001**, *28*, 123–150. [CrossRef]
41. Kim, Y.; Jung, S.K. Distance-weighted isovist area: An isovist index representing spatial proximity. *Autom. Constr.* **2014**, *43*, 92–97. [CrossRef]
42. Stamps, A.E., III. Isovists, enclosure, and permeability theory. *Environ. Plan. B Plan. Des.* **2005**, *32*, 735–762. [CrossRef]
43. Yang, Y.; Samaranayake, S.; Dogan, T. Using Open Data to Derive Local Amenity Demand Patterns for Walkability Simulations and Amenity Utilization Analysis. In Proceedings of the Blucher Design Proceedings, Porto, Portugal, 11–13 September 2016; Editora Blucher: Porto, Portugal, 2019; pp. 665–674. Available online: http://www.proceedings.blucher.com.br/article-details/34315 (accessed on 15 April 2022).
44. Koenig, R.; Treyer, L.; Schmitt, G. Graphical Smalltalk with My Optimization System for Urban Planning Tasks. In Proceedings of the Computer Aided Architectural Design in Europe (eCAADe 2013), Delft, The Netherlands, 18–20 September 2013; pp. 355–364. [CrossRef]
45. Koenig, R.; Miao, Y.; Knecht, K.; Buš, P.; Mei-Chih, C. Interactive Urban Synthesis. In *Computer-Aided Architectural Design Future Trajectories*; Çağdaş, G., Özkar, M., Gül, L.F., Gürer, E., Eds.; Springer: Singapore, 2017; pp. 23–41, (Communications in Computer and Information Science; vol. 724); Available online: http://link.springer.com/10.1007/978-981-10-5197-5_2 (accessed on 27 October 2022).
46. Koenig, R.; Schmitt, G. Backcasting and a New Way of Command in Computational Design. In *CAADence in Architecture, Back to Command*; Budapest University of Technology and Economics, Faculty of Architecture: Zurich, Switzerland, 2016; pp. 15–25. Available online: http://hdl.handle.net/10890/16274 (accessed on 27 October 2022).
47. Urbano-A New Tool to Promote Mobility-Aware Urban Design, Active Transportation Modeling and Access Analysis for Amenities and Public Transport. In Proceedings of the 2018 Symposium on Simulation for Architecture and Urban Design (SimAUD 2018), Delft, The Netherlands, 15 June 2018; Society for Modeling and Simulation International (SCS): Delft, The Netherlands, 2018. Available online: https://dl.acm.org/citation.cfm?id=3289778 (accessed on 15 April 2022).
48. Knecht, K.; König, R. *Automatische Grundstücksumlegung Mithilfe von Unterteilungsalgorithmen und Typenbasierte Generierung von Stadtstrukturen*; Springer Nature: Berlin, Germany, 2012.
49. Knecht, K.; König, R. Generating floor plan layouts with kd trees and evolutionary algorithms. In Proceedings of the Generative Art Conference, Milan, Italy, 15 December 2010; pp. 238–253.
50. Glen Huntly Activity Centre. Glen Eira City Council. 2017. Available online: https://www.gleneira.vic.gov.au/our-city/planning-for-the-future/from-project-to-policy/glen-huntly-activity-centre (accessed on 30 October 2022).

buildings

MDPI

Article

Green Roofs as an Approach to Enhance Urban Sustainability: A Study of Public Perception in Riyadh, Saudi Arabia

Ali Alqahtany

Department of Urban and Regional Planning, College of Architecture and Planning, Imam Abdulrahman Bin Faisal University, Dammam 31441, Saudi Arabia; amalqahtany@iau.edu.sa

Abstract: This study focuses on highlighting the major effects and challenges being faced in the implementation of the green roof technique in Riyadh, Saudi Arabia. Green roofs have proven to be energy efficient, environment friendly, and economical in a long run. Due to the increasing global environment temperature, it has become necessary to implement such sustainable methods that help in the achievement of urban sustainability. Saudi Arabia has seen some reluctance in the implementation of green roofs in buildings. The reasons for not adopting this system have not been reported as yet. To study the level of awareness among the public and the challenges they are facing regarding green roofs, this study was taken up. A survey questionnaire was designed with a high level of flexibility covering the key issues, including the related areas that are affected in the daily life of a resident and also the challenges faced by the general public in the installation of such systems in their existing or new buildings. An extensive literature review and a reconnaissance survey were performed before shortlisting the major factors and challenges to be included in the survey questionnaire. An overwhelming response was received from the people of Riyadh City. Almost 94% of people agreed to the fact that green roofs enhance the aesthetics of the building, and the same number of people agreed that they play a role in controlling the air quality. On the other hand, 91% of the respondents identified the climate of the area as the biggest challenge in implementing green roofs on the buildings. The study concludes with strong recommendations for the local authorities to plan quick actions. The study shall help the building owners, city planners, and policy makers in identifying the major hurdles being faced by the residents in adopting green roofs and will help them to provide solutions to these issues.

Keywords: green roofs; sustainable urban planning and design; urban development; public perception; urban policy and governance; Saudi Arabia

Citation: Alqahtany, A. Green Roofs as an Approach to Enhance Urban Sustainability: A Study of Public Perception in Riyadh, Saudi Arabia. *Buildings* **2022**, *12*, 2202. https://doi.org/10.3390/buildings12122202

Academic Editors: Liyin Shen, Jorge Ochoa and Haijun Bao

Received: 19 November 2022
Accepted: 7 December 2022
Published: 12 December 2022

1. Introduction

Humans have been interested in green elements since ancient times due to the close connection between them and their surrounding nature. Plants have been the main source of food and medicine, starting from the stages of grazing and picking fruits, then the beginning of agriculture, settlements, and then the formation of societies and urban areas. Green infrastructure approaches, whether natural or semi-natural, are often seen as common approaches to increasing green urban areas [1]. The green roofs technique is one of these approaches to enhance a range of ecosystem services that provide environmental, social, and economic advantages via natural solutions [2–4]. Among these services are the regulation services such as local climate regulation [5,6] and air quality improvement [7]; provisioning services including food and urban agriculture; the habitat services such as suitable living spaces for wild plants and animals; and cultural services, including aesthetic improvement and recreational spaces [4]. Nevertheless, although there are many advantages of the green roofs technique [2,8,9], it remains untapped on the urban scale [1].

The main structural part that determines the building's relationship with the surrounding nature is the roof of the building [10]. Green roofs are one of the strategic tools that can play an important role in creating sustainable and resilient cities [11]. Green roofs are also named roof gardens, living roofs, and eco-roofs and are roofs with plants in their final layer [12]. Green roofs can be defined simply as living vegetation installed on the roofs of buildings and can offer various environmental and social, as well as economical, advantages. They can be installed either by pre-cultivated systems, modular systems, or complete systems [13]. The classic features of various types of green roofs can be measured based on purpose, vegetation type, substrate thickness, irrigation requirement, supporting structural requirements, and maintenance requirement [13–15], as reproduced in Table 1 below. The concept of green roofs revolves around covering ordinary roofs with vegetation to improve thermal insulation, protect against climatic conditions, and help absorb rainwater [16]. It is a practical means of expanding the amount of vegetation in urban cities [13]. There are several types of green roofs, including intensive, semi-intensive, and extensive. The main differences between intensive and extensive green roofs are the type of vegetation planted and the depth of the substrate [17].

Table 1. Main features of green roof types [13–15].

Criteria	Specific Use	Semi-Specific Use	General Use
Purpose of Use	Parks and Gardens	Vegetation	Protection Layer
Depth of Growth Media	Deep (Min. 500 mm)	Medium (150 to 500 mm)	Shallow (20 to 150 mm)
Self-Weight Category (Saturated)	Heavy (200 to 500 kg/m^2)	Medium (120 to 200 kg/m^2)	Light (60 to 120 kg/m^2)
Self-Weight (Dry)	140 to 325 kg/m^2	90 to 140 kg/m^2	45 to 90 kg/m^2
Type of Plantation	Small Trees, Shrubs	Grass, Herbs, Shrubs	Low Growing
Installation Cost	High	Medium	Low
Irrigation Requirement	Regular	Periodic	Little to No Requirement
Water Holding Capacity	200 L/m^2	120 L/m^2	60 L/m^2
Maintenance Requirements	High	Periodic	Very High
Structural Requirements	Additional Structural Support	Additional Structural Support	Existing Structures

Generally, there are five major components of a green roof system, which include the grass, growth substrate, filtration layer, a layer for waterproofing, and root barrier [18]. A detailed green roof system and all its layers are shown in Figure 1.

The green roofs approach is now widely used as a tool in urban planning strategies due to its significant role in sustainable urban development [19]. Indeed, it has become an increasingly popular choice in urban planning over the past two decades [20]. In dense urban areas, the concept of green roofs has become one of the standard ways to introduce vegetation to these areas [21]. Green roofs provide numerous benefits to the urban built environment and offer a set of environmental, social, economic, and urban benefits [18]. The most prominent are the mitigation of urban air and noise pollution and increased air quality [19,22], reduction of the urban heat island effect in cities [23], reduction of building energy consumption [24–26], reduction of stormwater runoff [27,28], increase of biodiversity and habitats [21,29,30], and provision of more spaces for amenity and recreation [21]. Some executed examples of green roofs are shown in Figure 2.

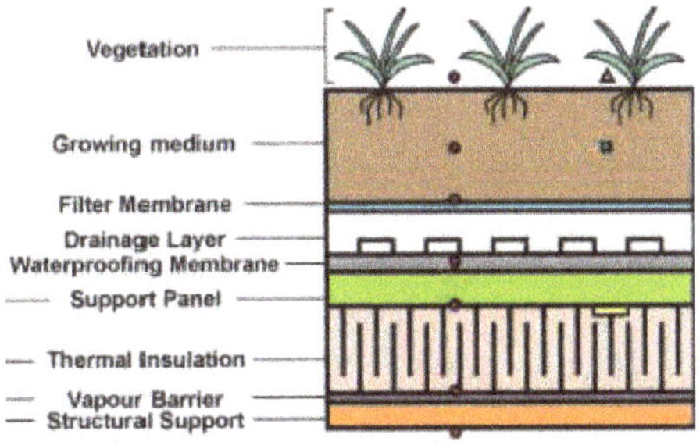

Figure 1. Typical cross-section of a green roof [31].

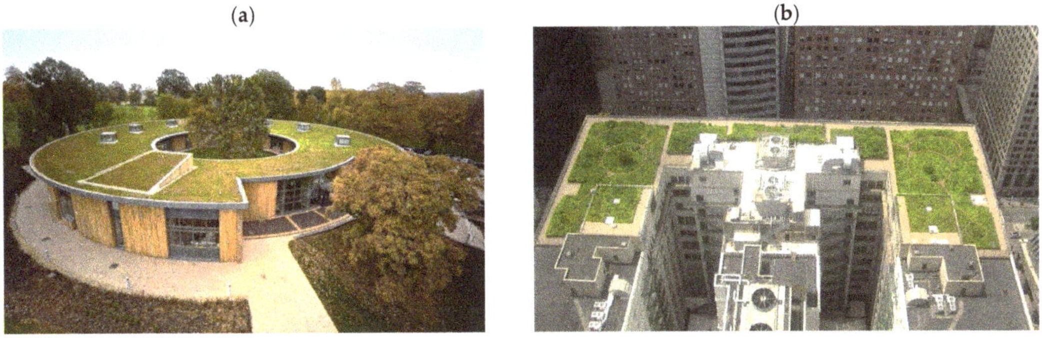

Figure 2. Examples of green roofs: (**a**) British Horse Society Headquarters, UK, and (**b**) Chicago City Hall, USA [31].

The high heat of the external air in the summer is transmitted into the building through the roof, which requires the use of a significant amount of energy to condition the building's interior [32]. Additionally, according to the laws of thermodynamics, in the winter, the internal heat of the building is lost and transferred into the cold external air surrounding the building [33,34]. Hence, energy consumption bills remain high irrespective of the weather [35,36]. Several studies have shown that green roofs can help reduce annual energy demand, which is either the demand for cooling in the summer or the demand for heating in the winter [10,37–40]. For instance, Jaffal et al. [40] pointed out that green roofs help to reduce the fluctuation amplitude of the roof slab temperature in the summer by 30 °C and decrease the summer indoor air temperature by 2 °C, in addition to reducing roof heat losses during the cold days in the winter and reducing the annual energy demand by 6%.

Green roofs have also appeared as an appropriate technique to fight the consequences of pollution, traffic, and lack of green spaces because of the numerous environmental problems facing today's society, particularly in urban areas [41]. Although the idea of green roofs is not new, as it was first used in Babylon and ancient Syria, it was not commonly used in modern cities until the beginning of the seventies of the last century [42]. It is considered one of the appropriate measures to increase the environmental resilience of cities that depend mainly on nature [43]. Several recent studies considered green roofs as one of the important aspects of mitigating the microclimate in urban areas. Berardi mentioned in his study that green roofs have positive effects both on the residents' thermal comfort, because it reduces the air temperature by 0.4 °C, and the building energy consumption, as it can also be reduced by 3% [44]. Moreover, the combination of greenery at the pedestrian level with green roofs can increase the advantage of the surrounding microclimate with an ambient temperature decline up to 2 °C, according to Alcazar et al. [45].

2. Literature Review

Numerous studies have explored the economic advantages arising from the application of the idea of green roofs. For instance, Wong et al. [46] compared the installation cost of green roof systems with traditional thermal and waterproofing roof treatments and found that the cost of a green roof system is lower considering the lifespan of the building. Other authors [47,48] concluded that the most effective benefit of green roof systems is energy saving, which results in an economical and sustainable environment inside and outside the building. Clark et al. [49] pointed out that the layers of green roofs protect the roof, which can increase the longevity of the roof from 20 to 40 years. Furthermore, green roofs can reduce exposure to sound inside and around the building [50] and, consequently, can increase the real estate value of the building from 6 to 15% [3]. In the sustainability context, Hegyi et al. [51] pointed out that green roofs successfully meet the principles of sustainable development. In a global context, there has been a growing interest in urban greenery in recent years, even in water-limited climatic regions [21]. As mentioned earlier, green roofs help in reducing energy consumption during hot climates, the energy consumption reduction values turned out to be between 6.5 and 17% for a case study in Guangzhou, China [52], a four-story representative building in Amman, Jordan [16], and a three-story building in Iran [53]. Another study in Madrid, conducted by Oberndorfer et al. [54], reported that green roofs could reduce the cooling requirement by 6% in the summer for an eight-story residential building. The study showed that the required cooling was reduced by 25%, 9%, 2%, and 1% for the first four floors, respectively, located just below the green roofs and was reduced by 10% for the entire building. Furthermore, green roofs have been recommended, required, and subsidized in several cities, including Tokyo, Stuttgart, Basel, Portland, and Toronto [12,18].

In many well-developed countries such as Singapore, the applications of green roofs in building construction are well established [13]. The first major green roof installed in Singapore was on the existing roof of a multistory car park. The project, sponsored by the Housing Development Board, was meant to encourage the application of green roofs in the country, in which the results showed that the installed green roof had to decrease the visible radiation significantly recorded on the facades of the residential area. Australia is also one of the developed countries that have adopted green roof implementation. Alexandri and Jones [55] reported that most major cities in Australia have hot and dry summers, which is very suitable for developing green roofs, as it will reduce the temperatures of these cities and reduce energy consumption as well. However, on the other hand, most developing countries are still exposed to many issues related to land constraints, which lead to increased competition for land between green areas and infrastructure developments [13]. Therefore, currently, there is interest in the subject of green roofs, and this interest is evident through associations, conferences, and competitions all over the world [12].

In the Kingdom of Saudi Arabia (KSA), most of the buildings use reinforced concrete on their roofs, which is not suitable for the air temperature in the region that reaches 50 °C, as it is considered a structural element with a high thermal conductivity coefficient. Therefore, it was found that 70% of the total electricity consumption in buildings in KSA is to meet the demand for air conditioning [10]. Several other studies [56–60] emphasized the need to review the requirements for the design and construction of the building roofs in KSA in terms of thermal conductivity and to identify the modifications and structural specifications necessary to improve its efficiency, especially concrete ones, whether it was according to the traditional methods using steel rebar, or it is strengthened according to modern methods using steel fiber reinforced concrete or nonmetallic fiber reinforced concrete. One of the environmentally preferred options is to convert traditional roof designs into green roofs that comply with the country's approved thermal conductivity standards and are compatible with the atmosphere of the region, with attention to the impact of that on the mechanical properties of the reinforced concrete or the plain concrete [10].

Although some nongovernmental or official bodies have called for the need to implement strategies that promote the creation of sustainable and resilient cities such as green roof systems, especially in residential buildings that represent the largest sector, there is still a significant delay in this field compared to other countries. Recently, the Saudi construction sector in general, and the residential sector, in particular, have witnessed steady and remarkable growth [61]. The residential sector is growing in parallel to the steady increase in the population, which has been proposed to be around 2.5% per year [62,63]. As a result of the region's climate, the residential sector in KSA consumes high levels of energy to meet the high demand for cooling and heating, which results in high rates of CO_2 emission [60]. According to Asif [64], nearly 50% of the total national energy generation is consumed by residential buildings alone. This can be attributed to the energy cost in KSA, which is relatively cheap when compared to other parts of the world due to its rich oil and gas reserves and government subsidies [61,65].

However, the situation has changed swiftly over the past few years, especially after the surfacing of the Saudi Vision 2030, approved by the Saudi Council of Ministers in 2016. The vision encompasses three major themes: a vibrant society, a thriving economy, and an ambitious nation. The energy conservation strategies are part of the first theme [64]. The vision has adopted many programs, initiatives, and construction projects that enhance the efforts to achieve the desired goals, and there were targets to remove about USD $53 billion of energy subsidies by 2020 [61,66]. KSA is now keen to reduce the increasing demand from the building sector, especially the residential sector, through the use of sustainable and energy-efficient strategies [61,65]. The concept of green roofs can be promoted as one of the options for energy saving in KSA through which energy consumption can be beneficially managed, along with the adoption of educational programs, to enhance people's perception and attitudes toward this option.

People's perception can be viewed as how people interpret, distinguish, critique, and analyze their environments according to their core values of adaptation to those environments [67]. People's expectations and preferences regarding green roof technology are very important especially for planners and designers when designing support systems for this type of technology or when setting up mandatory planning permissions [21]. Previous studies on people's perception of green roof technologies in urban areas have shown that it is highly correlated with people's socioeconomic factors, such as the level of income [68]. There are also some studies [69,70] that indicate that people's perception of the idea of green roofs in urban areas is related to the extent of knowledge about the system. However, this study hypothesizes that there are differences in the perception of green roof technologies and systems among different members of society due to other reasons, which the study seeks to discover.

The green roofs technique is relatively new in KSA, and it is believed that there is a lack of studies that shed light on the different aspects of this technique. Mahmoud et al. [61] pointed out that the green roofs technique is one of the sustainable building techniques that has not been appropriately explored and highlighted up to now. Therefore, the present study's target is to fill this research gap and build upon the literature. The present study aims to explore people's awareness of the green roof technique as a tool for urban sustainability and their willingness to adopt such a technique in KSA using Riyadh, the capital of KSA and the largest city, as a case study. Moreover, this study analyzes the relationship between demographic features and expectations of people concerning the contribution of green roofs to urban life quality and determines the benefits of such a technique. The first part of the study presents an overview of related concepts, such as green roofs, urban sustainability, and people's awareness, which will be discussed within the literature. This will be followed by describing the main methodology for data collection and analysis. Subsequently, the paper presents and discusses the main findings of the study and concludes with some recommendations for improvement and better planning.

3. Research Methodology

3.1. Study Area

The current study is focused on Riyadh, KSA. It is located in the eastern part of the central region, which lies in the middle of KSA, as shown in Figure 3. Riyadh is located between 34°38′ North and 46°43′ East [71]. The city is the capital of the country and is considered to be one of the fast-developing cities in the world [72].

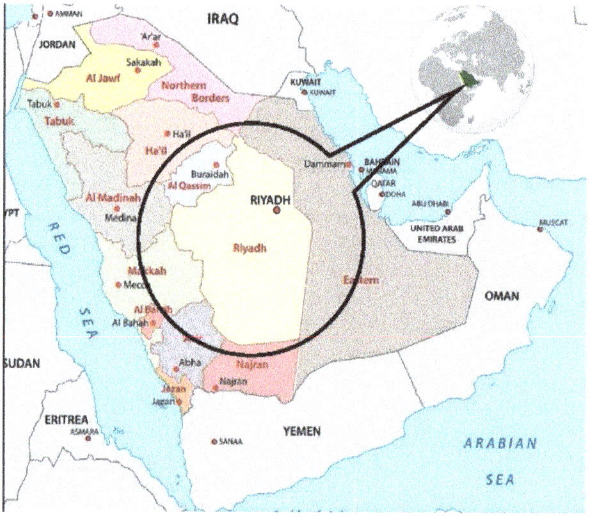

Figure 3. Location of Riyadh, Saudi Arabia, on a world map.

The population of Riyadh was estimated to be about 7.4 million in 2020, and it is expected to reach 10 million in the next few years, and they live in a total area of about 2435 km^2 [60]. Riyadh has an arid hot climate, where the average monthly temperature reaches 45 °C during the summer. This high temperature leads to high energy consumption for cooling indoor environments, which ultimately leads to high rates of carbon dioxide emissions, especially in residential buildings not only in Riyadh but in most major cities in the country.

In the past five decades, Riyadh has experienced significant demographic and physical growth and faced numerous issues in the process of urbanization. The rapid urban expansion of the city, in addition to the limited spaces in the built environment, led to a decrease in the percentage of green areas in Riyadh, which led to the emergence of many urban problems, including environmental and visual pollution, which, in turn, affected the rise in temperatures and the emergence of the so-called urban heat island phenomenon. Despite the presence of green spaces in Riyadh, represented by gardens and parks, it is relatively few compared to the size and expansion of the city, especially in light of the difficulty of creating additional spaces within the existing built environment. Therefore, due to the small amount of green space in Riyadh, as well as the lack and shortage of available land in the city and the issues of land use allocation, the development of green roofs is considered one of the important and useful approaches that can be adopted.

3.2. Methodology and Data Collection

This study aims to explore people's perceptions of the green roof technique as a tool for urban sustainability and their willingness to adopt such a technique in KSA using Riyadh as a case study; thus, the population interested in this study is Riyadh residents.

The questionnaire survey technique was employed for this study, which is considered to be one of the widely used methods for the collection of data, as already experienced by various researchers [73–75]. Alqahtany [60] indicated that the questionnaire survey is one of the useful tools for collecting data about people, their opinions, perceptions, and attitudes in a systematic way on a particular issue.

The basic data were collected by conducting a reconnaissance survey from the study site regarding the problems and challenges being faced by the residents related to green roofs and their applications. The residents included the general public who represent the domestic and commercial sectors of the area. The data included the list of problems being faced by the residents regarding green roofs. The shortlisted factors were obtained by comparing the response of the people recorded during the reconnaissance survey. The common factors found in both phases were considered to be the most important factors to be included in the online survey questionnaire.

The questionnaire was intended to be understandable for ordinary people and was designed around four key sections, including respondents' general social and demographic characteristics, characteristics of the respondents' houses, people's perceptions of the green roofs technique, and people's aspirations and willingness to adopt the technique. Open and closed-ended questions were designed for the questionnaire to achieve the required objectives. The survey was distributed randomly to the public coming from various walks of life. The respondents were given the opportunity of keeping their identity anonymous, and they were able to leave the survey at any time if they felt they could not answer any questions. Additionally, people had the opportunity to write additional responses that went beyond these predefined choices and expressed their opinions. The methodology followed for the study is shown in Figure 4.

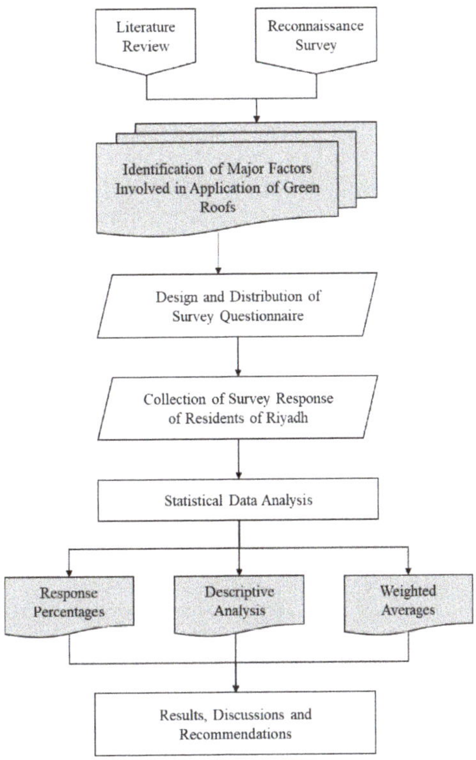

Figure 4. Research methodology followed for the study.

The survey questionnaire consisted of two types of questions. Both questions were based on a Likert scale, and the respondents were required to answer on a scale of 1 to 5 representing Strongly Disagree, Disagree, Do Not Know, Agree, and Strongly Agree, respectively, for Q-1, whereas 1 to 5 represented No Effect, Low Effect, Medium Effect, High Effect, and Very High Effect, respectively, for Q-2. The format of the online survey questionnaire is shown in Table 2.

Table 2. Survey questionnaire used for the study.

Sr. No.	Question	Scale				
		5	4	3	2	1
Q-1	**In your opinion what are the effects of adopting Green Roofs on the general environment of the building related to the following areas?**					
a	Increase in the Value of Building	○	○	○	○	○
b	Availability of Additional Space for Recreation and Amenities	○	○	○	○	○
c	Improvement in Aesthetic Features of Building	○	○	○	○	○
d	Reduction in Rainwater Runoff	○	○	○	○	○
e	Reduction in Electricity Bills	○	○	○	○	○
f	Reduction in Energy Consumption of Building	○	○	○	○	○
g	Enhancement of Ecology and Sustainability in Built Environment	○	○	○	○	○
h	Improvement of Air Quality and Reduction in Air & Noise Pollution	○	○	○	○	○
i	Positive Effect on City's Climate	○	○	○	○	○
Q-2	**To what extent do the following factors affect the application of green roof systems in buildings?**					
a	Safety and Security	○	○	○	○	○
b	Climate of the City	○	○	○	○	○
c	Irrigation System	○	○	○	○	○
d	System Weight	○	○	○	○	○
e	Maintenance	○	○	○	○	○
f	Installation Cost	○	○	○	○	○

For statistical analysis, the response mean and response standard deviation were calculated by using Equations (1) and (2), respectively [76].

$$\bar{x} = \frac{\Sigma x}{n} \quad (1)$$

$$\sigma = \sqrt{\frac{\Sigma(x-\bar{x})^2}{n-1}} \quad (2)$$

where x is the corresponding value provided by the respondent, and n is the total number of respondents for a specific question.

Moreover, the response percentage obtained for all questions was assessed separately, and the factor that received the highest number of selections was considered on highest priority. Along with this, the response to all questions was compared together as well, by using the method of weighted averages (WA). The following equation was used to calculate the WA of each factor.

$$A_w = \frac{\sum(R_i\, n)}{\sum R_i} \quad (3)$$

where A_w is the weighted average, R_i is the number of respondents for a specific level n of the Likert scale, and n ranges from 1 to 5.

4. Results and Discussions

A total of 380 people submitted their responses, which included people of all ages, gender, and professions living in Riyadh. The demographic data of the respondents, as shown in Figure 5, show that almost 65% of the respondents belong to the age group of 35–45 years, which is a young and experienced class of highly educated people who have a good understanding of the environmental sustainability and are well aware of advanced technologies and the effect of green roof buildings. More than 75% of the respondents are employed in various sectors, and almost 55% of them are earning USD 30,000 or more per annum.

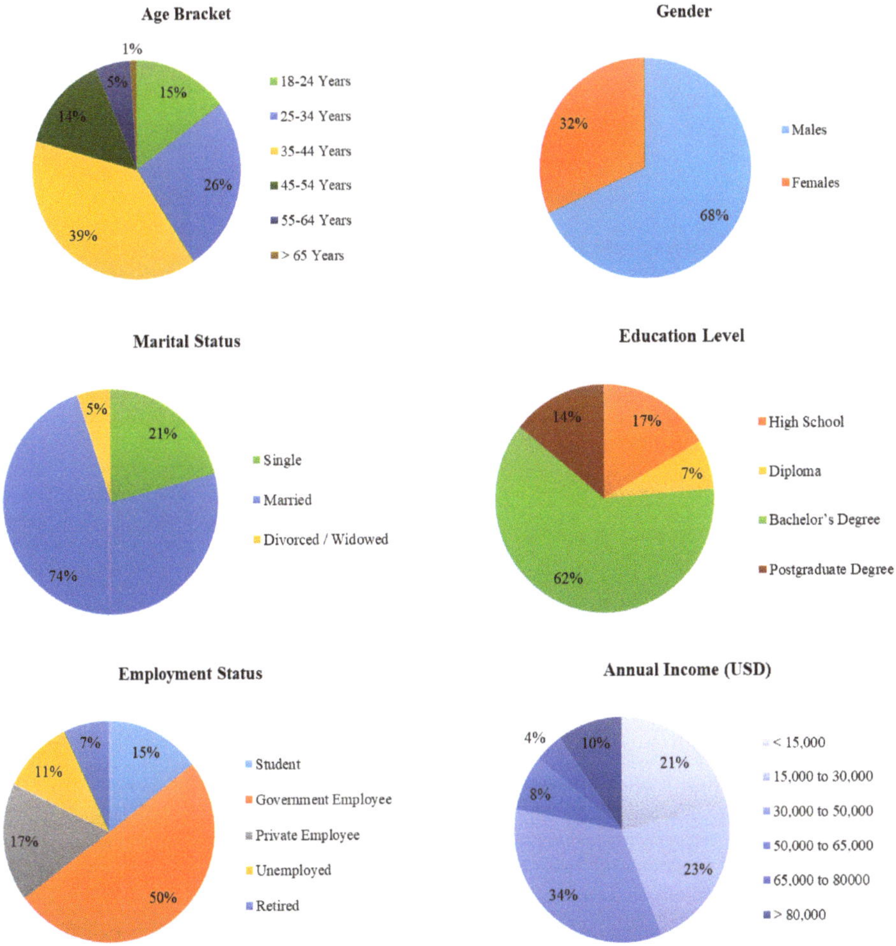

Figure 5. Demographic details of the respondents.

A few initial questions were designed to know the current status of residents regarding their living in Riyadh, as shown in Figure 6, and 73% of people were found to be living in comparatively bigger houses like villas or detached duplexes, while 64% of people disclosed that they own the property in which they are living. Regarding the size of the houses, 51% of people are having a house size of 250 to 500 sq. m., whereas 33% of the people living in a house having an area of more than 500 sq. m. These stats show that the respondents seem well settled and have a good standard of living and are well educated; hence, the acquired responses for Questions 1 and 2 are considered reliable and well justified.

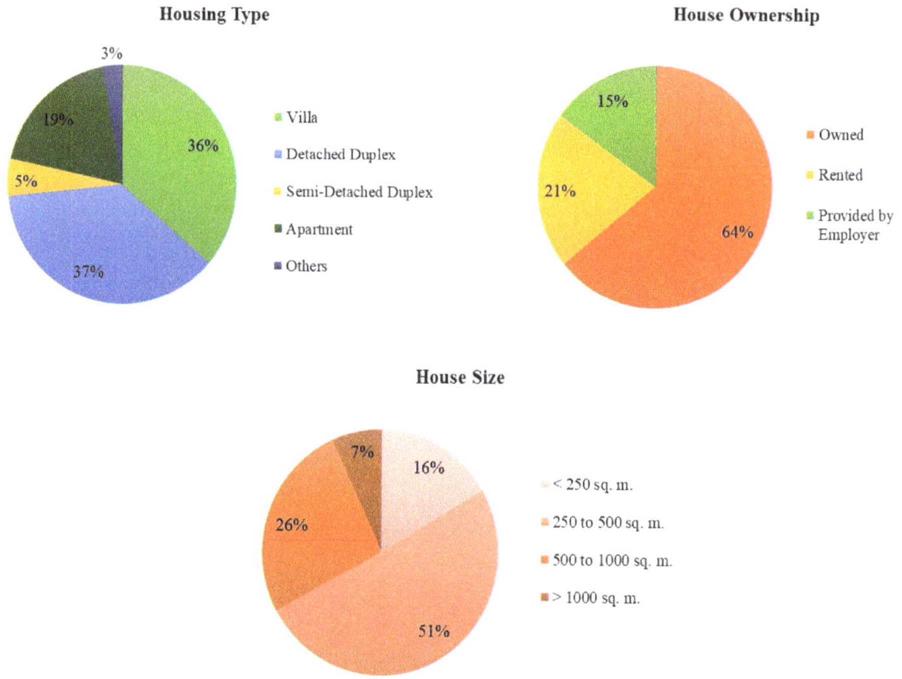

Figure 6. Existing housing stats of the respondents.

A descriptive statistical analysis was also performed for the demographic and existing housing stats of the respondents, as shown in Table 3. The values mentioned in the Response Mean column are the average of the Likert scale values opted by the respondents. For better clarification, the second column shows the interpreted average value of each parameter. The lower values of response standard deviations show that the responses are quite close to each other, which implies that the opinion of one resident does not deviate from the others to any larger extent.

The average values of the characteristics of the respondents in Table 3 show that the respondents are well mature, with an average age of 41 years, are well educated, and earn a good annual income. Additionally, the average number of respondents reside in duplex houses of suitable size. Hence, the data obtained from the sample of the population who completed the survey are eligible for further analysis.

Table 3. Descriptive statistical analysis results.

Parameter	Response Mean ($\bar{x}$)	Average Value	Response Standard Deviation (σ)
Age Bracket	2.72	41 Years	1.11
Education Level	2.74	Bachelor's Degree	0.9
Employment Status	2.45	Employed	1.08
Annual Income	2.79	USD 46,000	1.48
Housing Type	2.15	Detached Duplex	1.18
House Size	2.23	615 sq. m.	0.81

A brief discussion is presented on the response to the major questions of the survey. Question 1 was designed to get public opinion on the effects of adopting the concept of green roofs in the building. The overall study of the results obtained for Question 1 shows that people were excited and pleased with the concept. However, a significant trend can be seen in the results, shown in Figure 7, that the public is concerned with the aesthetics of the building enhanced by green roofs more than its technical benefits. The points related to the improvement in aesthetics of the building, availability of space for recreation, and improvement of air quality received more positive responses than any other options with a value of at least 94% of people agreeing to them. On the other hand, the points related to the technical aspects of the green roofs, including the increase in the value of the building, reduction in rainwater runoff, energy consumption, and electricity bills remained comparatively low opted points, with a value of almost 75% each. It is also necessary to mention that these points received a neutral response from almost 15–17% of people. The reason could be that 15% of people are less than 25 years of age, as they are students studying in high school and have not taken any technical studies yet, as shown in Figure 5, so this high percentage of neutral responses can be ignored, and the value of 75% is still considered reliable and comparative to all other options.

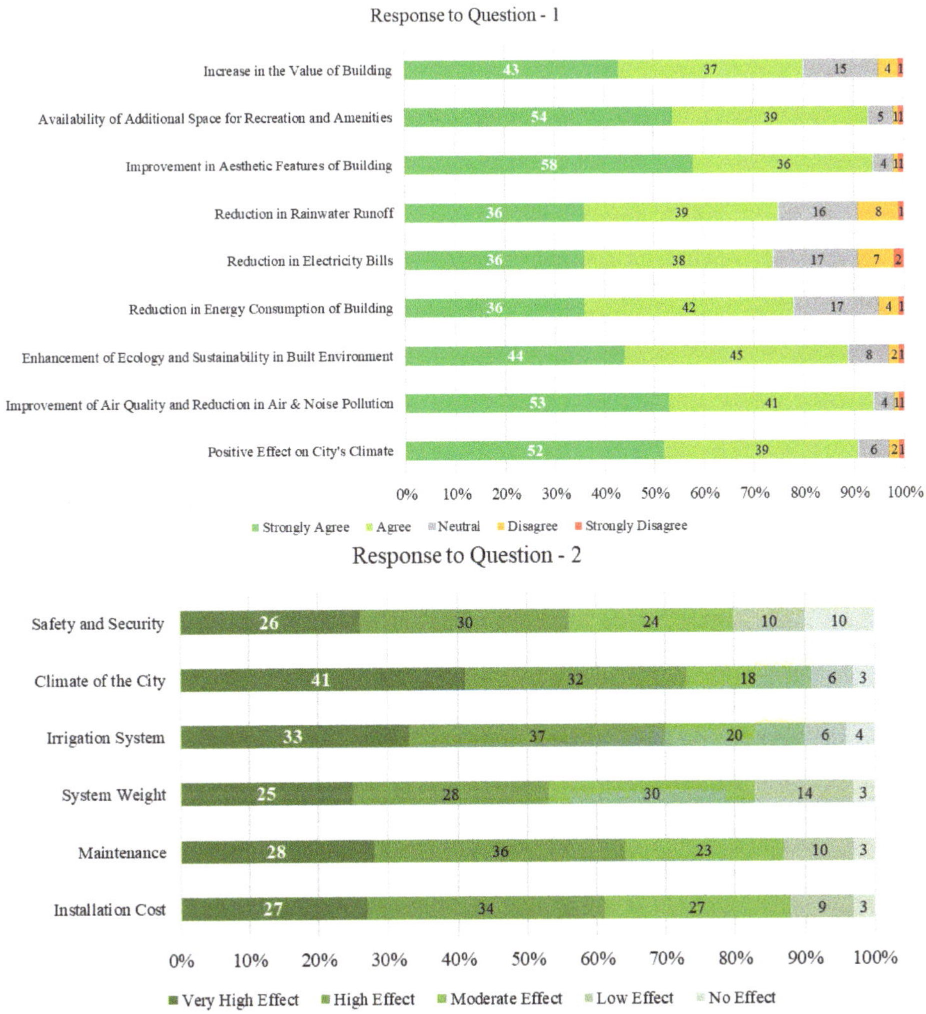

Figure 7. Response percentages for survey Questions 1 and 2.

Question 2 was designed to observe the public opinion on a few factors that they might take as a challenge in adopting the concept of green roofs in their houses. Almost 73% of people said that the climate of the city is the most challenging factor in Riyadh, as shown in Figure 7. As the city lies in an arid and hot climate zone, the environmental temperature genuinely affects various other factors related to it as well, including irrigation of green roofs and the selection of the type of grass and plants that can sustain the hot weather, including its maintenance. These both points stand second and third in the list with 70% and 64%, respectively. People are least concerned with the weight of the green roof system on the structural elements of the buildings. Only 53% of people showed this concern.

For a better comparison, the responses obtained for Questions 1 and 2 were converted to weighted average (WA) by using Equation (3) to obtain one of the listed factors having the maximum influence as per the public opinion, as shown in Figure 8. It can be seen that the WA for a few of the options is peaking as compared to others.

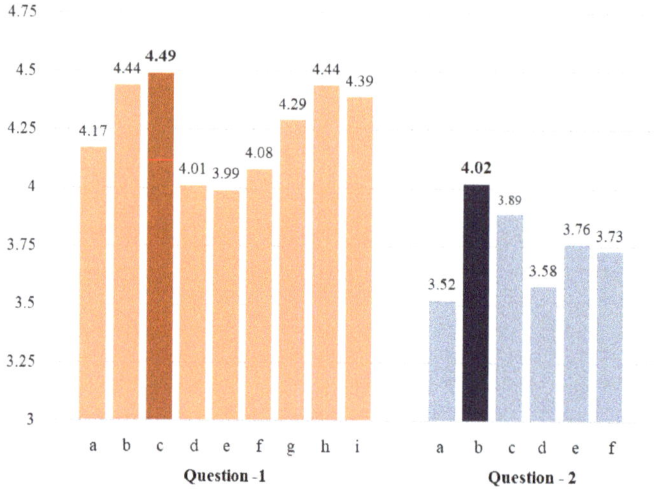

Figure 8. Weighted averages for responses on Questions 1 and 2.

These options having the highest WA were rated the highest priority by the respondents. The highest strength of response was found for Q-1(c) with a WA value of 4.49, where people agreed to the fact that green roofs increase the aesthetics of the building. As the second priority, people selected green roofs to provide additional space for recreation, and it also helps in decreasing air and noise pollution with a WA of 4.44. Figure 8 shows a peak WA value of 4.02 for Q-2(b) as well, where people consider the climate of the region as the biggest challenge in adopting green roofs.

At the end of the survey, two very direct but important supplementary questions were asked of the respondents. The first one was to get their willingness in installing green roofs on their houses, and the second was related to their opinion regarding recommending someone to install this system on their building. A very interesting response was obtained for these questions, as shown in Figure 9. Despite knowing all the benefits and positives of green roofs, people are hesitant to adopt this system in their homes as yet. Although the majority of the respondents are willing to adopt this system and were positive in recommending others to adopt it too, there is a significant number of people who are still confused and have opted for the third option of Do Not Know. The percentage of people who agreed to recommend green roofs to others was 61%, which is higher than the percentage of people who were willing to apply this system in their houses, which stands at 50%. This is completely understandable and shows that the people are aware of the benefits of such systems, but their financial liabilities are high and prevent them from applying it for themselves at their homes. Moreover, it was observed that many existing buildings have mechanical equipment fixed on the roofs, including outdoor units of split air conditioners, chillers, water pumps, and water tanks, which the owners think would be a huge task to relocate. This is counted as another reason for the comparatively low willingness level of owners to install green roofs at their existing buildings.

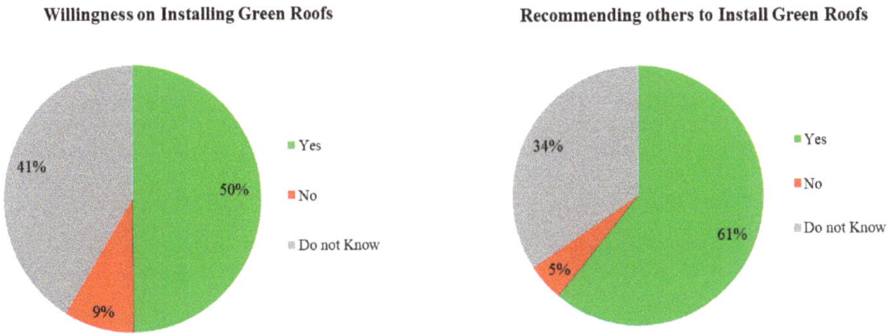

Figure 9. Response to supplementary questions.

5. Research Extension and Future Considerations

The study mentioned in this research article is completely extendable, and a lot more options can be included in future research of a similar kind. It was seen during the results and analysis phase that, although a good amount of people were highly educated who submitted their responses, there is an opportunity of including people with low education levels who own big houses or commercial properties in future research. More female respondents can also be targeted, or there may be separate analyses for male and female respondents, and research presenting analytical comparisons of the responses based on gender can be produced. The current research would help future researchers prepare a complex survey questionnaire for further study. Moreover, the current results are based on 380 responses, the target of minimum responses could be set to at least 600 responses for future works. Increasing the sample size would produce many reliable results.

6. Conclusions and Recommendations

In this study, an extensive literature review followed by a survey analysis was performed to explore the idea of implementing green roofs and the relevant challenges being faced by the general public. Based on the literature, the study found that the green roofs technique is a practical means of expanding the amount of vegetation in urban areas, and it has become a well-known approach in sustainable urban development approaches in recent decades. In this study, it is believed that green roofs can provide a lot of advantages, for instance, the mitigation of urban air and noise pollution, increase in air quality, reduction of the urban heat island effect in cities, reduction of building energy consumption, reduction of stormwater runoff, an increase of biodiversity and habitats, and provision of more spaces for amenity and recreation.

The public response received through the survey was a mix of different opinions. Clearly, the majority of the population of Riyadh understands the benefits related to green roofs, and they have shown a positive response to a few factors. Almost 94% of people agreed with the fact that green roofs enhance the aesthetics of the building, and the same number of people agreed that they play a role in controlling the air quality. Similarly, 93% of people that green roofs provide additional recreational space in the building. On the other hand, 91% of the respondents identified the climate of the area as the biggest challenge in implementing green roofs in the buildings. However, despite knowing the benefits, a good number of people are still hesitant in installing such systems in their houses with 41% of people who are still not sure if they should go for green roofs on their buildings or not. This is because there is still not much awareness in the general public and there is no applied example in the area as yet.

Based on the results, it is recommended that the local authorities must initiate strong campaigns in favor of such technologies at least for the new buildings or the buildings under construction. They must educate people about the benefits these green roofs can provide. In addition to this, the authorities must facilitate the residents and house owners in designing, executing, and installing such systems. With their help, the process shall progress quickly.

The study strongly believes that, in Riyadh and KSA in general, the possibilities of adopting the concept of green roofs are increasing, as there is awareness of the sustainable built environment and urban sustainability in general, especially in light of the Saudi Vision 2030. A little interest from the local authorities is required to provide it with a wider reach.

Funding: This research received no external funding.

Data Availability Statement: The datasets generated and analyzed during the research are included in the article and additional data is available for uploading to a repository on demand.

Conflicts of Interest: The author declares no conflict of interest.

References

1. Liberalesso, T.; Mutevuie, R.; Cruz, C.O.; Silva, C.M.; Manso, M. Users' Perceptions of Green Roofs and Green Walls: An Analysis of Youth Hostels in Lisbon, Portugal. *Sustainability* **2020**, *12*, 10136. [CrossRef]
2. Teotónio, I.; Silva, C.M.; Cruz, C.O. Eco-solutions for urban environments regeneration: The economic value of green roofs. *J. Clean. Prod.* **2018**, *199*, 121–135. [CrossRef]
3. Rosasco, P.; Perini, K. Selection of (Green) Roof Systems: A Sustainability-Based Multi-Criteria Analysis. *Buildings* **2019**, *9*, 134. [CrossRef]
4. Zhang, S.; Ramírez, F.M. Assessing and mapping ecosystem services to support urban green infrastructure: The case of Barcelona, Spain. *Cities* **2019**, *92*, 59–70. [CrossRef]
5. Dwivedi, A.; Mohan, B.K. Impact of green roof on micro climate to reduce Urban Heat Island. *Remote. Sens. Appl. Soc. Environ.* **2018**, *10*, 56–69. [CrossRef]
6. Herath, H.; Halwatura, R.; Jayasinghe, G. Modeling a Tropical Urban Context with Green Walls and Green Roofs as an Urban Heat Island Adaptation Strategy. *Procedia Eng.* **2018**, *212*, 691–698. [CrossRef]
7. Abdo, P.; Huynh, B.P.; Irga, P.J.; Torpy, F.R. Evaluation of airflow through an active green wall biofilter. *Urban For. Urban Green.* **2019**, *41*, 75–84. [CrossRef]
8. Perini, K.; Rosasco, P. Cost-benefit analysis for green façades and living wall systems. *Build. Environ.* **2013**, *70*, 110–121. [CrossRef]
9. Kumar, P.; Druckman, A.; Gallagher, J.; Gatersleben, B.; Allison, S.; Eisenman, T.S.; Hoang, U.; Hama, S.; Tiwari, A.; Sharma, A.; et al. The nexus between air pollution, green infrastructure and human health. *Environ. Int.* **2019**, *133*, 105181. [CrossRef]
10. Khabaz, A. Construction and design requirements of green buildings' roofs in Saudi Arabia depending on thermal conductivity principle. *Constr. Build. Mater.* **2018**, *186*, 1119–1131. [CrossRef]
11. Cristiano, E.; Deidda, R.; Viola, F. The role of green roofs in urban Water-Energy-Food-Ecosystem nexus: A review. *Sci. Total Environ.* **2021**, *756*, 143876. [CrossRef] [PubMed]
12. Berardi, U.; GhaffarianHoseini, A. State-of-the-art analysis of the environmental benefits of green roofs. *Appl. Energy* **2014**, *115*, 411–428. [CrossRef]
13. Chow, M.F.; Bakar, M.F.A. Environmental Benefits of Green Roof to the Sustainable Urban Development: A Review. In Proceedings of the 1st Global Civil Engineering Conference—GCEC17, Kuala Lumpur, Malaysia, 25–28 July 2017; Universiti Tenaga Nasional: Selangor, Malaysia, 2018; pp. 1525–1541.
14. Shafique, M.; Kim, R.; Rafiq, M. Green roof benefits, opportunities and challenges—A review. *Renew. Sustain. Energy Rev.* **2018**, *90*, 757–773. [CrossRef]
15. Chow, M.F.; Bakar, M.F.A. A Review on the Development and Challenges of Green Roof Systems in Malaysia. *Int. J. Archit. Environ. Eng.* **2016**, *10*, 16–20.
16. Goussous, J.; Siam, H.; Alzoubi, H. Prospects of green roof technology for energy and thermal benefits in buildings: Case of Jordan. *Sustain. Cities Soc.* **2015**, *14*, 425–440. [CrossRef]
17. Cavanaugh, L.M. Redefining the green roof. *J. Archit. Eng.* **2008**, *14*, 4–6. [CrossRef]
18. Vijayaraghavan, K. Green roofs: A critical review on the role of components, benefits, limitations and trends. *Renew. Sustain. Energy Rev.* **2016**, *57*, 740–752. [CrossRef]
19. Francis, L.F.M.; Jensen, M.B. Benefits of green roofs: A systematic review of the evidence for three ecosystem services. *Urban For. Urban Green.* **2017**, *28*, 167–176. [CrossRef]
20. Dunnett, N.; Kingsbury, N. *Planting Green Roofs and Living Walls*; Timber Press: Portland, OR, USA, 2008.

21. Fernández-Cañero, R.; Emilsson, T.; Fernandez-Barba, C.; Machuca, M.Á.H. Green roof systems: A study of public attitudes and preferences in southern Spain. *J. Environ. Manag.* **2013**, *128*, 106–115. [CrossRef]
22. Currie, B.A.; Bass, B. Estimates of air pollution mitigation with green plants and green roofs using the UFORE model. *Urban Ecosyst.* **2008**, *11*, 409–422. [CrossRef]
23. Schmidt, M. The evapotranspiration of greened roofs and façades. In Proceedings of the 4th North American Green Roof Conference: Greening Rooftops for Sustainable Communities, Boston, MA, USA, 11–12 May 2006; pp. 1–10.
24. Ip, K.; Lam, M.; Miller, A. Shading performance of a vertical deciduous climbing plant canopy. *Build. Environ.* **2010**, *45*, 81–88. [CrossRef]
25. Kontoleon, K.; Eumorfopoulou, E. The effect of the orientation and proportion of a plant-covered wall layer on the thermal performance of a building zone. *Build. Environ.* **2010**, *45*, 1287–1303. [CrossRef]
26. Wong, N.H.; Tan, A.Y.K.; Chen, Y.; Sekar, K.; Tan, P.Y.; Chan, D.; Chiang, K.; Wong, N.C. Thermal evaluation of vertical greenery systems for building walls. *Build. Environ.* **2010**, *45*, 663–672. [CrossRef]
27. Bengtsson, L.; Grahn, L.; Olsson, J. Hydrological function of a thin extensive green roof in southern Sweden. *Water Policy* **2005**, *36*, 259–268. [CrossRef]
28. Stovin, V. The potential of green roofs to manage Urban Stormwater. *Water Environ. J.* **2010**, *24*, 192–199. [CrossRef]
29. Fernández Cañero, R.; González Redondo, P. Green roofs as a habitat for birds: A review. *J. Anim. Vet. Adv.* **2010**, *9*, 2041–2052.
30. Francis, R.A.; Lorimer, J. Urban reconciliation ecology: The potential of living roofs and walls. *J. Environ. Manag.* **2011**, *92*, 1429–1437. [CrossRef]
31. Wikipedia, Green Roof. 2022. Available online: https://en.wikipedia.org/wiki/Green_roof (accessed on 20 November 2022).
32. Del Barrio, E.P. Analysis of the green roofs cooling potential in buildings. *Energy Build.* **1998**, *27*, 179–193. [CrossRef]
33. Liu, K.; Minor, J. Performance evaluation of an extensive green roof. In Proceedings of the 3rd North American Green Roof Conference: Greening Rooftops for Sustainable Communities, Washington, DC, USA, 4–6 May 2005; pp. 1–11.
34. Rakotondramiarana, H.T.; Ranaivoarisoa, T.F.; Morau, D. Dynamic Simulation of the Green Roofs Impact on Building Energy Performance, Case Study of Antananarivo, Madagascar. *Buildings* **2015**, *5*, 497–520. [CrossRef]
35. Getter, K.L.; Rowe, D.B.; Andresen, J.A.; Wichman, I.S. Seasonal heat flux properties of an extensive green roof in a Midwestern U.S. climate. *Energy Build.* **2011**, *43*, 3548–3557. [CrossRef]
36. Ma, X.; Liu, G.; Luo, Z.; Tan, Y.; Lei, J. Comprehensive Evaluation of Energy and Environmental Performances of an Extensive Green Roof of a Building in Subtropical Climate. *J. Arch. Eng. Technol.* **2017**, *6*, 192. [CrossRef]
37. Niachou, A.; Papakonstantinou, K.; Santamouris, M.; Tsangrassoulis, A.; Mihalakakou, G. Analysis of the green roof thermal properties and investigation of its energy performance. *Energy Build.* **2001**, *33*, 719–729. [CrossRef]
38. Santamouris, M.; Pavlou, C.; Doukas, P.; Mihalakakou, G.; Synnefa, A.; Hatzibiros, A.; Patargias, P. Investigating and analysing the energy and environmental performance of an experimental green roof system installed in a nursery school building in Athens, Greece. *Energy* **2007**, *32*, 1781–1788. [CrossRef]
39. Spala, A.; Bagiorgas, H.; Assimakopoulos, M.; Kalavrouziotis, J.; Matthopoulos, D.; Mihalakakou, G. On the green roof system. Selection, state of the art and energy potential investigation of a system installed in an office building in Athens, Greece. *Renew. Energy* **2008**, *33*, 173–177. [CrossRef]
40. Jaffal, I.; Ouldboukhitine, S.-E.; Belarbi, R. A comprehensive study of the impact of green roofs on building energy performance. *Renew. Energy* **2012**, *43*, 157–164. [CrossRef]
41. Velázquez, J.; Anza, P.; Gutiérrez, J.; Sánchez, B.; Hernando, A.; García-Abril, A. Planning and selection of green roofs in large urban areas. *Appl. Madr. Metrop. Area Urban For. Urban Green.* **2019**, *40*, 323–334. [CrossRef]
42. Getter, K.L.; Rowe, D.B. The Role of Extensive Green Roofs in Sustainable Development. *Hortscience* **2006**, *41*, 1276–1285. [CrossRef]
43. Ziogou, I.; Michopoulos, A.; Voulgari, V.; Zachariadis, T. Implementation of green roof technology in residential buildings and neighborhoods of Cyprus. *Sustain. Cities Soc.* **2018**, *40*, 233–243. [CrossRef]
44. Berardi, U. The outdoor microclimate benefits and energy saving resulting from green roofs retrofits. *Energy Build.* **2016**, *121*, 217–229. [CrossRef]
45. Alcazar, S.S.; Olivieri, F.; Neila, J. Green roofs: Experimental and analytical study of its potential for urban microclimate regulation in Mediterranean–continental climates. *Urban Clim.* **2016**, *17*, 304–317. [CrossRef]
46. Wong, N.H.; Tay, S.F.; Wong, R.; Ong, C.L.; Sia, A. Life cycle cost analysis of rooftop gardens in Singapore. *Build. Environ.* **2003**, *38*, 499–509. [CrossRef]
47. Perini, K.; Rosasco, P. Is greening the building envelope economically sustainable? An analysis to evaluate the advantages of economy of scope of vertical greening systems and green roofs. *Urban For. Urban Green.* **2016**, *20*, 328–337. [CrossRef]
48. Coma, J.; Perez, G.; Cabeza, L.F. Green roofs to enhance the thermal performance of buildings and outdoor comfort. In *Nature Based Strategies for Urban and Building Sustainability*; Butterworth-Heinemann: Oxford, UK, 2018; Chapter 3.2; pp. 109–117.
49. Clark, C.; Talbot, B.; Bulkley, J.; Adiaens, P. Optimization of green roofs for air pollution mitigation. In Proceedings of the 3rd North American Green Roof Conference: Greening Rooftops for Sustainable Communities, Washington, DC, USA, 4–6 May 2005; pp. 482–597.
50. Van Renterghem, T. Green roofs for acoustic insulation and noise reduction. In *Nature Based Strategies for Urban and Building Sustainability*; Butterworth-Heinemann: Oxford, UK, 2018; Chapter 3.8; pp. 167–179.

51. Hegyi, A.; Călătan, G.; Dico, C. The Green Roof-Partner In Sustainable Urban Development. In Proceedings of the 17th International Multidisciplinary Scientific GeoConference SGEM2017, Albena, Bulgaria, 29 June–5 July 2017; Volume 17, pp. 433–440.
52. Yang, W.; Wang, Z.; Cui, J.; Zhu, Z.; Zhao, X. Comparative study of the thermal performance of the novel green (planting) roofs against other existing roofs. *Sustain. Cities Soc.* **2015**, *16*, 1–12. [CrossRef]
53. Refahi, A.H.; Talkhabi, H. Investigating the effective factors on the reduction of energy consumption in residential buildings with green roofs. *Renew. Energy* **2015**, *80*, 595–603. [CrossRef]
54. Oberndorfer, E.; Lundholm, J.; Bass, B.; Coffman, R.R.; Doshi, H.; Dunnett, N.; Gaffin, S.; Köhler, M.; Liu, K.K.Y.; Rowe, B. Green Roofs as Urban Ecosystems: Ecological Structures, Functions, and Services. *Bioscience* **2007**, *57*, 823–833. [CrossRef]
55. Alexandri, E.; Jones, P. Temperature decreases in an urban canyon due to green walls and green roofs in diverse climates. *Build. Environ.* **2008**, *43*, 480–493. [CrossRef]
56. Alaidroos, A.; Krarti, M. Optimal design of residential building envelope systems in the Kingdom of Saudi Arabia. *Energy Build.* **2015**, *86*, 104–117. [CrossRef]
57. Taleb, H.M.; Sharples, S. Developing sustainable residential buildings in Saudi Arabia: A case study. *Appl. Energy* **2011**, *88*, 383–391. [CrossRef]
58. Khabaz, A. Determination of Friction Coefficient between Glass Fiber and the Concrete Fri (GF.C). *Int. J. Mater. Sci. Appl.* **2014**, *3*, 321. [CrossRef]
59. Khabaz, A. Analysis of sliding mechanism of straight steel fibers in concrete and determine the effect of friction. *Arch. Civ. Mech. Eng.* **2017**, *17*, 599–608. [CrossRef]
60. AlQahtany, A. People's perceptions of sustainable housing in developing countries: The case of Riyadh, Saudi Arabia. *Hous. Care Support* **2020**, *23*, 93–109. [CrossRef]
61. Mahmoud, A.S.; Asif, M.; Hassanain, M.A.; Babsail, M.O.; Sanni-Anibire, M.O. Energy and Economic Evaluation of Green Roofs for Residential Buildings in Hot-Humid Climates. *Buildings* **2017**, *7*, 30. [CrossRef]
62. Shaawat, M.E.; Jamil, R.; Al-Enezi, M.M. Analysis of Challenges in Sustainable Construction Industry by Using Analytic Hierarchy Process: A Case Study of Jubail Industrial City, Saudi Arabia. *Int. J. Sustain. Real Estate Constr. Econ.* **2018**, *1*, 109–122.
63. Alqahtany, A.; Jamil, R. Evaluation of Educational Strategies in the Design Process of Infrastructure for a Healthy Sustainable Housing Community. *Ain Shams Eng. J.* **2022**, *13*, 101665. [CrossRef]
64. Asif, M. Growth and sustainability trends in the buildings sector in the GCC region with particular reference to the KSA and UAE. *Renew. Sustain. Energy Rev.* **2016**, *55*, 1267–1273. [CrossRef]
65. Khan, H.S.; Asif, M. Impact of Green Roof and Orientation on the Energy Performance of Buildings: A Case Study from Saudi Arabia. *Sustainability* **2017**, *9*, 640. [CrossRef]
66. AlQahtany, A.M. Government regulation and financial support on housing delivery: Lessons learned from the Saudi experience. *Int. J. Hous. Mark. Anal.* **2021**, *15*, 613–631. [CrossRef]
67. Haksever, T.S.; Markoc, I. Social Perception of the Green Roofs in Contribution to Urban Sustainability: Istanbul. *Dev. Ctry. Stud.* **2020**, *10*, 74–81.
68. CJim, Y.; Chen, W.Y. Recreation–amenity use and contingent valuation of urban green spaces in Guangzhou, China. *Landsc. Urban Plan.* **2006**, *75*, 81–96.
69. Özgüner, H.; Kendle, A. Public attitudes towards naturalistic versus designed landscapes in the city of Sheffield (UK). *Landsc. Urban Plan.* **2006**, *74*, 139–157. [CrossRef]
70. Forbes, S.; Kendle, T. *Urban Nature Conservation: Landscape Management in the Urban Countryside*; Taylor & Francis: London, UK, 2013; ISBN 978-020-385-70-21.
71. MMRA; UNHSP. Riyadh City Profile, Ministry of Municipal and Rural Affairs and United Nations Human Settlements Program (UN-Habitat). 2019. Available online: https://unhabitat.org/sites/default/files/2020/03/riyadh.pdf (accessed on 15 November 2022).
72. Ali, A.; Yacine, R.; Haijiang, L. A Consensus-Based Framework for the Sustainable Urban Planning Development: As an Approach for Saudi Arabian Cities. *Int. J. Environ. Sci. Dev.* **2014**, *5*, 124–131.
73. Saunders, M.; Lewis, P.; Thornhill, A. *Research Methods for Business Students*, 7th ed.; Pearson Education: Harlow, UK, 2016; ISBN 9780273716860.
74. Dillman, D. *Mail and Internet Surveys: The Tailored Design Method*; John Wiley & Sons: Hoboken, NJ, USA, 2011.
75. Sekaran, U. *Research Methods for Business: A Skill-Building Approach*; Wiley: Chichester, UK, 2016; ISBN 978-111-994-22-52.
76. Bluman, A. *Elementary Statistics—A Step by Step Approach*; McGraw-Hill Education: New York, NY, USA, 2014; ISBN 978-007-353-49-85.

buildings

MDPI

Article

Post-Occupancy Evaluation of Sports Parks during the COVID-19 Pandemic: Taking Sports Parks in Beijing as Examples

Xianfeng Wu and Xiangyu Li *

Faculty of Architecture, Civil, and Transportation Engineering, Beijing University of Technology, No. 100 Pingle Yuan, Chaoyang District, Beijing 100124, China
* Correspondence: lixiangyu@bjut.edu.cn

Abstract: China fully built a wealthy society but faced a serious COVID-19 epidemic together with the rest of the world. The emergence of the epidemic highlights the importance of sports parks for physical activity. By reviewing national fitness policies and identifying several types of sports parks, this paper investigates urban dwellers' usage and preferences in sports parks by means of a questionnaire, with behavioural observation and interviews as complementary research methods. Taking the Beijing Olympic Forest Park, Sun Park, and Huilongguan Park as examples, this study reveals that participants present a high overall satisfaction with the sports parks. The factor analysis indicates that Sports Facilities and Maintenance & Management are the first and second most significant factors influencing residents' willingness to use sports parks. This research can guide the planning and construction of sports park in the future.

Keywords: post-occupancy evaluation; semantic differential method; sports parks

Citation: Wu, X.; Li, X. Post-Occupancy Evaluation of Sports Parks during the COVID-19 Pandemic: Taking Sports Parks in Beijing as Examples. *Buildings* **2022**, *12*, 2250. https://doi.org/10.3390/buildings12122250

Academic Editors: Liyin Shen, Jorge Ochoa, Haijun Bao and Nikos A. Salingaros

Received: 28 November 2022
Accepted: 14 December 2022
Published: 16 December 2022

1. Introduction

1.1. National Fitness Policies in China

Promoting the construction of a healthy China is the foundation for truly building a wealthy society and realizing socialist modernization. It is also a national strategy to improve the health of the Chinese nation and achieve coordinated development of people's health and the social economy. China also presents a vision for how it can participate actively in global health management and fulfill its international commitments in the 2030 Agenda for Sustainable Development [1]. With the influence of the Olympic spirit and advocacy for the national fitness movement, people have become more concerned about physical activity. The pursuit of personal physical and mental health and well-being has become a popular new value in relation to sports. Therefore, promoting the concept of a healthy lifestyle has brought about increased participation in fitness and exercise and has inspired many sports enthusiasts [2,3]. With the launch and implementation of a series of national fitness policies (see Table 1), the number of people who regularly participate in sports and exercise, the area of sports venues per capita, and the total scale of the national sports industry have all increased significantly (see Figure 1). With policy encouragement and continued capital investment, mass sports centres, sports parks, and other sports-related facilities were constructed for physical activity as well as for urban leisure lifestyles, which are of strategic importance for the quality of life in our increasingly urbanized society [4].

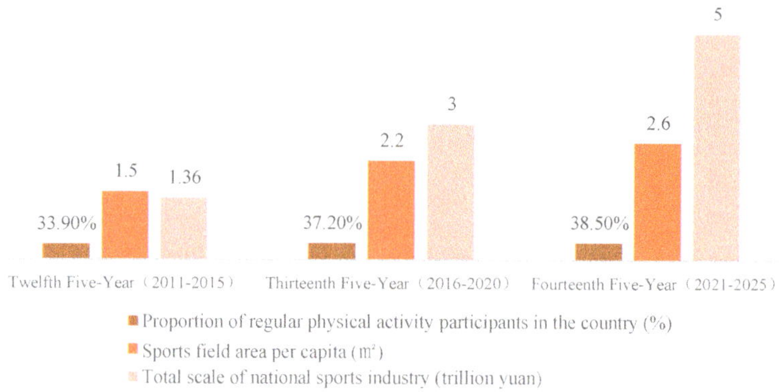

Figure 1. Summary of the development of national fitness and trends in China.

Table 1. Summary of key National Fitness policies in China.

Report	Issue Department	Issue Number	Release Date
The National Fitness Program (2021–2025) [5]	China's State Council	[2021] No.11	3 August 2021
The implementation plan for the national fitness facilities to supplement the shortcomings during the 14th Five-Year Plan period [6]	National Development and Reform Commission	[2021] No. 555	20 April 2021
Opinions on Strengthening the Construction of National Fitness Venues and Facilities to Develop Mass Sports [7]	China's State Council	[2020] No. 36	10 October 2020
Opinions on promoting national fitness and sports consumption and promoting the high-quality development of the sports industry [8]	China's State Council	[2019] No.43	17 September 2019
Health China Action Task (2019–2030) [9]	Health China Action Promotion Committee	N/A	9 July 2019
Outline of the "Healthy China 2030" Plan [10]	China's State Council	N/A	25 October 2016
The National Fitness Program (2016–2020) [11]	China's State Council	[2016] No. 37	15 June 2016
The National Fitness Program (2011–2015) [12]	China's State Council	[2011] No. 5	15 February 2011
National Fitness Regulations [13]	China's State Council	National Order No. 560	13 August 2009
Outline of the National Fitness Program [14]	China's State Council	[1995] No. 14	20 June 1995

1.2. Sports Parks—A New Place for National Fitness

From leisure urban parks and national fitness centres to gymnasiums, a variety of places for physical activity have been provided to urban dwellers in China. Sports parks not only bring vitality to existing urban parks, but also provide a new testing ground for inter-disciplinary integration and interactive applications of technology, and they upgrade and transform the sports industry. Sports parks are parks that are themed around physical fitness. They are built on green land with vegetation, provide facilities for competitive sports and physical exercise, and are open to the public for free or at a low cost, to meet the needs of residents for rest, excursions, and exercise [15]. Promoting the construction of sports parks is of great significance in meeting the people's growing demand for sports and fitness and in improving the quality of people's lives. The National Development and Reform Commission asserts that around 1000 more sports parks will be constructed by 2025 [16]. As an important space for conducting physical activity, the spatial planning of sports parks has become a prominent issue in the transformation of China into a strong sporting nation [17]. The people's increasing demand for healthy lives, national fitness as a national goal, diversified integration, and upgrading of the sports industry, etc., all provide important support for the design and construction of sports parks in China.

Even though the official report on sports park design and planning guidelines remains unpublished, researchers and designers have started to consider the classification of sports parks in their own ways and attempt to summarise the rules and past experiences in sports park planning. As a means of practicing the concept of a healthy China, construction of the sports park is one of the key measures to relieve the pressure of urban land construction [18]. Existing urban public spaces and communal social spaces are all ideal places for adding sports elements. In general, sports parks can be classified into three types: (1) Legacy Sports Park (LSP): This is a place where at least one major sports event occurred before, and which was transformed into a park with a legacy for urban dwellers' tourism as well as for their daily physical activity. Unlike other categories of sports parks, one or more professional-level stadiums exist here and are in use for hosting sporting competitions [19,20]. (2) Urban Leisure Sports Park (ULSP): In response to the National Fitness Program, existing urban leisure parks have been upgraded with extra sports facilities for urban dwellers' physical activity. In addition to holding sports competitions regularly, these parks are mainly open to citizens for daily physical and leisure activities [15,21]. (3) Community Sports Park (CSP): This is a new type of community park with exercise through sports as the main function, using landscaping combined with various outdoor sports fields (including basketball courts, badminton courts, table tennis courts, etc.) on separate land [22–24].

The sports park in China was identified and developed through a process of transformation from high-speed growth to high-quality development. The number of sports parks in China has been increasing in the last decade. The State Council of China issued the National Fitness Plan (2021–2025) to explain that China will continue to construct new sports parks, expand more than 2000 existing sports parks, and add fitness venues and facilities in urban parks to promote physical activity and improve public health [5]. Meanwhile, how to design layouts and improve service quality at sports parks to promote people's involvement in the national fitness program is a new challenge for the development of sports parks.

Research on spatial environments as well as evaluations of sports parks were previously conducted by international academics. Theoretical research and practical exploration of sports parks in Japan [25], the United States [26,27], and other countries [28–30] have explored different sports park management and operation models.

Evaluation systems such as the Physical Activity Resource Assessment (PARA) [22], the Recreation Facility Evaluation Tool (RFET) [31], the Environmental Assessment of Public Recreation Spaces Tool (EAPRS) [32], and the Bedimo-Rung Assessment Tools (BRAT) [33] have been applied to focus on park environmental characteristics along with non-physical factors, including park facilities, leisure time available, aesthetics, sense of security, and proximity to the park, etc. [34] Many scholars in China have studied the classification, characteristics, and management modes of sports parks in the form of case study analysis [17,24,35–37]. They have conducted practical work on sports parks based on sports industry policy planning to explore sports park design strategies [23,24,38–40].

More research on sports parks in China should be conducted in advance of publishing the national policies, guidelines, and programs, especially at the beginning of the period of their high-quality development. The quality of sports parks here refers to the significance of their contributions in improving the urban living environment and increasing residents' expectations for better lives [24]. The COVID-19 pandemic has made people more concerned about their health. People chose a "slow life" model and were limited to public places to avoid being infected. Consequently, it has been necessary but challenging for researchers to do field studies during the pandemic. How people perform physical activity, what their subjective preferences are for existing sports parks, and what the determining factors are in people's willingness to select and use sports parks remain unclear. The objectives of the study are: (1) to record physical activity behaviour patterns; (2) to examine users' subjective perceptions of existing sports parks based on the Semantic Differential method; (3) to explore the factors that influence users' willingness to use sports parks. The findings of this study will provide a spatial optimization strategy for sports parks planning, construction, and management.

2. Materials and Methods

2.1. Study Area

The Beijing Olympic Forest Park, Sun Park, and Huilongguan Park were selected as case studies (see Figure 2) to conduct a quantitative survey on behavioural demand and functional space of sports parks in China.

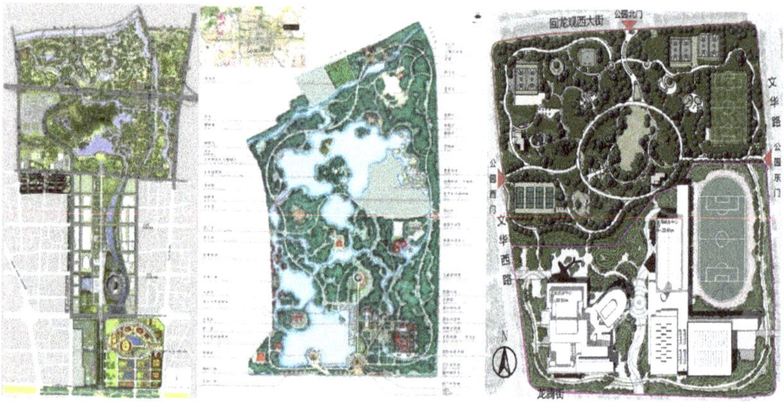

Figure 2. Site plan of the Beijing Olympic Forest Park (**left**), Sun Park (**middle**), and Huilongguan Park (**right**).

The Beijing Olympic Forest Park is the legacy of the 2008 Beijing Olympic Games as well as the 2022 Beijing Winter Olympic Games. As a large, manufactured nature park situated at the north end of the Olympic Green in Beijing, the park consists of the south, central, and north parts, with many walking paths, competition venues, and leisure facilities for urban dwellers. It has a strong brand effect that attracts tourists from all over the world. Meanwhile, it is also a place for public fitness and leisure use.

Sun Park is a ULSP built in 1984. Over 85% of it is green space, with a total area of 288.7 ha, which includes 68.2 ha of water surface area. The layout of the park has changed over time. In 2008, Sun Park was part of the Beijing 2008 Olympic Games and was the venue for the beach volleyball competition. After the competition, a beach volleyball theme park was built to serve as a model of post-game utilization. Now, a well-designed landscape and pedestrian walkway is proposed as part of the National Fitness program, which would be open to the public and mainly used for regular recreation and sports exercise by locals.

Huilongguan Park is a CSP with sports facilities, green spaces, and recreational footpaths built in the last two years. With over 50 ha of green space, the total area of Huilongguan Park is 80 ha, which includes a variety of sports facilities: four outdoor tennis courts, four full basketball courts, 30 badminton courts, 3000 m^2 of roller-skating space, 10 table tennis tables, as well as leisure pathways. In response to the call of the national fitness program to meet the requirements of people's physical activities, an innovative commercial management and operation model was proposed to support leisure and exercise spaces for the surrounding residents.

2.2. Data Collection

The main data collection tool is a questionnaire. Behavioural observations and interviews were used as complementary research methods, mainly during the pilot study to understand how urban dwellers used the sports park as part of our search for key places to disseminate the questionnaires. The questionnaire was divided into three aspects: basic information on respondents (including gender, age, education level, income status, occupation, etc.), sports park usage (including the distance between residence and sports park, time, mode and frequency of visit, purpose of visit, how to get information about sports park, etc.), and a scale with evaluation factors (including evaluation of overall park perception, sports facilities, and park facilities).

All questionnaires were distributed and collected on-site. When the respondents filled out the questionnaires anonymously, we explained the parts of the questionnaires that were not clear to the respondents to ensure that they understood and filled out the questionnaires accurately. In response to the epidemic prevention and control requirements, all researchers wore masks throughout the process, kept a safe distance of more than one meter from the interviewees, and completed data collection in the form of speaking out the questions and filling in the questions on the respondents' behalf. A pilot study was done to find ways to improve the design of the questionnaire in advance of its formal distribution. The researchers studied three representative sports parks of diverse types, the Beijing Olympic Forest Park, Sun Park, and Huilongguan Park, covering five time periods on weekdays as well as weekends between August and September 2021. The time slots were 6 a.m.–9 a.m., 9 a.m.–12 a.m., 12 a.m.–3 p.m., 3 p.m.–6 p.m., and 6 p.m.–9 p.m. The location of the questionnaire distribution covered, as much as possible, all physical activity areas, including the square spaces, specific exhibition areas, fitness footpaths, children's playgrounds, sports facilities, stadium areas, etc. Respondents were selected carefully to involve all age groups to ensure the representativeness of the sample.

2.3. Analysis Tools

Valid responses to the questionnaires were analysed according to the following steps (see Figure 3). Firstly, the basic information on respondents and sports park usage in the first two parts of the questionnaires were analysed statistically to gain insight into urban dwellers' daily usage of the sports parks. Secondly, the mean scores of the evaluation factors in the overall perception of sports parks, sports facilities, and park facilities were calculated. A Semantic Differential score method (SD) evaluation line chart for assessment of sports park facilities was drawn to indicate participants' subjective preferences for the sports parks. The SD method is a research method created by American psychologist Charles E. Osgood and his colleagues, which uses semantic differentiation scales to study the meaning of things [41]. By focusing on subjective evaluation, with the advantage of easy administration and relatively fast Question & Answer sessions, this method is especially suitable for measuring emotional and behavioural aspects of attitude [42] and has been applied to research in the fields of architecture and environment [43–45]. The method quantitatively measures human perception through linguistic scale analysis, clearly reflecting the research objectives. We assigned a semantic scale to sports park-related factors by using adjectives and their antonyms that describe the users' preferences for sports park usage. The scale measures respondents' psychological feelings by counting and analysing the differences between the two adjectives chosen by the respondent, thus transforming the respondents' perceptual evaluation of space into a value that can be analysed quantitatively [46,47].

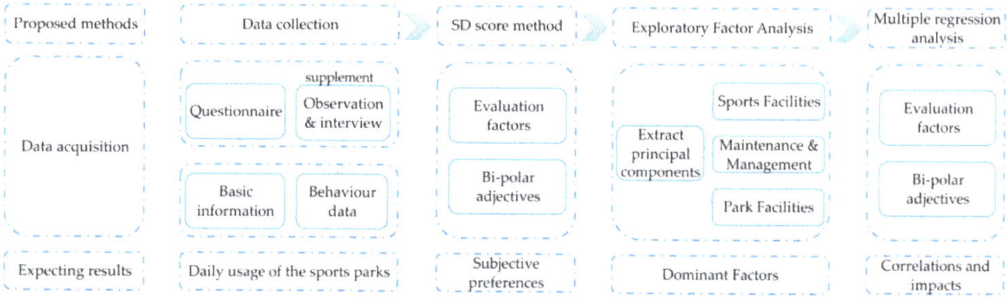

Figure 3. Research design.

The evaluation factors of the scale were generated based on the literature from two databases, the Web of Science (WoS) and the China National Knowledge Infrastructure (CNKI). Consequently, 26 evaluation factors were first selected as the indicators to evaluate the sports parks. According to Lenno, the sources of bi-polar adjectives about the affective dimension of evaluation factors are both the literature and the participants [48]. Then, by summarizing the views of scholars as well as the results of the pilot tests, the affective dimension of three major categories, namely the overall perception of sports parks, sports facilities, and park facilities, 14 pairs of adjectives were finally designated to report through a five-point rating Likert scale: unpleasant–pleasant, inconvenient–convenient, monotonous–diverse, dangerous–safe, dirty–clean, uncomfortable–comfortable, crowded–spacious, insufficient–sufficient, gloomy–bright, undemanding–demanding, bad–good, disordered–ordered, inapparent–apparent, difficult–easy. Semantic differential scores were transformed to fit a scale ranging from -2 to $+2$, which are easier to interpret with a neutral point at zero (0). The system is divided into three major categories, including the overall perception of sports parks, sports facilities, and park facilities, containing a total of 17 evaluation factors (see Table 2).

Table 2. Semantic evaluation factors.

Category	No.	Evaluation Factors	Adjectives Pair
overall perception of sports park	1	Fitness and leisure atmosphere	Unpleasant—Pleasant
	2	Convenience and accessibility	Inconvenient—Convenient
	3	Types of activities	Monotonous—Diverse
	4	Sense of security	Dangerous—Safe
	5	Cleanliness	Dirty—Clean
sports facilities	6	Types of sports facilities	Monotonous—Diverse
	7	Comfort of sports facilities	Uncomfortable—Comfortable
	8	Space between sports facilities	Crowded—Spacious
	9	Number of sports facilities	Insufficient—Sufficient
	10	Brightness	Gloomy—Bright
park facilities	11	Commercial facilities	Undemanding—Demanding
	12	Children's facilities	Unpleasant—Pleasant
	13	Landscape design and greening	Bad—Good
	14	Maintenance and Management	Disordered—Ordered
	15	Safety signs	Unapparent—Apparent
	16	Public restroom arrangement	Different—Easy
	17	Lounge seating arrangement	Insufficient—Sufficient

Thirdly, the Exploratory Factor Analysis (EFA) method was employed using IBM SPSS Statistics 26 to reduce the dimensionality of the main factors affecting the willingness of people to use sports parks. The EFA was conducted to define the underlying constructs and identify possible factors using the Principal Component method with promax rotation.

Finally, a multiple linear regression method was employed to analyse the impact of the factors on the willingness to use sports parks. Multiple linear regression analysis is a process to find the linear relationship between two or more independent variables and a dependent variable [49]. The method determines the direction of the relationship between the independent variable with the dependent variable, whether each independent variable can predict the value of the dependent variable.

3. Results

3.1. The Usage of the Sports Parks

In total, 270 responses to the questionnaire were collected with a 100% return rate and 241 valid questionnaires. Among them, 99 were collected from the Beijing Olympic Forest Park (valid number: 91; validity rate: 91.92%), 90 from Sun Park (valid number: 77; validity rate: 85.56%), and 81 from Huilongguan Park (valid number: 73; validity rate: 90.12%). The ratio of male to female participants is 1.1:1. Young people aged between 18 and 35 years and older people aged 56 years and above were the main respondents, accounting for about 71% of all respondents (see Table 3).

Table 3. Basic information and the number of respondents in three parks.

Category	Classification	Olympic Park	Sun Park	Huilongguan Park
Gender	Male/Female	41/50	47/30	39/34
Age	18 years old and below/18–35/36–55/56 years old and above	7/40/21/23	5/36/13/23	9/32/15/17
Educational level	Junior high school and below/ high school/college/undergraduate/ graduate and above	6/14/15/36/20	4/7/15/41/10	8/11/13/33/8
Working Status	Retired/Working	25/66	24/53	16/57

The distance from residence of the participants to the sports park and the number of participants in different age groups at different time periods are shown in Figure 4. As one of the most famous tourist attractions in Beijing, the LSP had a magnetic power over urban dwellers be like tourists; the same was true for visiting and engaging in physical activity at the Beijing Olympic Forest Park. Nearly half of the respondents lived more than 5 km away from the Beijing Olympic Forest Park (see Figure 4). Meanwhile, over 30% of people who were in the middle-aged group, 36 to 55 years old, lived around the park less than 2 km away, and chose to run, walk, and engage in other leisure activities between 18:00 and 21:00 at night (see Figure 4).

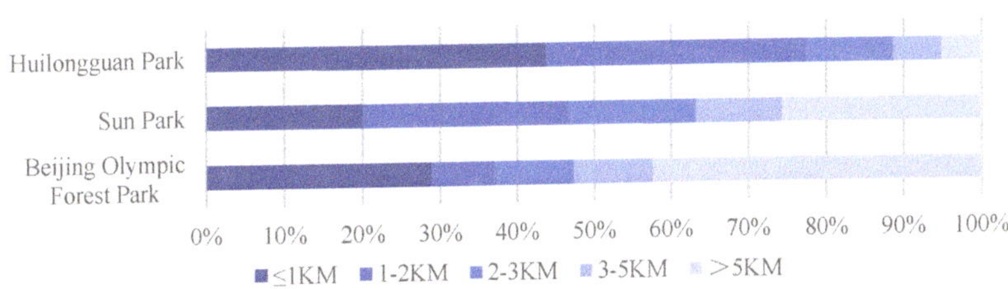

Figure 4. The distance from the users' residences to the sports park.

According to the statistics, the age composition of participants is significantly different between morning and afternoon times at Sun Park. In the morning, between 6:00 and 9:00, retired people over 55 years old make up 70% of the total number of participants. In the afternoon, between 15:00 and 18:00, the number of young people aged 18–35 years old reached a peak, accounting for over 60% of the total number of participants (see Figure 4).

As a CSP serving the local community, nearly 90% of the participants lived within three km of the Huilongguan Park. The park has become the main place for doing morning exercise for the elderly nearby (up to 70% of the participants) between 6:00 and 9:00 in the morning (see Figure 5). Yet, during the lunch break and after work hours, over 90% of the participants are customers who pay for the physical education training and the rental of Sports Venues.

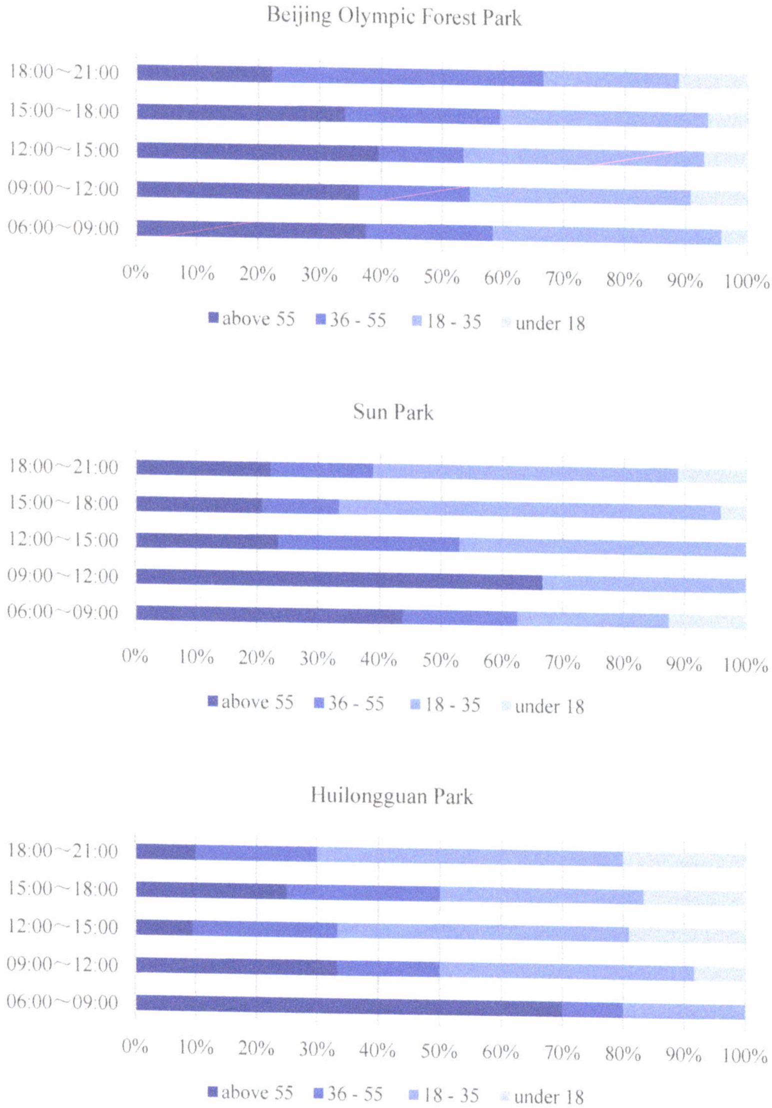

Figure 5. Changes in population age ratio in different periods of a day.

3.2. SD Evaluation Results

Following the statistical analysis of the sports park questionnaire responses, the table of evaluation indicators based on the SD scale method for sports parks is presented in Table 4. The SD evaluation curve was plotted on the vertical axis of the average scores of each factor of the 241 valid questionnaire responses (see Figure 6). It is an intuitive way to assess subject's impressions of the usage of sports parks. The results obtained have no negative values and all the factors received favorable comments. The mean scores for most factors were greater than one for the three sports parks. This indicates that the factors of overall perception, sports facilities, and park facilities of the three sports parks investigated are quite high from an overall perspective. Relatively speaking, the mean values of the commercial facilities and children's facilities were only 0.62 and 0.88 at LSP, indicating that more commercial and children's facilities were required in the park. The mean value of the commercial facilities was only 0.91 at ULSP, indicating that participants seek to be served with more commercial facilities in the park. Finally, the standard deviations for 17 pairs of adjectives had statistically insignificant difference, which were approximately 0.2. This result indicates that although some differences exist among individuals' perceptions of the sports park, their choices of adjectives as a whole present the same opinion on indicators.

Table 4. Statistical results of the evaluation indexes of the three sports parks.

	Questionnaire Content		LSP	ULSP	CSP	Mean Score
	Evaluation Indicators	**Adjectives Pairs**				
overall perception of sports park	Fitness and leisure atmosphere	Unpleasant—Pleasant	1.48	1.48	1.96	1.64
	Convenience and accessibility	Inconvenient—Convenient	1.58	1.61	1.47	1.55
	Types of activities	Monotonous—Diverse	1.22	1.30	1.81	1.44
	Sense of security	Dangerous—Safe	1.41	1.49	1.89	1.60
	Cleanliness	Dirty—Clean	1.44	1.17	1.19	1.27
Evaluation of sports facilities	Types of sports facilities	Single—Diverse	1.09	1.30	1.58	1.32
	Comfort of sports facilities	Uncomfortable—Comfortable	1.27	1.19	1.27	1.25
	Space between sports facilities	Crowded—Spacious	1.35	1.39	1.66	1.47
	Number of sports facilities	Insufficient—Sufficient	1.34	1.09	1.53	1.32
	Brightness	Gloomy—Bright	1.40	1.38	1.78	1.52
Evaluation of park facilities	Commercial facilities	Undemanding—Demanding	0.62	0.91	1.53	1.02
	Children's facilities	Unpleasant—Pleasant	0.88	1.21	1.56	1.22
	Landscape design and greening	Bad—Good	1.64	1.61	1.10	1.45
	Maintenance & Management	Disordered—Ordered	1.56	1.34	1.44	1.45
	Safety signs	Inapparent—Apparent	1.45	1.14	1.75	1.45
	Public restroom arrangement	Different—Easy	1.20	1.18	1.62	1.33
	Lounge seating arrangement	Insufficient—Sufficient	1.05	1.09	1.70	1.28

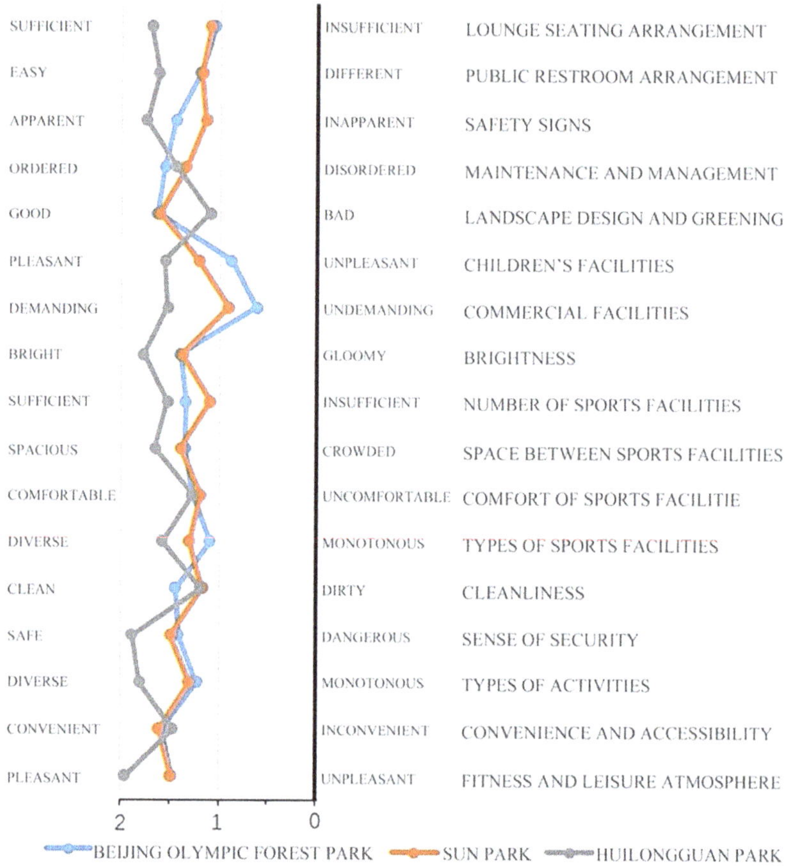

Figure 6. SD evaluation curves of three sports park spaces.

3.3. Factor Analysis

To determine the relationship between willingness to use sports parks and SD evaluation factors, an EFA was employed using the Principal Components method, and the reproduced rotational correlation matrix represented 53.156% of the original correlation matrix, which indicates good construct validity of the scale (KMO = 0.776, $p < 0.000$). The reliability was tested via Cronbach's coefficient. The α coefficient for all the questionnaire data is 0.803, which is greater than 0.8, indicating acceptable internal consistency [50,51]. Therefore, the questionnaire is useable and reliable. It indicates that the data are suitable for factor analysis, which can be employed to reduce the number of variables and explain the same amount of variance with fewer variables. Three extracted principal components are presented in Table 5, with the value of only those items above 0.5 being presented. Factor 1 was renamed Sports Facilities (X1), with five items with a factor loading from 0.676 to 0.814. Factor 2 was renamed Maintenance & Management (X2), with four items with a factor loading from 0.566 to 0.708. Factor 3 was renamed Park Facilities (X3), with three items with a factor loading from 0.510 to 0.701.

Table 5. The rotated component matrix.

SD Factor	Factor 1	Factor 2	Factor 3
Comfort of sports facilities	0.814		
Number of sports facilities	0.769		
Space between sports facilities	0.712		
Types of sports facilities	0.683		
Brightness	0.676		
Lounge seating arrangement		0.708	
Public restroom arrangement		0.686	
Safety signs		0.642	
Maintenance & Management		0.566	
Children's facilities			0.701
Commercial facilities			0.666
Landscape design and greening			−0.510

3.4. *Multiple Regression Analysis*

The correlations between the three factors obtained, namely Sports Facilities X1, Maintenance & Management X2, and Park Facilities X3, and the willingness of urban dwellers to use sports park, were analysed (Table 6).

Table 6. Results of multiple regression variables.

Dependent Variable	Independent Variables	Unstandardized Coefficient		Standardization Factor	t	sig
		B	Standard Deviation			
Willingness to use	**(Constant)**	**4.507**	**0.026**	—	174.510	0.000
	Sports Facilities	0.194	0.026	0.431	7.515	0.000
	Maintenance & Management	0.162	0.024	0.359	6.809	0.000

The degree of willingness of urban dwellers to use sports parks is positively correlated with the degree of two of the three independent variables—Sports Facilities and Maintenance & Management ($p < 0.05$). The Park Facilities factor did not have a significant effect on the respondents' intentions to use the sports parks. A multivariate linear regression between the degrees of willingness to use the parks and two principal component factors was established, as shown in Equation (1):

$$Y = 0.194\ X1 + 0.162\ X2 + 4.507 \quad (1)$$

where X1 and X2 are the key factors affecting the willingness of residents to use sports parks, Sports Facilities, and Maintenance & Management. The weights of the impact of each independent variable on the dependent variable were determined by comparing their coefficients in the multivariate linear regression equation [52]. In Equation (1), Sports Facilities, and Maintenance & Management have coefficients of 0.194 and 0.162, respectively. Therefore, urban dwellers' selection of sports parks was dependent on Sports Facilities first, followed by their Maintenance & Management.

4. Discussion

The differences in core service functions and facility configurations among the three types of sports parks resulted in different usage patterns and preferences of the respondents. Visited by surrounding residents as a regular exercise place for physical activity, LSP was generally selected to be visited by tourists with a strong intention of visiting venues. It provides not only a place where users can be physically active but is an important photogenic location that is part of the tourist experience for some, as well as a symbol of self-confidence for China. The latter may be one of the reasons why people treat it as one of the most famous tourist attractions [53]. Meanwhile, participants have a contrary view in terms of commercial facilities. Obviously, allocating proper commercial facilities such as retail, souvenir stores, and vending machines in the sports park could increase income from the manager's perspective. Meanwhile, one of the participants indicates that necessary commercial facilities would increase the joyful experience of visiting LSP. However, participants who live close to LSP and do regular exercises there indicate that too many commercial facilities will impact their experience of using sports and park facilities. Compared with LSP, ULSP is a more inclusive and popular place for urban dwellers for leisure and physical activity. Urban dwellers tend to invite friends and families together to ULSP for a better quality of life. Not only can ULSP provide sports facilities for physical activity but can serve as a place for leisure and socialising. In ULSP, people of different ages choose to visit ULSP at separate times. ULSP provides a variety of sports and park facilities for a more diverse range of users. Even though CSP also provides services to different age groups, it is more like a place for business operation where fees are charged for physical education training for adolescents, and a social and sports place for the middle-aged. In response to the National Fitness Program and national goal to improve the urban quality of life, CSP is also built with green spaces and entry is free of charge to the elderly.

The study finds that the selected sports parks have a suitable number of staff, and satisfactory level of maintenance and management. Although many visitor gathering points are scattered throughout the parks, there is no obvious crowding situation. The COVID-19 pandemic severely impacts the social economic development and limits population mobility in China, which has resulted in slightly different findings in this work compared with research conducted before the pandemic [54,55]. Compared with the findings in previous work, participants expressed their pleasure and satisfaction with the sports parks when they have fewer people. This satisfaction is reflected in the evaluation of the characteristics of the sports parks. In terms of individual preferences, the overall SD average score is above one for all the characteristics of sports parks except for children's and commercial facilities of LSP and commercial facilities of ULSP. With a fine overall atmosphere, urban dwellers prefer to choose sports parks as their leisure and sports places on weekends and holidays, especially during the pandemic. The whole family can benefit from the sports-related and leisure atmosphere and their time and economic costs are relatively low. Regularly visiting sports parks for physical activity is gradually becoming a lifestyle for families to provide them with physical and mental health benefits [2].

Even though three distinct types of sports parks were selected as case studies, the results of the multiple regression indicate that the key factors influencing the willingness of residents to use sports parks were Sports Facilities and Maintenance & Management. As the dominant factor affecting respondents' willingness to use sports parks, the provided Sports Facilities could support people who are in different age groups to engage in physical activity and thus have a significant positive effect on community attachment [23,56]. Furthermore, the Sports Facilities of the sports park must also meet certain requirements and specified standards to meet participants' sports-related needs. The respondents assert that comfortable, bright, and spacious sports courts, and the quality of the sports facilities were the determining factors in whether they will come to a sports park.

The Maintenance & Management of the sports parks is not related to their architectural design and spatial planning but is related to the long-term maintenance for a high-quality sports and leisure environment. The quality of the sports environment is not only determined by the physical facilities such as casual seating, restrooms, etc., but also key characteristics of the overall spatial environmental quality such as cleanness, convenience, safety, and so on. It is the responsibility of the sports park managers to ensure that there is no long-term damage to equipment [57]. The Maintenance & Management could improve the user experience and impression of the parks, which will attract more urban dwellers to do regular physical fitness activities in the parks.

5. Conclusions

People's demand for physical activity is booming, and the construction of sports parks is the most effective and direct way to meet these needs. This research takes three sports parks in Beijing as examples and uses the Semantic Differential score method as well as statistical analysis to understand how urban dwellers use sports parks and their subjective perceptions of sports parks. Furthermore, this research identifies the two significant factors—sports facilities, and Maintenance & Management—that impact participants' willingness to use sports parks. The sports park is one of the important places for citizens to do leisure activities as well as physical exercise. During the planning and construction of the sports park, these are the two factors that require consideration in order to support the high-quality development of the sports parks and better serve urban dwellers. The sports facilities, key elements of the sports parks, play a dominant role in the willingness of the participants selecting to use sports parks for physical activity. This paper stresses strengthened communication between architects and sports park decision-makers. How to allocate sports facilities within the overall layout of the sports parks, how to quantify the number and types of sports facilities to better serve urban dwellers, and even how to satisfy participants who immerse themselves in the atmosphere of leisure and physical activity in sports parks, can all be tailored and reshaped by architects' technique.

Furthermore, an interdisciplinary collaboration between managers and decision-makers was required for the sports park. A value co-creation for the stakeholders of the sports park, including designers, managers, urban dwellers, and decision-makers, can shed light on the spatial organization and design quality of the sports park, which also helps the sports park better serve the urban dwellers. Meanwhile, the biophilic design of the sports park should be considered in advance of its design and construction. Especially, as proposed by the government, the proportion of green land in newly built sports parks should not be less than 65% of the land area of the park [16] to achieve sustainability as framed through the UN Sustainable Development Goals. Empirical research is unique during the pandemic. With the end of the pandemic, a comparison of sports park usage during and after the pandemic can be studied in the future.

Author Contributions: Conceptualization, X.W.; methodology, X.W. and X.L.; software, X.W.; validation, X.W. and X.L.; formal analysis, X.W.; investigation, X.W.; resources, X.W.; data curation, X.W.; writing—original draft preparation, X.W.; writing—review and editing, X.W. and X.L.; visualization, X.W.; supervision, X.L.; funding acquisition, X.W. and X.L. All authors have read and agreed to the published version of the manuscript.

Funding: This research was funded by China Postdoctoral Science Foundation, grant number 2021M693038.

Acknowledgments: We would like to acknowledge Weijue Wang and Ang Li for helping conduct field study data.

Conflicts of Interest: The authors declare no conflict of interest.

References

1. General Assembly. *United Nations Transforming Our World: The 2030 Agenda for Sustainable Development*; Division for Sustainable Development Goals: New York, NY, USA, 2015.
2. Hanani, E.S. The study on value of recreational sports activity of urban communities. *KEMAS J. Kesehat. Masy.* **2017**, *12*, 286–291. [CrossRef]

3. Zhuo, L.; Guan, X.; Ye, S. Quantitative evaluation and prediction analysis of the healthy and sustainable development of China's sports industry. *Sustainability* **2020**, *12*, 2184. [CrossRef]
4. Tyrväinen, L.; Väänänen, H. The economic value of urban forest amenities: An application of the contingent valuation method. *Landsc. Urban Plan.* **1998**, *43*, 105–118. [CrossRef]
5. China's State Council. The National Fitness Plan 2021–2025. 2011. Available online: http://www.gov.cn/zhengce/content/2021-08/03/content_5629218.htm (accessed on 1 November 2022).
6. National Development and Reform Commission. The Implementation Plan for the National Fitness Facilities to Supplement the Shortcomings during the 14th Five-Year Plan Period e. 2021. Available online: https://www.ndrc.gov.cn/xxgk/zcfb/tz/202104/t20210427_1277520.html?code=&state=123 (accessed on 3 November 2022).
7. China's State Council. Opinions on Strengthening the Construction of National Fitness Venues and Facilities to Develop Mass Sports. 2020. Available online: http://www.gov.cn/zhengce/content/2020-10/10/content_5550053.htm (accessed on 3 November 2022).
8. China's State Council. Opinions on Promoting National Fitness and Sports Consumption and Promoting the High-Quality Development of the Sports Industry. 2019. Available online: http://www.gov.cn/zhengce/content/2019-09/17/content_5430555.htm (accessed on 3 November 2022).
9. HCA Promotion Committee. Health China Action Task (2019–2030). 2019. Available online: http://www.gov.cn/xinwen/2019-07/15/content_5409694.htm (accessed on 3 November 2022).
10. China's State Council. Outline of the 'Healthy China 2030' Plan. 2016. Available online: http://www.gov.cn/zhengce/2016-10/25/content_5124174.htm (accessed on 3 November 2022).
11. China's State Council. The State Council Issued the National Fitness Program (2016–2020). 2016. Available online: http://www.gov.cn/zhengce/content/2016-06/23/content_5084564.htm (accessed on 3 November 2022).
12. China's State Council. The National Fitness Program (2011–2015). 2011. Available online: http://www.gov.cn/zwgk/2011-02/24/content_1809557.htm (accessed on 3 November 2022).
13. China's State Council. National Fitness Regulations. 2009. Available online: http://www.gov.cn/flfg/2009-09/06/content_1410716.htm (accessed on 3 November 2022).
14. China's State Council. Outline of the National Fitness Program. 1995. Available online: http://www.scio.gov.cn/xwfbh/xwbfbh/wqfbh/2015/33862/xgzc33869/Document/1458253/1458253.htm (accessed on 3 November 2022).
15. Zhang, F. Research on the Interactive Promotion Mechanism of Urban Parks and Leisure Sports. In Proceedings of the 4th International Conference on Innovative Development of E-commerce and Logistics (ICIDEL 2018), Sanya, China, 28–30 September 2018; Volume 22, p. 17. [CrossRef]
16. National Development and Reform Commission. Guidelines on Promoting the Construction of Sports Parks. 2021. Available online: http://www.gov.cn/zhengce/zhengceku/2021-10/30/content_5647758.htm (accessed on 5 November 2022).
17. Chen, T.; Hui, E.C.M.; Lang, W.; Tao, L. People, recreational facility and physical activity: New-type urbanization planning for the healthy communities in China. *Habitat Int.* **2016**, *58*, 12–22. [CrossRef]
18. Jeanes, R.; Spaaij, R.; Farquharson, K.; McGrath, G.; Magee, J.; Lusher, D.; Gorman, S. Gender Relations, Gender Equity, and Community Sports Spaces. *J. Sport Soc. Issues* **2021**, *45*, 545–567. [CrossRef]
19. Kaziadrumis, A. Athens 2004 Olympic Legacy: Sport Infrastructure and General Aftereffects. Masters' Thesis, University of Peloponnese, Tripoli, Greece, 2020.
20. Preuss, H. A framework for identifying the legacies of a mega sport event. *Leis. Stud.* **2015**, *34*, 643–664. [CrossRef]
21. Peters, K. Being together in urban parks: Connecting public space, leisure, and diversity. *Leis. Sci.* **2010**, *32*, 418–433. [CrossRef]
22. Lee, R.E.; Booth, K.M.; Reese-Smith, J.Y.; Regan, G.; Howard, H.H. The Physical Activity Resource Assessment (PARA) instrument: Evaluating features, amenities and incivilities of physical activity resources in urban neighborhoods. *Int. J. Behav. Nutr. Phys. Act.* **2005**, *2*, 1–9. [CrossRef]
23. Luo, R.; Wang, J. Interactive Landscape Design and Application Effect Evaluation of Community Sports Park by Wireless Communication Technology. *Wirel. Commun. Mob. Comput.* **2022**, *2022*, 9334823. [CrossRef]
24. Zhang, Z.; Wang, M.; Xu, Z.; Ye, Y.; Chen, S.; Pan, Y.; Chen, J. The influence of Community Sports Parks on residents' subjective well-being: A case study of Zhuhai City, China. *Habitat Int.* **2021**, *117*, 102439. [CrossRef]
25. Takagi, D.; Kondo, N.; Tsuji, T.; Kondo, K. Parks/sports facilities in local communities and the onset of functional disability among older adults in Japan: The J-shaped spatial spillover effects. *Health Place* **2022**, *75*, 102801. [CrossRef] [PubMed]
26. Wen, M.; Zhang, X.; Harris, C.D.; Holt, J.B.; Croft, J.B. Spatial disparities in the distribution of parks and green spaces in the USA. *Ann. Behav. Med.* **2013**, *45* (Suppl. 1), S18–S27. [CrossRef] [PubMed]
27. Rigolon, A.; Browning, M.; Jennings, V. Inequities in the quality of urban park systems: An environmental justice investigation of cities in the United States. *Landsc. Urban Plan.* **2018**, *178*, 156–169. [CrossRef]
28. Boone, C.G.; Buckley, G.L.; Grove, J.M.; Sister, C. Parks and people: An environmental justice inquiry in Baltimore, Maryland. *Ann. Assoc. Am. Geogr.* **2009**, *99*, 767–787. [CrossRef]
29. Mäntymaa, E.; Jokinen, M.; Louhi, P.; Juutinen, A. Visitors' heterogeneous preferences for urban park management: The case of a city park in Oulu, Finland. *Urban For. Urban Green.* **2022**, *77*, 127751. [CrossRef]
30. Miaux, S.; Garneau, J. The sports park and urban promenade in the quais de Bordeaux: An example of sports and recreation in urban planning. *Loisir Soc.* **2016**, *39*, 12–30. [CrossRef]

31. Kirtland, K.A.; Evans, M.H.; Wilson, D.K.; Williams, J.E.; Mixon, G.M.; Henderson, K.A. Evaluating the Quality of Recreation Facilities: Development of an Assessment Tool. *Spring* **2004**, *22*, 96–114. Available online: https://search.ebscohost.com/login.aspx?direct=true&profile=ehost&scope=site&authtype=crawler&jrnl=07351968&asa=Y&AN=19626690&h=Vh9rpMl%2FPIziX5o5iWrjJaps91K2SekoZcoPSpYf78tbRKVjwcfIZnUu1se8QPCfKgDmiBYAuQ2D5nnFxSI20g%3D%3D&crl=c (accessed on 3 November 2022).
32. Saelens, B.E.; Frank, L.D.; Auffrey, C.; Whitaker, R.C.; Burdette, H.L.; Colabianchi, N. Measuring Physical Environments of Parks and Playgrounds: EAPRS Instrument Development and Inter-Rater Reliability. *J. Phys. Act. Health* **2016**, *3*, S190–S207. [CrossRef]
33. Bedimo-Rung, A.L.; Mowen, A.J.; Cohen, D.A. The significance of parks to physical activity and public health: A conceptual model. *Am. J. Prev. Med.* **2005**, *28* (Suppl. 2), 159–168. [CrossRef]
34. Wang, D.; Brown, G.; Liu, Y. The physical and non-physical factors that influence perceived access to urban parks. *Landsc. Urban Plan.* **2015**, *133*, 53–66. [CrossRef]
35. Ye, Y.; Pan, S. Research on the Evolution of Sports Park Model and the Development of Space System Based on the Logic of Competition, Scenery and Catalyst. 2019. Available online: http://www.jchla.com/ch/reader/view_abstract.aspx?file_no=20190911 (accessed on 1 November 2022).
36. Ran, L.; Tan, X.; Xu, Y.; Zhang, K.; Chen, X.; Zhang, Y.; Li, M.; Zhang, Y. The application of subjective and objective method in the evaluation of healthy cities: A case study in Central China. Sustain. *Sustain. Cities Soc.* **2021**, *65*, 102581. [CrossRef]
37. Wu, Y.; Guo, X.D. Integration of architecture, people and environment-A case of sports park design in Beijing Huangcun satellite town. *Appl. Mech. Mater.* **2013**, *409-410*, 410–414. [CrossRef]
38. Tian, Y.; Ning, H.; Ren, H.; Liu, J.; Wang, K.; Hong, B. National Fitness Evaluation of Urban Parks in the National Ecological Garden City: A Case Study in Baoji, China. *Land* **2022**, *11*, 889. [CrossRef]
39. Ministry of Housing and Urban-Rural Development of the People's Republic of China. Standard for Classification of Urban Green Space. 2017. Available online: https://scholar.google.com/scholar?hl=en&as_sdt=0%2C5&q=Standard+for+Classification+of+Urban+Green+Space&btnG= (accessed on 1 November 2022).
40. Li, B. Research on the Construction Layout of Urban Sports Park Based on Constraint Graph Model. *Open House Int.* **2019**, *44*, 24–27. [CrossRef]
41. Osgood, C.E. Semantic Differential Technique in the Comparative Study of Cultures. *Am. Anthropol.* **2009**, *66*, 171–200. [CrossRef]
42. Hewstone, M.; Stroebe, W. Sociální Psychologie. 2006. Available online: https://is.slu.cz/el/fvp/leto2022/UPPVJP008/um/Skopal_-_socialni_psychologie_-_studijni_text_k_testu.pdf (accessed on 9 November 2022).
43. Kang, J.; Zhang, M. Semantic differential analysis of the soundscape in urban open public spaces. *Build. Environ.* **2010**, *45*, 150–157. [CrossRef]
44. Schlag, P.; Yoder, D.; Sheng, Z. Words Matter: A Semantic Differential Study of Recreation, Leisure, Play, Activity, and Sport. *Sch. A J. Leis. Stud. Recreat. Educ.* **2015**, *30*, 25–38. Available online: https://www.tandfonline.com/doi/abs/10.1080/1937156X.2015.11949724 (accessed on 1 November 2022). [CrossRef]
45. Carroll, J.B.; Osgood, C.E.; Suci, G.J.; Tannenbaum, P.H. The Measurement of Meaning. *Language* **1959**, *35*, 58. [CrossRef]
46. Cao, M.F.; Zhang, J.J. Evaluation of Urban Waterfront Landscape Quality Based on Semantic Differential Method: A Case of Zhonghuamen Section of Qinhuai River in Nanjing. *J. Nanjing For. Univ. (Nat. Sci. Ed.)* **2020**, *44*, 221–227. Available online: https://scholar.google.com/scholar?hl=en&as_sdt=0%2C5&q=Evaluation+of+urban+waterfront+landscape+quality+based+on+semantic+differential+method%3A+a+case+of+Zhonghuamen+section+of+Qinhuai+River+in+Nanjing&btnG= (accessed on 1 November 2022).
47. Boarin, P.; Besen, P.; Haarhoff, E. Post-Occupancy Evaluation of Neighbourhoods: A Review of the Literature. 2018. Available online: www.buildingbetter.nz (accessed on 1 November 2022).
48. Lenno, G.W. Electronic Portfolios as High-Stakes Assessments of Teacher Candidates: A Semantic Differential of the California State University Teacher Education Faculty. Doctoral Thesis, Pepperdine University, Malibu, CA, USA, 2006.
49. Black, W.; Babin, B.J. Multivariate Data Analysis: Its Approach, Evolution, and Impact. In *The Great Facilitator*; Springer International Publishing: Berlin/Heidelberg, Germany, 2019; pp. 121–130.
50. Raykov, T.; Marcoulides, G.A. *Introduction to Psychometric Theory*; Routledge: New York, NY, USA, 2011.
51. Moalemi, S.; Kavoosi, Z.; Beygi, N.; Deghan, A.; Karimi, A.; Parvizi, M.M. Evaluation of the Persian Version of Maslach Burnout Inventory-Human Services Survey among Iranian Nurses: Validity and Reliability. *Galen Med. J.* **2018**, *7*, e995. [CrossRef]
52. Xu, H.; Huang, Q.; Zhang, Q. A study and application of the degree of satisfaction with indoor environmental quality involving a building space factor. *Build. Environ.* **2018**, *143*, 227–239. [CrossRef]
53. Jinxia, D.; Mangan, J.A. Beijing Olympics Legacies: Certain Intentions and Certain and Uncertain Outcomes. *Int. J. Hist. Sport* **2008**, *25*, 2019–2040. [CrossRef]
54. Lee, O.; Park, S.; Kim, Y.; So, W.Y. Participation in Sports Activities before and after the Outbreak of COVID-19: Analysis of Data from the 2020 Korea National Sports Participation. *Healthcare* **2022**, *10*, 122. [CrossRef]
55. Huh, M.K.; Park, M.S. A Study on the Use of Living Sports Facilities at Dalseong-Gun in Korea after Covid-19. Volume 9, p. 2021. Available online: http://www.idpublications.org/wp-content/uploads/2021/11/Full-Paper-A-STUDY-ON-THE-USE-OF-LIVING-SPORTS-FACILITIES-AT-DALSEONG-GUN-IN-KOREA-AFTER-COVID-19.pdf (accessed on 17 November 2022).

56. Kim, M.C.; Park, S.; Kim, S. The perceived impact of hosting mega-sports events in a developing region: The case of the PyeongChang 2018 Winter Olympic Games. *Curr. Issues Tour.* **2021**, *24*, 2843–2848. [CrossRef]
57. Sun, G.; Fong, D.; Liu, Y. The comparison between China and UK of the construction of city community sports service system in the scope of eco-civilization. *J. Fac. Eng. Cent. Univ. Venez. (UCV)* **2017**, *32*, 500–506.

MDPI
St. Alban-Anlage 66
4052 Basel
Switzerland
Tel. +41 61 683 77 34
Fax +41 61 302 89 18
www.mdpi.com

Buildings Editorial Office
E-mail: buildings@mdpi.com
www.mdpi.com/journal/buildings

www.ingramcontent.com/pod-product-compliance
Lightning Source LLC
Chambersburg PA
CBHW061439210926
51850CB00008B/1552
* 9 7 8 3 0 3 6 5 7 3 5 6 4 *